A guide to effective care in pregnancy and childbirth

Third Edition

Murray Enkin
Marc J. N. C. Keirse
James Neilson
Caroline Crowther
Lelia Duley
Ellen Hodnett and
Justus Hofmeyr

OXFORD
UNIVERSITY PRESS

OXFORD
UNIVERSITY PRESS

Great Clarendon Street, Oxford OX2 6DP

Oxford University Press is a department of the University of Oxford.
It furthers the University's objective of excellence in research, scholarship,
and education by publishing worldwide in

Oxford New York

Auckland Cape Town Dar es Salaam Hong Kong Karachi
Kuala Lumpur Madrid Melbourne Mexico City Nairobi
New Delhi Shanghai Taipei Toronto

With offices in

Argentina Austria Brazil Chile Czech Republic France Greece
Guatemala Hungary Italy Japan South Korea Poland Portugal
Singapore Switzerland Thailand Turkey Ukraine Vietnam

Oxford is a registered trade mark of Oxford University Press
in the UK and in certain other countries

Published in the United States
by Oxford University Press Inc., New York

© Oxford University Press 2000

The moral rights of the author have been asserted

Database right Oxford University Press (maker)

First edition published 1989
Second edition published 1995
Reprinted (twice) 1998, 1999
Third edition published 2000
Reprinted 2002, 2003, 2004, 2006

A catalogue record for this title is available from the British Library

Library of Congress Cataloguing in Publication Data
A guide to effective care in pregnancy and childbirth / Murray Enkin . . . [et al.].–3rd ed.
(Oxford medical publications)
Includes bibliographical references and index.

ISBN 978 0 19 263173 2   ISBN 0 19 263173 X

1. Prenatal care. 2. Obstetrics. I. Enkin, Murray II. Series.
[DNLM: 1. Prenatal Care. 2. Labor WQ 175 G946 2000
RG940 .E55 2000 618.2′4–dc21 00–021832

Printed in Great Britain on acid-free paper by Biddles Ltd, King's Lynn, Norfolk

OXFORD MEDICAL PUBLICATIONS

A guide to effective care in pregnancy and childbirth

ʒ‧ ‧‧ʒ‧ital, Guildford

Authors

Murray W. Enkin MD, FRCS(C), LLD
Professor Emeritus, Departments of Obstetrics and
Gynecology, Clinical Epidemiology and Biostatistics,
McMaster University, Canada.

Marc J. N. C. Keirse MD, DPHIL, DPH, FRANZCOG, FRCOG
Professor and Head, Department of Obstetrics, Gynaecology
and Reproductive Medicine, The Flinders University of
South Australia.

James P. Neilson BSC, MD, FRCOG
Co-ordinating Editor, Cochrane Pregnancy and Childbirth
Group. Professor of Obstetrics and Gynaecology,
University of Liverpool, UK.

Caroline A. Crowther MD, DCH, DDU, FRCOG, FRANZCOG, CMFM
Associate Professor, Department of Obstetrics and
Gynaecology, University of Adelaide, South Australia.

Lelia Duley MD, MSc(Epid), MRCOG
Obstetric Epidemiologist, Institute of Health Sciences,
Oxford, UK.

Ellen D. Hodnett RN, PHD
Professor and Heather M. Reisman Chair in Perinatal
Nursing Research, University of Toronto, Canada.

G. Justus Hofmeyr MBBCH, MRCOG
Professor of Obstetrics and Gynaecology,
Coronation Hospital and University of the Witwatersrand,
Johannesburg, South Africa.

To the individuals who conscientiously and selflessly prepare the systematic reviews for The Cochrane Library, on which the updates in this book are mainly based.

Preface

Work towards *A guide to effective care in pregnancy and childbirth* started over a quarter-century ago, when Iain Chalmers, later joined by Murray Enkin and Marc Keirse, began to assemble a register of controlled trials in perinatal medicine. Together they established explicit criteria to identify studies that were likely to provide the best evidence for evaluating care, and began a comprehensive and systematic search for those studies. They then, with the help of content experts in each field, brought the results of this research together into two major publications: *Effective care in pregnancy and childbirth*, a 1500 page, two-volume book; and a regularly updated electronic database. The electronic database, which consisted of a register of controlled studies and systematic reviews of their results, was first published as the *Oxford database of perinatal trials*, and continued as *The Cochrane pregnancy and childbirth database*. It was then incorporated in *The Cochrane Library* and is now maintained and kept up to date by the editors of the Cochrane Pregnancy and Childbirth Group, Jim Neilson, Caroline Crowther, Lelia Duley, Ellen Hodnett, and Justus Hofmeyr, and their editorial team. At the time of writing, there are over 9000 controlled trials on the register, from almost 400 medical journals in 18 different languages, from 85 different countries.

A guide to effective care in pregnancy and childbirth was prepared to make the conclusions of these larger publications more readily available, in a more portable format, to all who are involved in the care of childbearing women. The first edition appeared in 1989. It was widely acclaimed as a landmark publication, which made readable, evidence-based information on the effects of pregnancy and childbirth care accessible to all who need and want it. The second edition won first prize in the British Medical Association's 1995 Medical Book Competition in the Primary Health Care category, and was translated into several languages. The success of the first two editions has confirmed the importance of accurate, up to date information to guide the decisions that must be made by those who plan, provide or receive care during pregnancy and childbirth.

Research has continued to add new information, which is regularly incorporated into the electronic *Cochrane Library*. But the printed word stands still, and must be brought up to date. This third edition of *A guide to effective care in pregnancy and childbirth* has been prepared by the editors of the Cochrane Pregnancy and Childbirth Group, along with two of the authors of the first edition. It has been extensively revised and rewritten to incorporate new research and new understandings.

Annotation of reference sources is a particular problem for a book of this type. To cite all primary sources would make the book far too long. Most new references are listed in *The Cochrane Library* (Update Software Ltd, Summertown Pavilion, Middle Way, Oxford OX2 7LG, England, or 936 La Rueda Drive, Vista, California 92084, USA. Internet: 'http://www.update-software.com'); older sources will be found in *Effective care in pregnancy and childbirth* (1989, Oxford University Press, Oxford). We have noted for each chapter the relevant reviews from the *Cochrane Library* and chapters from *Effective care in pregnancy and childbirth*, plus a few key additional sources.

We hope that the information in this book will help those who provide or receive care during pregnancy and childbirth to make the right decisions for themselves, in the context of their own circumstances and priorities.

June 2000

Murray Enkin, Marc Keirse, Jim Neilson, Caroline Crowther, Lelia Duley, Ellen Hodnett, Justus Hofmeyr.

References

Please note, that the reference sources for the information at the end of each chapter, can be found in the following:

Chalmers, I., Enkin, M.W. and Keirse, M.J.N.C. (1989) *Effective care in pregnancy and childbirth.* OUP, Oxford.

The Cochrane Library, Issue 4 (1999) Update Software: Oxford.

Pre-Cochrane reviews refer to:

Cochrane pregnancy and childbirth database (1995) Update Software: Oxford.

Acknowledgements

We owe particular thanks to the authors of each chapter of *Effective Care in pregnancy and childbirth*, and to those who prepared the systematic reviews for *The Cochrane Library*. Most of this book is derived from, and extensively quotes, their contributions. We are well aware and appreciative of the countless hours that they spent in reviewing and analyzing the data on which those contributions were based. The credit for the review and analysis is theirs; the blame for any errors that may have crept into our condensation of their work rests with us.

We are grateful to Iain Chalmers, who first conceived this project, and to Mary Renfrew, who contributed so much to the second edition of this book, and the chapter on breastfeeding for this edition. We would like to thank the many colleagues who read chapter manuscripts and gave valuable comments and suggestions, in particular: Zarko Alfirevic, Eva Rebecca Bild, Beverley Chalmers, Iain Chalmers, Peter Choi, Patricia Crowley, Anita Gagnon, Adrian Grant, Phil Hall, Mary Hannah, Michael Helewa, David Henderson-Smart, Eileen Hutton, Charlotte Howell, Karyn Kaufman, James King, Michael Kramer, Nancy Lowe, Judith Lumley, Laura Magee, Deana Midmer, Patrick Mohide, Renato Natale, Cheryl Nikodem, Sally Pairman, Jeffrey Robinson, Greg Ryan, Carol Sakala, Penny Simkin, Jack Sinclair, Fiona Smaill, Patricia Smith, John Smith, Gordon Stirrat, Joan Tranmer, Chris Wilkinson,

Current funding for the Cochrane Pregnancy and Childbirth Group is provided by the UK NHS Research and Development Programme; previous funding was received from the NHS Executive (North West), and the Department of Health, UK. The World Health Organization provided the initial funding for the register of controlled trials in perinatal medicine on which much of this work is based, and the Rockefeller Foundation provided the opportunity to work on the first edition at their study center in Bellagio. McMaster University, The

Flinders University of South Australia, the University of Liverpool, the University of the Witwatersrand, the University of Adelaide, the UK Medical Research Council and Department for International Development, and the University of Toronto allowed the authors the time necessary to work on this project.

Alison Langton of Oxford University Press was helpful and encouraging at all times; thanks also goes to Hannah Kenner. Additional thanks to Sonja Henderson, Lynn Hampson, Claire Winterbottom, for their help in the Pregnancy and Childbirth Group office; to Clive Adams and Barbara Farrell, Sue Gibbons, Lyn Brown, and Myriam Hanssens, for providing the essential behind the scenes support. And a very special thanks to Eleanor Enkin, who critically checked over every page, every paragraph, and every word.

Murray Enkin, Marc Keirse, Jim Neilson, Caroline Crowther, Lelia Duley, Ellen Hodnett, Justus Hofmeyr.

Contents

Care after childbirth

Synopsis

Basic care

CHAPTER 1

What do we mean by 'effective care'?

Women who receive care, professionals who provide care, and those who pay for care, all want that care to be effective. Although everyone agrees with this in principle, there is much less agreement about what actually constitutes effective care in pregnancy and childbirth. Controversies arise from differences in opinion both about what we want to achieve and about the best way to achieve it.

What we most want to achieve depends on what we think is most important. Different communities, groups, and individuals may have different opinions about this. Some may give priority to each woman's personal experience of childbirth, even if this might mean some sacrifice in terms of safety. Others may aim to minimize perinatal morbidity and mortality no matter how much this may increase the mother's risk or discomfort. Still others, primarily concerned about the rising costs of care and the limited resources available, consider efficiency and cost savings to be the most important objectives. All of these goals are important, but often they involve trade-offs. Not surprisingly, the diversity of aims and priorities has resulted in widely differing recommendations for care during pregnancy and childbirth.

This variety of views about the objectives of care helps to explain the different ways in which the effects of care can be measured. Some choose ratings of women's satisfaction with their care as the most important measure of its effectiveness, while others concentrate on direct measures of death, disease, and disability. Still others focus on surrogate or indirect measures of the baby's well-being, such as fetal heart-rate tracings or estimates of the acid-base status of umbilical cord blood, in the belief that they can be translated into indices of real health.

These differences of opinion are clearly revealed by the widely differing care practises seen among otherwise similar countries, communities, and institutions, from one care-giving discipline to another, and from individual to individual. Countless examples come to mind: the different methods used to assess the risk status of the mother and the well-being of the fetus; the place, if any, for routine iron or vitamin supplements during pregnancy; the usefulness of cervical examination at each antenatal visit; the value of routine ultrasound visualization of the fetus; the need for bed-rest for women with an uncomplicated twin pregnancy; the appropriate indications for the use of forceps, vacuum extraction, or cesarean section. The list is endless.

A number of other factors may help to explain these variations in practice. Some relate to differences in the populations served, or in the needs or circumstances of childbearing women and their babies. Others result from differences in resources, including personnel, hospital beds, and equipment. Still others reflect differences in culture, tradition, status, fashion, and political correctness. There may be differences in the need to provide opportunities for clinicians in training to gain experience; in the extent to which malpractice litigation is feared; in the way that caregivers are paid. Commercial pressures from pharmaceutical companies, equipment manufacturers, and others, may also influence practice.

This *Guide to Effective Care in Pregnancy and Childbirth* relates to none of these factors. Rather, the information it contains refers to the specific effects, beneficial or harmful, of the various elements of care that may be carried out during pregnancy and childbirth. Knowledge about these effects is required by everyone who provides or receives that care. It is essential for making informed choices among the available alternatives.

Evidence-based care has been defined as the 'conscientious, judicious, and explicit use of current best evidence in making decisions about the care of individual patients'. In the next chapter, we outline the rationale, the materials, and the methods that we used to find and relate the current best evidence, and how we arrived at the conclusions we present in the rest of this book.

CHAPTER 2

Evaluating care in pregnancy and childbirth

1 Introduction

There are many ways of learning about the effects of different care policies and practices. Sometimes the belief that one form of care is better than another is based on an informal impression, gained from personal experience, the experience of others, or previous teaching. A number of factors contribute to the powerful effect of this informal learning. Primary among these is the emotional interest of the information. Events that happen to us personally are more interesting than those that happen to others; those that happen to people we know or care about are more persuasive than those that occur to strangers. 'I saw it myself' is more personal and more vivid than a second-hand report. The experience of people whom we admire and respect influences us more strongly than that of those we regard less highly.

There can be little question about the ability of anecdotes, examples, and informal observations to convey information or modify behavior. Their role in determining a cause-and-effect relationship is much more controversial. When we make inferences from observations or examples, we use simple rules of thumb that allow us to define and interpret the data of every-day life. For the most part, these rules of thumb lead us to correct conclusions. They are essential for rapid decision-making under normal circumstances.

Unfortunately, while our informal impressions are often right, they are sometimes wrong. The impression that women were less likely to sustain injury during delivery with the vacuum extractor than with forceps, originally gained from informal observation, has been confirmed by the results of formal studies. Other beliefs, such as the once widely held conviction that diethylstilboestrol could prevent miscarriages and fetal death, have been refuted by the results of properly controlled studies.

Because individual experience is haphazard, and sometimes mis-leading, it must be supplemented by the results of formal research studies. Unless the validity of informal impressions about the effects of care is assessed by formal evaluation, effective forms of care will not be recognized as such, and may not be brought into general use as promptly as possible. Similarly, ineffective or harmful forms of care will not be detected efficiently, and may do harm on a wider scale than necessary. All too often the necessary confirmation or refutation happens only after a great deal of damage has already been done.

An overwhelming number of research studies have been mounted in attempts to resolve uncertainties about the effects of many elements of care during pregnancy and childbirth. Not all of these studies, however, provide reliable information. If judgements about the effects of care based on research studies are to be valid, we must pay careful attention to the strengths and weaknesses of the methods used by the investigators. In this way we can establish a rational basis for selecting those studies that are most likely to provide useful information.

There are two main types of error that can occur in all research studies: systematic errors, in which results are consistently skewed in one direction or another (technically referred to as bias); and chance or random errors, which reduce the precision of the results. Studies can be arranged in a hierarchy that reflects the likelihood that biases (systematic errors) will result in misleading conclusions. In addition, it is possible to estimate the extent to which the play of chance (random errors) may be misleading.

2 Minimizing systematic errors (biases)

The results of any intervention – any element of care – can only be evaluated by comparing them with the results of some other course of action or of no action at all. Sometimes past experience is enough for us to be confident in assessing the effects of care. This is certainly the case when these effects are dramatically different from what would have been expected on the basis of past experience. For example, cesarean section can save the lives of both mother and baby when a central placenta praevia covers the cervix and prevents vaginal delivery. Case reports have shown that prostaglandin administration may be life-saving when used to treat otherwise uncontrollable hemorrhage caused by the uterus failing to contract after the baby is delivered. The effectiveness of penicillin to prevent the transmission of syphilis to the fetus is clear, because when women with the infection are treated, the baby is very rarely infected, whereas without treatment of the mother, infection rates in the baby are high.

Situations like this, where the results of one form of treatment are dramatically better than those of another, are gratifying but not common. Usually, the best we can expect are more modest differences, which may still be important, in the effects of alternative forms of care. Single case reports, and case series without comparison groups (controls), are not enough to let us make valid judgements about the effects of care. Studies of this type are subject to a number of biases that may either mask real differences between alternative forms of care, or suggest that differences exist when, in fact, they do not.

These biases are not, as a rule, made consciously. In fact, the researcher is often not aware of them, and they are not always readily apparent to others. In the sections that follow we discuss two of the most important sources of bias. The first of these occurs during the selection process that leads people to receive one form of care over another; the second can result when those providing, receiving, or evaluating care, know which one of two or more alternative forms of care has been received.

2.1 Minimizing bias in the selection of controls

Uncontrolled observations of events after a particular form of care has been given usually do not tell us what might have happened if a different form of care had been provided. Judgements about the effects of care require comparisons of what happens to people who have received one form of care with what happens to the 'controls' who have received an alternative form of care (or no care at all).

Differences found between the outcomes for people who have received alternative forms of care can be due either to real differences in the effects of the different forms of care, or to differences in the pretreatment characteristics (prognoses) of the people who received these forms of care. The extent to which the differences in results are due to the effects of the treatment thus depends on the extent to which the people who received the different forms of care are similar in every other respect that matters. The challenge, therefore, is to select comparison groups that are comparable in every important respect.

2.1.1 Studies using historical controls

One approach to the selection of controls involves comparing the results for people who have received a recently introduced form of care with similar people who received a different form of care in the past. The use of such 'historical controls' sometimes leads to valid conclusions, but at other times it can be seriously misleading. For example, studies with historical controls suggested that administration of diethylstilboestrol during pregnancy dramatically decreased the risk of miscarriage and stillbirth, thus giving rise to one of the best known examples of harmful treatment.

Even when the outcome, following the use of a new treatment, appears to differ substantially from the outcome after earlier forms of care, the difference may simply reflect changes in other, undocumented factors that may have occurred over time. Without concurrent comparisons between alternative forms of care, there is no way of knowing which of the studies using historical controls reliably reflect the true effects of care, and which do not. The most useful role for comparisons using historical controls may, therefore, be as 'screening tests' for promising new forms of care, which can then be assessed in properly controlled, prospective experimental studies.

2.1.2 Case-control studies

The underlying principle of a case-control study is straightforward: groups of people who have, and who have not, experienced a particular outcome are assembled. Then the frequencies with which each group has received the form of care in question are compared. This approach is particularly valuable when the postulated outcome of care is rare, or when it cannot be ascertained for some months or years after the particular care has been received. For example, when cases of cerebral palsy were compared with controls, no difference in the frequency of substandard care during labor and delivery was detected, thus casting further doubt on the widespread belief that the quality of intrapartum care is an important factor in the etiology of cerebral palsy.

Although case-control studies may sometimes offer the only practicable research strategy for evaluating some of the postulated effects of care during pregnancy and childbirth, they are subject to a variety of biases that restrict their value. Some of these biases may be eliminated by careful matching of cases and controls, but it is never possible to know how successful such measures to reduce selection and other biases have been. No amount of matching based on information about known confounding factors can ever eliminate the effect of unrecognized confounding factors. Thus, conclusions about causes and effects based upon case-control studies are often insecure.

Like the results of studies using historical controls, the results of case-control studies are sometimes supported and sometimes not supported by those of studies that are less subject to bias. In many instances, however, there are simply no unbiased comparisons available. In these circumstances, consistent findings from a number of well-designed, case-control studies may provide the best evidence that is ever likely to be available.

2.1.3 Studies using non-randomized concurrent controls
Another common approach to controlled evaluation involves comparing two or more groups of individuals who have received different forms of care over the same period of time. Before accepting a cause-and-effect relationship about the results of care on the basis of such studies, one must be convinced that 'like has been compared with like'.

There are a number of ways in which bias can affect comparisons between non-randomized, concurrent groups (cohorts) who have been chosen to receive different forms of care. For example, many studies have compared the results for very low-birthweight infants delivered by cesarean section with those for other such babies delivered vaginally. In most reports of these comparisons, infants delivered by cesarean section were more likely to survive than those delivered vaginally. This does not mean, however, that cesarean section is a safer method of delivery for very low-birthweight babies. This conclusion would not be justified, unless the two groups of babies could be shown to be at comparable risk of death and morbidity before delivery. These risks may be very different. Cesarean section is less likely to be used to deliver babies whose chances of survival are judged to be minimal anyway; vaginal delivery is more likely to have occurred when labor has been precipitate, in itself a risk factor for poor outcome. These and other factors that can influence the result, can introduce bias in the non-randomized comparisons of these two methods of delivery. As in studies using historical controls and in case-control studies, the conclusions drawn from non-randomized cohort studies may be invalid because important, but sometimes unknown, selection biases have not been controlled adequately.

2.1.4 Studies using randomized controls

There is only one certain way to overcome the bias that results from people at different prior risk being selected to receive one of the alternative forms of care that are being compared. This is to conduct a prospective experimental study, in which chance (randomization) is used to determine which of the alternative forms of care a particular woman or baby should receive. By giving each woman and each baby an equal chance of receiving the alternative treatments, randomization not only controls selection biases from factors known to be important (which could, in theory at least, be controlled for by matching those factors in the two groups); it is the *only* known way to control for *unknown* selection biases.

Randomization does not guarantee, nor does it need to guarantee, that the comparison groups will be exactly matched in respect of all characteristics that may affect the outcome. What randomization does guarantee is that the members of the groups being compared will be selected by chance, rather than by any biased form of selection. The statistical test procedures used to compare the outcomes in the two groups take into account the probabilities that chance imbalances may affect the study results.

The logic underlying the use of randomized controls in prospective experiments to create comparable groups of people for comparing alternative forms of care has great force once it is clearly perceived. Indeed, the randomized controlled trial has become widely accepted as the methodological 'gold standard' for comparing alternative forms of care.

The fact that a formal comparison of two or more forms of care is reported to be a randomized, controlled trial is not, however, a guarantee that selection bias has been eliminated. Knowledge of the group to which the woman would be allocated may influence the caregiver's decision about whether or not to enter a potential participant into a study, or may change the decision of the woman herself. Even after enrolling in a trial, participants may be selectively withdrawn from the study, because of knowledge of the group to which they have been assigned. The selection bias that results from tampering with the make-up of the randomized groups in these ways is sometimes a more important determinant of the differences in outcome than the effects of the forms of care that are compared; comparisons of the groups can then be misleading. For these reasons it is important to assess the likelihood of selection bias in studies purporting to be randomized comparisons of alternative forms of care, when trying to decide whether the results should be used to guide practice.

2.2 Minimizing other biases

The second major source of bias results when those receiving, providing, or evaluating care know which of the alternative forms of care has been received. This bias can be reduced and sometimes eliminated by 'masking' or 'blinding' (keeping those administering or receiving care unaware of the particular form of care that is being used).

Masking is particularly important when one or more of the forms of care being compared is likely to have psychologically-mediated effects on the outcomes of interest. The expectation that a form of care will have certain effects may result in a self-fulfilling prophecy. This phenomenon is known as the 'placebo effect' (literally, 'I will please'), when the effects are pleasant or beneficial in some other way. When the effects are unpleasant or unwanted, it is referred to as 'symptom suggestion'. In either case, it would be wrong to ascribe an outcome to a specific effect of a treatment, when the effect observed is actually an effect of the expectation.

Another reason for trying to keep caregivers unaware of the forms of care that are compared is to reduce the extent to which they may adjust other aspects of their care in the light of this knowledge. This 'co-intervention' may make the results of the comparison more difficult to interpret.

Lastly, knowledge of which form of care has been received can affect people's perception of the outcomes. This can occur, for example, if the people assessing the outcome of treatment consciously or unconsciously believe that one of the forms of care is better than the other; they may tend to record the outcomes in ways that confirm their expectations.

Protection against these observer biases is not a problem when the outcome in question is unambiguous; death is the clearest example. Observer biases among those assessing more ambiguous outcomes of care, such as, for example, pain in the mother or jaundice in the newborn, can be reduced, and sometimes abolished, by masking what care has been received. When it is either not feasible or not possible to mask the identity of the alternative forms of care, observer bias may be reduced by having the outcomes assessed by independent observers who are not aware of the treatment allocation.

It is important to remember that the number of participants in the trial (sample size) does not in any way correct for systematic (bias) errors. Indeed, if there is a bias in the selection of participants or in the assessment of outcomes, the larger the trial the greater, in absolute terms, will be the error.

3 Minimizing random errors (the play of chance)

Even after successful control of selection biases and other biases that can distort comparisons of alternative forms of care, the results of such comparisons may still be misleading because of random, or chance, errors. Unlike systematic errors, which will influence the apparent effect in one direction, random errors result from the play of chance, and can affect the results in either direction, haphazardly. Unlike errors due to bias, the larger the number of participants in the trial (sample size), the lower the risk of random errors.

Tests of statistical significance are used to assess the likelihood that the observed differences between alternative forms of care may simply be a reflection of random errors. If the differences are not statistically significant, these tests will prevent people from inferring that a real difference exists, when in truth it does not. Unfortunately, the failure to find a statistically significant difference between alternative forms of care often tends to be misinterpreted as meaning that there really is no difference. Failure to detect a difference does not mean that a difference does not exist. Estimating the range within which the true differential effects of alternative forms of care is likely to lie, by calculating a confidence interval for the statistically estimated differences in the outcome of care, provides further protection against being misled by random error.

Random errors will be reduced as samples yielding larger numbers of the outcomes of interest are studied. This can be achieved both by conducting larger trials than has been usual in the past, and by incorporating all the available data from broadly similar trials within a particular field of enquiry in systematic reviews (meta-analyses).

4 Ethics of randomized, controlled trials

The ethical principles of randomized trials are: that the trial should address an important question in a way that can contribute to the answer; that the answer is not already known; and that all who participate in the trial do so willingly, free from any coercion, and with as much information as they wish to have about the purpose of the trial and about all the proposed alternatives under study.

The essence of the randomized trial is fairness. Should one of the alternative forms of care tested prove to be better than the other, all participants have an equal chance of receiving it. Similarly, should one of the forms prove to be less effective, or even harmful, all have an equal chance of avoiding it. Thus, in addition to helping women and babies in the future, women who participate in randomized trials are improving their own likelihood of receiving the best care.

5 Applying the results of research

Even when one is reasonably certain that systematic and random errors have been adequately controlled in a particular study, or in a review of similar studies, questions still remain about the extent to which this research evidence should determine care for each individual woman or baby. There may be crucial differences between the women who participated in the research studies and women who receive care in other contexts; there may be important differences between the nature of the care given within the studies and that provided in usual clinical practice. These differences may limit the applicability of the results in different contexts. It would be rare, however, for a particular form of care to have opposite effects in different groups of individuals. Any real differences in the effects of care between participants in controlled trials and apparently similar people seen in every-day clinical practice, are more likely to be differences in the size, rather than in the direction, of the effects.

The results of formal research apply to groups of people. They cannot and should not be mechanistically applied to individuals. People may interpret risks differently, may value certain outcomes more than others, may have their own preferences, their personal sense of what is right or wrong for them. Individuals have a right to the most accurate, up-to-date information available, and the right to make an informed choice among the available alternatives.

6 Conclusions

The consequences of being misled by systematic errors (biases) and random errors (the play of chance) in research studies are that some women and babies will be denied effective care during pregnancy and childbirth, while others will receive care that is ineffective or actually harmful. In the hierarchy of evidence that we have adopted for arriving at the conclusions presented in this book, we have given less credence to the results of studies comparing groups of people who happened, for one reason or another, to have received one or other form of care (observational evidence), than to evidence derived from comparisons of people who have been randomized, in prospectively planned trials, to alternative forms of care (experimental evidence).

The distinction between these two kinds of evidence is crucial. Uncontrolled case series and studies using non-randomized controls so frequently lead to biased estimates of the effects of different forms of care that they should usually be seen as 'screening tests' to identify forms of care that *may* prove to be effective, rather than be used as a basis for guiding clinical practice.

Although well-designed, small, randomized trials may offer protection against the possibility of being misled by bias (systematic error), they provide little protection against being misled by the play of chance (random error). In the analyses on which this book is based, this problem has been addressed, whenever possible, by grouping similar studies together in systematic reviews (meta-analyses).

Our objectives in this book have been to use the strongest available evidence, and to bring that evidence together in a way that will help those who wish to give or receive effective care in pregnancy and childbirth. As we quoted in the previous chapter, and reiterate here:

> Evidence-based care is the conscientious, judicious, and explicit use of current best evidence in making decisions about the care of individual patients.

Evidence from research studies should be used to guide care, not to dictate it.

Sources

Effective care in pregnancy and childbirth

Chalmers, I., Evaluating the effects of care during pregnancy and childbirth.

Chalmers, I., Hetherington, J., Elbourne, D., Keirse, M.J.N.C., Enkin, M. Materials and methods use in synthesizing evidence to evaluate the effects of care during pregnancy and childbirth.

Mugford M, Drummond MF. The role of economics in the evaluation of care.

Robinson, J., The role of social sciences in evaluating perinatal care.

Support for pregnant women

1 Introduction

Outcomes of pregnancy and childbirth depend to a large extent on the social policies and health-care organization of the country in which the woman lives. Her health, her use of and response to health services, and her ability to follow the advice that she is offered, are affected by her own social circumstances and by the wider social, financial, and health-care policies.

Public and private concerns meet in many aspects of maternity care. Antenatal advice about rest or admission to hospital during pregnancy, for example, often does not take into account a woman's circumstances. The woman must weigh the benefits that she may gain from following the advice against its financial and social costs. Soundly based dietary advice may be ineffective if women are unable to follow it because of cost, or because it fails to take into account the constraints of cultural or family customs about food.

There is an association between a woman's social situation and both her health and her utilization of health services. This can be modified to only a limited extent by policies of social and financial support for childbearing families. In complex societies, fiscal, economic, social, and other policies all interact.

2 Social policy

National social policies have a direct and important effect on the well-being of childbearing women. When women have inadequate resources of money, time, and energy, they may not be able to make the choices that promote health. People may behave in a way that seems irrational to an outsider, but which is the best choice for them. Pregnant women may have other priorities besides care, such as finding the time and money to provide for children already in the household. A pregnant woman does not leave her work, community, and family responsibilities behind when she steps into the clinic or doctor's office.

Most industrialized countries provide direct financial aid to childbearing families, although the amount of aid women receive varies dramatically among countries. In addition to maternity benefits, there are other aspects of the welfare and taxation systems to be considered, such as family or tax allowances. In the Netherlands, for example, provision for 'maternity aides' is an integral part of the maternity system. These specially trained women provide support for up to five days postpartum for the substantial proportion of women who are at home for some or all of this period.

Most industrialized countries also have legislation intended to protect the fetus, newborn, and mother from the general and specific harmful effects of work, to protect employment by enabling parents to keep jobs while caring for children, and to provide income maintenance for parents during breaks in employment. Many countries have laws that restrict the type of work that pregnant women can do. Contact with low temperatures, lead, ionizing radiation, and other hazards may be controlled by law. Pregnant women may be barred from night work or long working hours. In some countries, employers may not be allowed to employ a woman in the period just before or just after delivery.

There has been considerable debate about this type of legislation. While it has laudable aims, it can restrict women's employment opportunities and result in them losing earnings during the childbearing period. Legislation of this nature, in the absence of adequate unemployment benefits or alternative work, may lead some women to conceal their pregnancies and to avoid seeking care. One way to avoid some of this effect is to have laws that protect women from dismissal on the grounds of pregnancy and that offer alternative work or compensation to women if their usual jobs are thought to be dangerous.

The other main area of legislation concerns leave, reinstatement, and income maintenance during maternity or parental leave. Most industrialized countries allow all employed women to have paid leave around the time of birth. For legislation to be effective in protecting parents and infants from stress and hardship, the level of income replacement during leave must be adequate. In some countries the maternity allowance is the same as, or close to, the woman's usual earnings, while in others it is fixed at a lower rate. If benefits are too low, women will be more likely to work during their period of maternity leave.

There is no evidence at present that would allow one to determine the optimal timing or length of leave. Some types and aspects of work seem more likely than others to compromise health during pregnancy. Different women may have different requirements, and more flexible leave arrangements are needed to allow some pregnant women to take time off earlier in pregnancy.

3 Antenatal care

Antenatal care programs, as currently practised, originated from models developed in Europe, in the early decades of the twentieth century. The core of these early models remains practically unchanged in current programs. Although new technologies, mostly diagnostic, have been added to routine antenatal care, these new components have often been introduced without proper scientific evaluation. The contents of antenatal care visits are more ritualistic than rational. The frequency of antenatal care visits and the interval between the visits have not been adequately tested.

Epidemiological and observational studies tend to show that women who receive antenatal care early in pregnancy, and who have more antenatal visits, tend to have lower maternal and perinatal mortality, and better pregnancy outcomes. Because of this, some antenatal care programs seek to increase the quantity of care provided, without considering the fact that by and large it is low-risk women who tend to attend for antenatal care earlier in pregnancy. Few attempts have been made to evaluate antenatal care programs for low-risk women by comparing models of antenatal care that differ in the quantity of care or type of care provider.

The trials that have been carried out suggest that, in both developed and developing countries, small reductions in the number of prenatal visits are compatible with good perinatal outcomes. Effective diagnostic and preventive interventions during pregnancy can be provided with fewer visits than are usually recommended. Until further evidence becomes available, four antenatal visits appears to be the minimum that should be offered to pregnant women without identified risk factors. The best care will not be effective if it is not available to those who need it. The cost of getting care can be a major impediment to access. For low-income people there is a close association between the lack of support for medical costs and low uptake of medical services. In many countries, teenagers, immigrants, and socially marginal women, may delay seeking care because of feeling ill at ease in conventional care settings. They are made uncomfortable by the difficulties they experience in communicating with the staff, the frequent impossibility of following the advice they are given, and, often, the reactions of caregivers. Partly because of problems of access and communication, women from lower social classes, as well as women from ethnic minorities, tend to be less well informed about the progress of pregnancy and birth, about potential problems, and about preventive and curative care. In giving greater priority to the preventive aspects of care than to the alleviation of symptoms, the current system of antenatal care is more adapted to the usual behavior of middle- and upper-class women.

4 Social and professional support during pregnancy

The interests of mothers are sometimes forgotten by those who profess an interest in promoting maternal and child health. The social, psychological, and physical problems experienced by pregnant women are often substantial. Those providing care must be sufficiently aware of them. Social and psychological support should be an integral element of all care provided for pregnant women.

During the 1980s and 1990s, considerable attention was given to trials of support during pregnancy for women who were believed to be at increased risk of adverse outcomes, in particular the risk of giving birth to a baby of less than 2500 g. Data from 12 trials, mostly of excellent quality, involving over 9000 women in nine countries on five continents have been reported. Most of the participants in the trials were socially disadvantaged, and most had one or more pre-existing medical risk factors for preterm birth or low birthweight. In general, the social support intervention was comprehensive and fairly intensive from the second trimester to the end of pregnancy. It included emotional support (e.g. counseling, reassurance, sympathetic listening) and information/advice, either in home visits or during clinic appointments, and could include tangible assistance (e.g. transportation to clinic appointments, assistance with the care of other children at home).

The results have been disappointing. Despite the quality of the additional support provided, and the fact that individual trials have found a few improvements in immediate psychosocial outcomes (lessened anxiety, fewer worries about the baby, increased satisfaction with care), no substantial improvements in medical outcomes were found. Specifically, when compared with women receiving standard care, women at high risk who received enhanced support during pregnancy experienced similar rates of stillbirth, neonatal death, preterm delivery, cesarean section, low-birthweight babies, babies with low Apgar scores, and babies who required admission to neonatal intensive care units. The results of different trials, in different places, were remarkably similar. Programs that offer additional support to women who are at high risk during pregnancy are unlikely, on the evidence available so far, to improve the outcome of the current pregnancy in clinical terms.

An argument could be made that, given the immense social deprivation experienced by most of the women in these trials, it would be surprising if social support could have such an immediate and powerful effect. While the theoretical rationale for links between social support, stress, and health is strong, it may be that social support (regardless of the quality and quantity) is not sufficiently powerful to improve the outcomes of the pregnancy during which it is provided. An important question remains about the potential benefits for subsequent pregnancies, since the benefits of additional pregnancy support may be long-term.

5 Control

Giving women more control during pregnancy may have an inherent value. Two small trials have evaluated allowing women to carry their own case-notes. This simple reversal of the usual practice had no apparent harmful effects, and was associated with an increased likelihood of feeling in control during pregnancy. The results of these trials suggest that consideration should be given to a policy of allowing women to carry their own records during pregnancy, and also that other forms of care, which offer women greater control during the childbearing period, should be evaluated.

6 Caregivers

Both access to care, and the extent to which care meets the social and psychological needs of women, depend to a large extent on the nature and training of those who provide care during pregnancy and childbirth.

As technical advances have become more complex, in many countries care has come to be increasingly controlled by, or even carried out by, specialist obstetricians. The benefits of this trend can be seriously challenged. It is inherently unwise, and perhaps unsafe, for women with normal pregnancies to be cared for by obstetric specialists, even if the required personnel were available. Because of time constraints, obstetricians caring for women with both normal and abnormal pregnancies have to make an impossible choice: to neglect the normal pregnancies in order to concentrate their care on those with pathology, or to spend most of their time supervising biologically normal processes. Midwives and general practitioners, on the other hand, are primarily oriented to the care of women with normal pregnancies, and are likely to have more detailed knowledge of the particular circumstances of individual women. The care that they can give to the majority of women, whose pregnancies are not affected by any major illness or serious complication, will often be more responsive to their needs than that given by specialist obstetricians. Industrialized countries in which midwives are the primary caregivers for healthy childbearing women have more favorable maternal and neonatal outcomes, including lower perinatal mortality rates and lower cesarean delivery rates, than countries in which many or most healthy women receive care from obstetricians during pregnancy.

Women have repeatedly stressed the importance of receiving care during pregnancy and childbirth from the same caregiver, or from a small group of caregivers with whom they can become familiar. The effects of continuity of care have been evaluated in two randomized, controlled trials – one in the UK and one in Australia – which compared care given by a small team of midwives with that given by a variety of midwives, obstetricians, and general practitioners during pregnancy and childbirth. Women who received care from the small team were less likely to experience prolonged antenatal clinic waiting times or antenatal admission to hospital. They were more likely to attend antenatal classes, were more able to discuss their worries during pregnancy, and to feel well-prepared for labor. They used less intrapartum analgesia or anaesthesia, and experienced fewer other intrapartum medical interventions. They felt more in control during labor, perceived the labor staff as more supportive, and felt more prepared for child care. They had fewer babies who required resuscitation at birth.

It was not possible, however, to determine from these trials whether these benefits were due to midwifery care or to continuity of care. Large-scale, randomized trials comparing care given by a team of midwives with physician-led shared care are currently in progress, and these may provide an answer to this question.

7 Conclusions

Persons providing maternity care share the collective responsibility for ensuring that effective care is not only known, but is also available, accessible, and affordable to all women who require it. Programs that provide special support to women considered to be at high risk have not been shown to reduce adverse clinical outcomes. Nevertheless, social and psychological support of pregnant women should be an integral part of all forms of care for childbearing women.

Women with normal pregnancies should be cared for by midwives or family doctors who are primarily oriented towards normal pregnancy, and who are likely to have a more detailed knowledge of the individual woman and her particular circumstances.

Sources

Effective care in pregnancy and childbirth

Kitzinger, S., Childbirth and society.

Shearer, M., Maternity patients' movements in the United States.

Reid, M. and Garcia, J., Women's views of care during pregnancy and childbirth.

DeVries, R., Caregivers in pregnancy and childbirth.

Robinson, S., The role of the midwife: opportunities and constraints.

Klein, M. and Zander, L., The role of the family practitioner in maternity care.

Parboosingh, J., Keirse, M.J.N.C. and Enkin, M.W., The role of the obstetric specialist.

Keirse, M.J.N.C., Interaction between primary and secondary care during pregnancy and childbirth.

Garcia, J., Blondel, B. and Saurel-Cubizolles, The needs of childbearing families: social policies and the organization of health care.

Elbourne D, Oakley A, Chalmers I. Social and psychologic support during pregnancy.

Cochrane Library

Brown H., Women carrying their own case-notes during pregnancy [registered title].

Bigirimana, P-C., Midwifery-led versus medical-led care for low-risk women during pregnancy and childbirth [Protocol].

Hodnett, E.D., Support during pregnancy for women at increased risk. Continuity of caregivers for care during pregnancy and childbirth.

Villar, J. and Khan-Neelofur, D., Patterns of routine antenatal care for low-risk pregnancy.

Other sources

Hodnett, E. (1993). Social support during pregnancy: does it help? *Birth*, **20**, 218–9.

Marmor, T.R., Barer, M.L. and Evans, R.G. (1994). The determinants of a population's health: What can be done to improve a democratic nation's health status? In *Why are some people healthy and others not?* (ed. Evans, R.G., Barer, M.L. and Marmor, T.R.), pp.217–30. New York: Aldine De Gruyter.

McClain, C.S. (1983). Perceived risk and choice of childbirth service. *Social Science and Medicine*, **17**, 1857–65.

Schramm, W.F. (1992). Weighing costs and benefits of adequate prenatal care. *Public Health Reports*, **107**(6), 647–52.

Wilkins, R., Sherman, G. and Best, P. (1991). Birth outcomes and infant mortality by income in urban Canada, 1986. *Health Report*, **3**, 7–31.

CHAPTER 4

Antenatal education

1 Antenatal classes

1.1 Introduction

In the 1950s and 1960s in Europe and North America, 'natural childbirth' and 'psychoprophylaxis' began as alternatives to what was perceived as over-medicalized obstetrics, with its liberal use of pain-relieving drugs and operative delivery. Many different programs appeared at about the same time, all with a single common aim: the use of psychological or physical, non-pharmaceutical modalities for the prevention of pain in childbirth.

Modern antenatal classes have expanded their horizons beyond that simple objective. Most classes today have additional goals including good health habits, stress management, anxiety reduction, enhancement of family relationships, feelings of empowerment, enhanced self-esteem and satisfaction, successful infant feeding, smooth postpartum adjustment, and advice on family planning. A major objective is to enhance the woman's sense of confidence as she approaches childbirth.

Because of their complex, often disparate goals and ideologies, one cannot make general statements about the effects of antenatal classes as if they were a single entity. Research on the effectiveness of antenatal classes over the years reflects their changing emphasis. The early studies focused on the effects of class attendance on labor pain, use of medication, and other qualities of labor. Later the emphasis shifted to study of the psychological effects, parenting behaviors, and the effectiveness of specific teaching, counseling, or labor-coping techniques.

1.2 Content of antenatal classes

The information content of modern antenatal classes may include the relation of pregnancy symptoms to underlying mechanisms, and suggest ways of alleviating these symptoms. The emotional shifts of pregnancy may be explored, and issues of sexuality, and relations with the partner and other children may be discussed as well.

Antenatal classes allow an opportunity to review the mechanisms of labor and birth in adequate detail, and to explain medical and obstetrical terminology, as well as the use of tests, medications, and other interventions. Information need not come from the instructor alone. Discussion with other participants allows for the reassurance and sense of community that comes from sharing experience and information.

In addition to knowledge and information, most antenatal classes attempt to impart skills for coping with the stress and pain of labor. These often include a variety of physical and mental relaxation techniques, various forms of attention-focusing and distraction, controlled breathing patterns, the teaching of comfort measures and labor-support skills to the birth partners of the pregnant woman, and discussions of both pharmacologic and non-pharmacologic methods of pain relief (see Chapter 34).

Finally, antenatal classes can be a vehicle for attitude modification. On the one hand they may foster increased self-reliance and questioning of professional routines and recommendations. On the other hand, they may lead towards increased acceptance of, and compliance with, prescribed medical regimens.

1.3 Effects of antenatal classes

Antenatal class attendance results in the use of significantly less pain-relieving medication. A Canadian trial of antenatal classes with a special focus on changes in the marital relationship concluded that such classes may enhance marital adjustment post-birth; however the trial was too small to draw definitive conclusions. No other important effects of antenatal classes have been clearly demonstrated. Non-randomized cohort studies have reported a variety of other beneficial effects of antenatal classes, but the self-selection of the study and control groups introduces such major biases that the results of these studies must be largely discounted.

There are few studies comparing the pain-relieving effects of different methods of childbirth preparation. Two methods that were popular in the 1960s and 1970s, Read's natural childbirth and Lamaze's psychoprophylaxis, have never been compared systematically. Because today's antenatal educators learn from a variety of sources, they are less likely to identify themselves with a particular method. Thus it is unlikely that direct comparisons of alternative methods will be carried out. The benefits of antenatal education are difficult to document in a systematic manner. The adverse effects and potential hazards are even more elusive. The extent to which fear is created rather than alleviated by classes, and whether women succumb to peer or educator pressures to conform, or to refuse needed medication or intervention, is completely unknown. There has been little systematic evaluation of the extent to which negative feelings of anger, guilt, or inadequacy are engendered when a woman's or her partner's expectations, possibly raised by the antenatal classes, are not met. There has been equally little evaluation of the potential hazards of classes that teach women to comply with their caregivers' routines, without adequate information.

While in years past, antenatal classes appealed primarily to middle-class women or couples, they are now routinely offered free of charge or at low cost in many clinics, health departments, and schools in developed countries. The effects of antenatal classes depend not only on the characteristics of those who attend, and the competence and skills of the teacher, but also, to a large extent, on the underlying objectives of the program. Some classes are taught by independent childbirth educators or co-ordinated by large consumer groups. Others are offered by official health agencies; still others by doctors for their own patients, or by hospitals for the women who plan to deliver there. The curricula outlined for these classes may be similar, and there may be little difference in the information taught, or the skills imparted. Nevertheless, there may be great differences in the attitudes that are encouraged. As a general rule, community-sponsored childbirth education classes are structured to incorporate the interests of parents into the curriculum. Hospital-based classes may be directed at explaining and justifying, rather than questioning, existing policies, offering alternatives, or helping parents decide their own birth plans.

It is possible that the actual existence of antenatal classes is more important than the details of what is taught. The full impact of childbirth education cannot be assessed solely by its effect on the individual woman giving birth, for there may be indirect effects that engender significant changes in the ambience in which all women give birth. Once a critical mass of mothers becomes aware of the fact that options are available to them, major changes in obstetrical practice may ensue.

If information on risks, benefits, and alternatives to conventional care remains a major focus among a large proportion of antenatal classes, we may expect increasingly influential and well-informed consumer involvement in the future patterns of childbirth practices. If, on the other hand, the ideology of classes shifts toward an acceptance of conventional obstetric practices, the group consciousness among expectant parents may fade, reducing their impact and their influence on the direction of maternity care.

2 Print, audio-visual, and electronic media

There are thousands of books and pamphlets, as well as many magazines and videotapes, aimed at childbearing women and their families, and even more Internet websites offering information and advice. The quality of information and advice varies widely, from excellent to inaccurate and potentially dangerous. There is a clear need to develop strategies to help consumers to evaluate the quality of the information in these resources.

There is limited evidence of the impact of mass media on consumer behavior, and none that specifically focuses on childbearing women and their families. A review of 17 studies of the impact of mass-media campaigns on health services utilization, concluded that mass-media campaigns can be an important influence on primary and secondary preventive health behavior. The burgeoning worldwide use of the Internet as a resource for information, as well as contact with others with similar health problems, particularly by adolescents and young adults (e.g. those entering their childbearing years), suggests that the Internet may soon become a powerful influence on the health-related decisions of childbearing women and their families.

3 Conclusions

In developed countries, the widespread popularity of antenatal classes testifies to the desire of expectant parents for childbirth education and peer support. As there are benefits in terms of amount of analgesic medication used and in some aspects of satisfaction with childbirth, and as significant adverse effects have not been demonstrated, such classes should continue to be available. The objectives of the classes must be made clear to the participants and unrealistic expectations of what the classes can achieve must be avoided. A variety of different types of classes, whose goals are explicitly stated, may help women or couples choose the program most likely to meet their needs. The quality of information and advice found in printed, audio-visual, and electronic media varies widely, from excellent to inaccurate and potentially dangerous. There is an urgent need to develop strategies to help consumers to evaluate the quality of the information in these resources.

Sources

Effective care in pregnancy and childbirth

Simkin, P., Non-pharmacological methods of pain relief during labour.

Simkin, P. and Enkin, M., Antenatal classes.

Cochrane Library

Gagnon, A., Antenatal education for childbirth/parenthood [protocol].

Grilli, R., Freemantle, N., Minozzi, S., Domenghetti, G. and Finer, D., Mass media interventions: effect on health services utilisation.

Other sources

Jadad, A.R. and Gagliardi, A. (1998). Rating health information on the Internet: navigating to knowledge or to Babel? *JAMA*, **279**, 611–4.

Lifestyle in pregnancy

1 Introduction

A pregnant woman is subject to a variety of prescriptions and proscriptions to modify her customary or desired lifestyle, in the guise of 'advice'. Unlike ordinary advice, however, there is frequently no option of refusal. Those believed to be authorities on reproduction, such as physicians, midwives, and childbirth educators, can give advice that appeals powerfully to the pregnant woman's desire for a perfect pregnancy and a perfect child. The effectiveness of this advice must be questioned and evaluated as rigorously as must every other intervention carried out during pregnancy.

2 Prepregnancy advice

The appeal of prepregnancy advice is easy to understand. Whether a fetus is normally formed or malformed is usually determined by the time of the first antenatal visit. Antenatal care may permit detection of an abnormality, but preconceptional precautions may help to avoid it. Other major complications of pregnancy, such as preterm labor, which have proven difficult to influence during pregnancy, may also be influenced by prepregnancy advice. It would seem plausible that care should start earlier, even before pregnancy begins.

A few measures have been found to be effective and useful. The most important among these is the use of folic acid supplementation to prevent neural tube defects and, possibly, conotruncal and limb defects (see Chapter 6). Prepregnancy assessment and advice can be vitally important for women with known problems, such as diabetes (see Chapter 20), a family history of, or genetic predisposition to, congenital abnormalities (see Chapter 9), or to screen for conditions that may affect the decision to become pregnant (e.g. HIV infection).

Except for these, and ensuring that the woman has been immunized against rubella and will not be taking any unnecessary drugs, what sensible advice can be given? Smokers need practical assistance for quitting rather than advice. Suggestions to adopt a prudent diet, although probably beneficial as general dietary guidelines, have not been shown to prevent malformations or low birthweight. Supplementation with trace minerals and vitamins other than folic acid cannot be justified in the present state of knowledge. Evidence on the effects of physical activity, work, exercise, and travel is still inconsistent.

The possible unwanted side-effects of prepregnancy advice include reduced self-confidence, reduced self-reliance, and increased anxiety for the woman. For advice-givers the side-effects may be a reduced awareness of the social factors that underlie individual health behaviors associated with adverse pregnancy outcomes, and a misguided though sincere belief that they have the answers.

It would be ill advised to make any judgements about routine prepregnancy advice (with the above exclusions) except to say that, on the basis of present knowledge, its beneficial effects are likely to be modest, and that it cannot automatically be regarded as harmless.

3 Sexual activity

Advice on the subject of sexual activity in pregnancy is often poorly given: inexact, inexplicit, euphemistic, misleading, allowing no opportunity for clarification and discussion of alternatives. Moreover, there are few or no data to support the various forms of advice given. The many studies reported on the effects of sexual activity in pregnancy are methodologically unsound and contradictory. On the basis of available evidence, any prohibition of sexual activity is inappropriate. A wide range of changes in sexual feelings occur normally during pregnancy, including a marked increase or a marked decrease in desire.

With respect to postulated benefits of sexual activity, the possibility that coitus near term may reduce the incidence of post-dates pregnancy has not been adequately investigated.

4 Smoking

The evidence that cigarette smoking has harmful effects on the fetus is strong. Maternal smoking reduces birthweight. The effect of smoking on pre-eclampsia, other perinatal outcomes, and subsequent child development, is more controversial.

Between one in five and one in three pregnant women in developed countries report smoking. Up to a quarter of women who smoke before pregnancy stop before their first antenatal visit. Smoking is more common among women with social disadvantage, high parity, no partner, low income, or receiving Medicaid-funded maternity care. Women with psychosocial problems, such as depression, job strain, excessive workload, and low levels of practical support, are also likely to smoke more than women without these disadvantages.

Smoking remains one of the few potentially preventable factors associated with low birthweight, very preterm birth, and perinatal death. For this reason it is an important public health issue in pregnancy. Smoking is also associated with low rates of initiation of breastfeeding, and reduced duration, although whether this is a causal relationship is still uncertain.

Smoking cessation programs have a definite place in antenatal care. They can be effective for a small minority of smokers in terms of reducing the amount smoked, in decreasing the proportion of women who continue to smoke, and in increasing mean birthweight, and reducing the proportion of low-birthweight babies. Of 100 women still smoking at the time of recruitment to a program (typically the time of the first antenatal visit), about 10 will stop smoking with 'usual care' and a further six or seven will stop as the result of a formal smoking cessation program. No trials have reported any assessment of the impact of smoking cessation programs on the method of delivery, breastfeeding, maternal psychological well-being, or the well-being of other family members.

Behavioral strategies in particular significantly reduce the proportion of smokers who continue smoking through pregnancy, compared with standard antenatal care. They are much more effective than personal advice supplemented by written material, than additional group sessions, or than advice and feedback.

Nicotine administered as transdermal patches, gum or nasal spray, or inhaled, has been shown to be effective in the reduction of smoking in non-pregnant subjects. There are currently package warnings not to use these preparations during pregnancy, though the appropriateness of this has been argued. The only trials carried out in pregnancy to date are small 'physiological' studies. Use of a nicotine patch in pregnancy resulted in similar blood nicotine levels and possibly similar effects on fetal middle cerebral artery resistance index and fetal heart-rate pattern as continued smoking. Short-term use of nicotine gum was associated with lower serum nicotine levels than continued smoking . The safety or effectiveness of nicotine substitutes in pregnancy has not been established.

One trial showed that simple change in question format (from yes or no to multiple options including 'I used to smoke', and 'I have cut down') will increase smoking disclosure.

Women's fears about smoking reduction have only rarely been taken into account. They may have fears that stopping smoking will, by increasing fetal size, increase the probability of a difficult labor or an operative delivery. They may worry about the effects on their psychological well-being and their capacity to cope with adverse circumstances, with flow-on detrimental effects to the well-being of other family members.

The possible adverse effects of smoking-cessation interventions have not been given adequate consideration. The campaign against smoking in pregnancy has sometimes had unwanted side-effects. Many smokers spend the whole of their pregnancy in a state of guilt and feelings of inadequacy. We do not know what the effects of such chronic stress and anxiety might be on the course of pregnancy and labor, or on the ultimate relationship with the child. We do know that more than half of the women who smoke worry about smoking during pregnancy and that 10% of smokers actually smoke more heavily in pregnancy. The global nature of much anti-smoking exhortation means that any bad outcome of pregnancy (including malformations and mental retardation) may be retrospectively blamed on smoking, even when this could not have been the cause. Sometimes health professionals unwittingly reinforce the self-blame.

The effectiveness of smoking-cessation programs, particularly those using behavioral strategies, has been clearly demonstrated. Such programs must, however, be used with understanding, sensitivity, and compassion. Much anti-smoking 'advice' and propaganda ignores the problem of physical and psychological addiction, the meaning of smoking for the women involved, and the guilt and anxiety felt by those who continue to smoke in the face of exhortations to give it up. Much health promotional material for use in pregnancy is characterized by its particularly strident tone.

Recognition of the social and environmental context in which individuals take up or continue certain behaviors has led some people to condemn health-education activities addressed to individuals as 'victim blaming'. Interventions that focus on self-help and behavioral strategies are less likely to be perceived in this way, and, in relation to quitting smoking, are soundly based. They are more effective than advice.

Obstetricians, family physicians or general practitioners, and midwives should support the population strategies towards a progressive reduction in cigarette smoking in the whole of society: to increase cigarette excise taxes; to ban all forms of tobacco advertising; to make public areas non-smoking; and to develop non-smoking policies for institutions and workplaces. The aim should be to make healthy choices easy choices.

5 Alcohol

The damaging effects of excessive alcohol consumption in pregnancy are well known. They include: fetal growth restriction; mental retardation and a dysmorphic syndrome with variable features (at high levels of consumption); and altered neonatal behavior. Developmental abnormalities are associated only with regular consumption of at least 28.5 ml alcohol (two standard drinks) per day, though one case has been reported following a single massive exposure to alcohol in the early weeks of pregnancy. Moderate alcohol consumption has not been associated with adverse perinatal and infant outcomes.

Campaigns to increase public awareness of the dangers of alcohol during pregnancy run the risk of arousing anxiety in some women already pregnant, partly because of the uncertainty about the safe lower limit for alcohol intake and also because of the possibility that the most dangerous time for dysmorphic effects may be the first trimester, sometimes even before women know that they may be pregnant. The very first weeks of pregnancy are often reported to be a period of high anxiety and depression that may increase drinking to relieve tension.

Policy development on alcohol and pregnancy requires, first of all, clarification as to the degree of risk around conception for low levels of regular alcohol consumption (fewer than two standard drinks a day), and for regular but infrequent 'binge' drinking. The rates of alcohol cessation during pregnancy are far higher than for smoking, and may be further increased by specific interventions, though in one study a program of home visits with advice, including advice about alcohol consumption, failed to affect alcohol use. It may be that better detection of heavy drinkers should be the priority.

6 Marijuana (cannabis)

There is limited information on the effects of marijuana use in pregnancy. A fair appraisal of the public health significance of cannabis use has been hampered by the polarized opinions about its health effects expressed by partisans on both sides of the debate on its legal status. A meta-analysis of the 10 published studies in which the results were adjusted for smoking, found no evidence that cannabis, at the amount typically consumed by pregnant women, causes low birthweight. In newborn infants, maternal marijuana use was associated with mild withdrawal symptoms. Between 6 months and 3 years of age, however, no behavioral consequences of marihuana exposure were noted.

No effects on motor development, including balance and ball-handling items at 3 years, have been identified. Longer term studies also failed to demonstrate important adverse effects prenatal marijuana exposure, which was not significantly related to reading or language outcomes in 9–12 year olds

This general failure to demonstrate important adverse effects should not lead to complacency, however. Sleep disturbance in the offspring has been suggested. Other long-term studies suggest that as children become older, certain aspects of neuropsychological functioning, such as increased behavioral problems and decreased performance on visual perceptual tasks, can discriminate between *in utero* exposed and unexposed children.

7 Work

Professional guidelines on work during pregnancy too often neglect any mention of housework and childcare as work, whether in regard to exposure to toxic chemicals (e.g. pesticides, household cleaners) or lifting heavy weights (e.g. a toddler plus a folding push chair or stroller). For example, although women who have previously given birth to infants weighing less than 2 kg are often advised not to work, we have not seen any official recommendations that such women be provided with free childcare and daily household help throughout pregnancy. Equally, discussions of whether pregnant women should work usually pay scant attention to the implications for family health and welfare of the concomitant reduction in family income. In fact, the benefits of paid employment are rarely mentioned.

The main cause of confusion results from regarding paid employment as a single category, lumping together women working with much less physical effort or stress than they would have at home with women whose work involves standing all day, carrying heavy loads, or exposure to extremes of temperature or humidity.

General advice on employment in pregnancy is clearly inappropriate. Where working conditions involve occupational fatigue, women's requests for a change of work during pregnancy should be supported by those providing antenatal care. Apart from this situation, it is extremely difficult to weigh up the net benefits and risks.

8 Aerobic exercise

Aerobic exercise in pregnancy improves or maintains physical fitness. Possible benefits or risks with respect to the outcome of pregnancy have not been adequately evaluated, though data regarding a postulated shortening of pregnancy is reassuringly negative.

9 Conclusions

Prepregnancy counseling for specific indications has a definite place, but there is no evidence at present to warrant routine preconceptional visits. Prepregnancy advice about routine folate supplementation can be important, for reducing the risk of neural tube defects.

There is no evidence to warrant any restriction on sexual activity during pregnancy.

Smoking-cessation programs should be routinely offered to pregnant women who smoke, but should be used with sensitivity and consideration for each woman's individual circumstances.

The dangers of moderate use of alcoholic beverages during pregnancy have been exaggerated. Women should be warned against excessive use of alcohol.

With the implied promise that it will help her have a perfect birth, a perfect baby, and become a perfect mother, a pregnant woman is exhorted to lead a selfless, healthy life, uncontaminated by sex, cigarettes, alcohol, employment, or anxiety. The evidence for most of these exhortations is slight. Where the evidence is stronger, the flaw has been in the way that research and prescription fail to take into account the real lives and responsibilities of women.

Sources

Effective care in pregnancy and childbirth

Lumley, J. and Astbury, J. Advice for pregnancy.

Cochrane Library

Kramer, M., Regular aerobic exercise during pregnancy.

Lumley, J., Interventions for promoting smoking cessation during pregnancy.

Lumley, J., Watson, L., Watson, M. and Bower, C., Periconceptional supplementation with folate and/or multivitamins for preventing neural tube defects.

Silagy, C., Nicotine replacement therapy.

Physician advice for smoking cessation.

Other sources

Belizan, J.M., Barros, F., Langer, A., Farnot, U., Victora, C. and Villar, J. (1995). Impact of health education during pregnancy on behavior and utilization of health resources. Latin American Network for Perinatal and Reproductive Research. *Am. J. Obstet. Gynecol.*, **173**, 894–9.

Benowitz, N.L. (1991). Nicotine replacement therapy during pregnancy. *JAMA*, **266**, 3174–7.

Borrelli, B., Bock, B., King, T., Pinto, B. and Marcus, B.H. (1996). The impact of depression on smoking cessation in women. *Am. J. Prev. Med.*, **12**, 378–87.

Campion, P., Owen, L., McNeill, A. and McGuire, C. (1994). Evaluation of a mass media campaign on smoking and pregnancy. *Addiction*, **89**, 1245–54.

Mullen, P.D., Carbonari, J.P. and Glenday, M.C. (1991). Identifying pregnant women who drink alcoholic beverages. *Am. J. Obstet. Gynecol.*, **165**, 1429–30.

Reynolds, K.D., Coombs, D.W., Lowe, J.B., Peterson, P.L. and Gayoso, E. (1995). Evaluation of a self-help program to reduce alcohol consumption among pregnant women. *Int. J. Addict.*, **30**, 427–43.

CHAPTER 6

Dietary modification in pregnancy

1 Introduction

The relation between the diet of the mother and the well-being of the fetus and infant continues to be a matter of controversy. Observational studies have generated uncertain and conflicting conclusions because they encompass many other aspects of the pregnant woman's life that vary along with diet and nutrition. Limits to nutritional intake imposed by economic, educational, social, or other constraints, are likely to be accompanied by additional stresses, such as exposure to infection, the need for physical labor, inadequate housing, or family disruption. Controlled studies of dietary interventions have not, for the most part, been large enough to allow firm conclusions to be drawn; nevertheless, much important information has been obtained.

2 Pre- and periconceptional nutrition

The protective effect of folate supplementation against neural tube defects (spina bifida and anencephaly) was first suggested by cohort and case-control studies, and has been confirmed by randomized, controlled trials. Periconceptional supplementation with folic acid can reduce the risk of neural tube defect by more than two-thirds, both for women who are at increased risk (because of a previously affected fetus), and for women at normal risk. Multivitamin preparations without folate have not been shown to prevent neural tube defects. All women who have had a fetus with a neural tube defect in a previous pregnancy need to be given information about the risk of recurrence. They should be advised of the substantial (although not complete) protective effect of folate supplementation, and offered continuing folate supplementation (4 mg/day) as long as there is any possibility of pregnancy. At a minimum, supplementation should begin at least two months before a planned conception, and continue for the first three months of pregnancy. Epileptic women who are receiving anticonvulsant medication, particularly valproic acid, may require larger doses of folate to counter the antifolate action of the medication.

There is also a clear preventive effect of added folate for women with no known risk factors for neural tube defect. Because as many as half of all pregnancies are unplanned, and folate supplementation must begin at least two months before conception, there are special challenges in the application of this evidence. In some countries, basic food stuffs, such as flour, are now supplemented with folate, for the benefit of women who might become pregnant. This practice is still controversial, because not enough is known about the balance of benefits and risks of additional folic acid to the entire population.

An alternative strategy would focus on women in the childbearing age. Health-care providers can take advantage of contacts with these women, such as at routine examinations or the provision of contraception, as an opportunity to inform them about the benefits of periconceptional folate supplementation, of the protective effects of a folate-rich diet, and about how this can be achieved. It is still unclear whether adequate folate to maximize the preventive effect can be provided by diet alone. The only primary prevention trial employed a dose of 0.8 mg folic acid, a level difficult to achieve by diet alone. Trials of lower doses of folic acid are required. If a lower dose is found to be effective, it might be possible to achieve it by dietary change, and avoid the need for supplementation.

3 Diet and fetal growth

Two main conclusions can be drawn from studies on dietary modification in pregnancy. First, severe dietary restriction can cause marked decreases in birthweight. During famine, average birthweight can be depressed by as much as 500 g; dietary manipulation and restriction as a result of well-meaning advice can have almost as marked an effect. The low birthweight observed in these studies resulted from impairment of fetal weight gain, as no effect was found on gestational age or on the rate of preterm birth. Trials of dietary restriction in pregnant women with high weight-for-height or high weight gain suggest that such restriction impairs fetal growth; they have been too small to demonstrate any significant effect on other outcomes. Although the extent to which major suppression of fetal weight causes perinatal mortality and morbidity is not known, there can be no justification for allowing pregnant women to go hungry, or for imposing dietary restriction or major manipulation of dietary constituents upon them.

Second, attempts at nutritional supplementation, while well-intentioned, have not always had the desired effect. Trials of high-protein nutritional supplements provide no evidence of benefit on fetal growth; on the contrary, the evidence suggests they may be harmful. Comparisons of supplements with equivalent energy content but different protein concentrations, also show lower average birthweights and a higher incidence of small-for-gestational-age births in the higher protein intervention groups.

In contrast, balanced energy and protein supplementation decreases the incidence of small-for-gestational-age birth, and the likelihood of stillbirth or neonatal death. These effects are important, although rather difficult to explain, because it results in only a small (about 30 g) increase in mean birthweight, unless the energy content of the supplement is very high (around 1000 kcal per day). Such supplementation has no demonstrated effect on mean gestational age at birth, although a non-significant reduction in the frequency of preterm birth is suggested by the available data. No long-term benefits for child growth and development have been demonstrated. Surprisingly, there is no evidence that supplementation has a larger effect on mean birthweight in women who are clearly undernourished before or during pregnancy. One cannot exclude the possibility that the small size of the effect may result from women sharing their meagre diets with other hungry members of their families (see Chapter 16).

Specific supplementation to enhance fetal growth has been investigated with several nutrients, such as carnitine, calf blood extract, amino acid, and glucose solutions. Although the results of two trials show some benefit in terms of the outcomes studied, both have small sample sizes. At present, there is inadequate evidence to support the routine use of nutrient therapy for suspected impaired fetal growth in clinical practice, and further, well-controlled trials are needed.

Nutritional advice appears to be moderately effective in increasing pregnant women's energy and protein intakes, but the implications for fetal, infant, or maternal health, cannot be judged from the available trials. Furthermore, advice is not benign. Efforts to encourage women to eat well during pregnancy, however well-intentioned, often include explicit statements that women can reduce their risk of having a preterm birth through attention to their diet and other lifestyle issues. Such statements are not only misleading, but can engender guilt, anxiety, and a false sense of responsibility for untoward pregnancy outcomes.

4 Diet and pre-eclampsia

Attempts to prevent pre-eclampsia by modification of protein or calorie intake continue to influence antenatal care, despite the fact that the evidence and arguments on which they are based are far from convincing. Presently available evidence provides no justification for telling women to restrict their diet in an effort to limit weight gain. Equally, there is no evidence to support the alternative view that eating sufficient amounts of a good diet will reliably protect against pre-eclampsia.

Controlled trials of prophylactic fish oil in pregnancy show a promising increase in the length of gestation and birthweight, but there are insufficient data to show a decrease in the incidence of hypertension, or any measure of perinatal mortality or morbidity.

The available trials of salt restriction are insufficient to provide reliable information about the effects of salt restriction during normal pregnancy. Salt consumption should remain a matter of personal preference. No trials have included women with pre-eclampsia. The effects of calcium supplementation are discussed below in Section 7 (see also Chapter 15).

5 Special diets to avoid antigens

Special diets to avoid antigens have been prescribed for women at high risk of giving birth to an atopic child (based on a history of atopy in the mother, the father, or a previous child). The evidence available from controlled trials shows that prescription of an antigen-avoidance diet to a high-risk woman during pregnancy is unlikely to reduce her risk of giving birth to an atopic child substantially. It is also possible that such a diet might have adverse effects on maternal and/or fetal nutrition. A firm conclusion on this issue would require further trials, involving larger numbers of women and babies, with longer follow-up.

6 Hematinic supplements

As pregnancy proceeds, most women show hematological changes that suggest iron and folate deficiency; the hemoglobin, serum iron, serum folate, and red cell folate concentrations fall and the total iron-binding capacity rises. In developed countries, the decrease in blood values is rarely sufficient to be serious, especially in women who receive an adequate diet. Despite this, it is common practice for women to routinely receive iron and folate supplementation during pregnancy. The available data from controlled trials provide clear evidence that normal (for non-pregnant women) values can be restored by this supplementation, but there is no evidence that it has any effect, beneficial or harmful, on clinical outcomes for mother or baby.

In developing countries the amount of iron and folate available from dietary sources may not meet the additional demands placed on maternal iron and folic acid stores by the growing fetus, the placenta, and the increased maternal red cell mass, even though the increased demands are partially offset by the amenorrhea and increased absorption of iron and folate during pregnancy. Anemia in pregnancy is a major health problem in many developing countries. Routine iron supplementation raises and maintains serum ferritin above 10 g/l, and results in a substantially lower proportion of women with a hemoglobin level below 10 or 10.5 g per cent (below 6–6.5 mmol/l) in late pregnancy. Routine folate supplementation after the first few weeks of pregnancy substantially reduces the prevalence of low serum and red cell folate levels, and of megaloblastic hematopoiesis, but has no apparent effect on the frequency of hypertension, maternal infection, placental abruption, preterm birth, cesarean birth or stillbirth. However, few of the data relate to communities in which nutritional anemia from either iron or folate deficiency is common. Trials are needed in these populations to establish the most appropriate strategies for combating the deficiencies.

There is cause for concern in the findings of a well-conducted trial involving over 2300 pregnant women in Finland, in whom iron supplementation resulted in an increase in perinatal mortality, as well as a substantial number of adverse side-effects from iron in the last month of pregnancy. However, this trial also showed a decrease in the rates of cesarean section and blood transfusion; the latter may be particularly important in areas where HIV infection is prevalent. An individual's hemoglobin concentration depends much more on the complex relation between red-cell mass and plasma volume than on deficiencies of iron or folate. A low hemoglobin, without other evidence of iron deficiency, requires no treatment. If there is evidence of genuine iron deficiency, iron treatment is needed, and the usual approach is to give iron salts by mouth. There is no convincing evidence that the addition of copper, manganese, or molybdenum improves the efficiency with which the iron is used.

The cause of megaloblastic anemia in pregnancy is almost always folate deficiency, and treatment with folic acid supplementation is rapidly effective.

7 Other vitamin or mineral supplementation

Vitamin D deficiency may occur in women whose diet is relatively low in the vitamin, such as vegetarians and those who either remain indoors or whose clothing leaves little exposed skin, particularly in relatively sunless climates. Controlled trials in vulnerable populations show a reduction in neonatal hypocalcemia (leading to hyper-irritability) with vitamin D supplementation. No significant effects on other substantive outcomes have been reported.

The little evidence available on vitamin B6 supplements in pregnancy suggests that they may protect against dental decay in the mother when given in the form of lozenges, but no effect has been found on other clinical outcomes.

A number of well-designed trials have assessed the effects of calcium supplementation on important measures of maternal morbidity, and perinatal morbidity and mortality. Calcium supplementation during pregnancy appears to produce a modest reduction in the risk of high blood pressure in normal pregnancy, and a substantial risk reduction among those at high risk of hypertension and those with low baseline dietary calcium. The pattern is the same for pre-eclampsia. There was no overall effect on the risk of preterm birth, but a reduction in risk among women at high risk of pre-eclampsia. There is no evidence of any effect on perinatal mortality.

Several trials have concluded that oral magnesium treatment from before the 25th week of gestation resulted in a lower incidence of preterm birth, less maternal hospitalization during pregnancy, fewer cases of antepartum hemorrhage, as well as lower incidences of low birthweight and small-for-gestational-age infants compared with placebo treatment. However, because nearly all of the trials were of poor methodological quality, dietary magnesium supplementation of pregnant women cannot be recommended for routine clinical practice.

The available data from five controlled trials of routine zinc supplementation during pregnancy show no effect, either beneficial or harmful. Iodine supplementation in a population with high levels of endemic cretinism results in an important reduction in the incidence of the condition, with no apparent adverse effects.

8 Conclusions

There is no evidence that dietary restriction of any sort confers any benefit to pregnant women or their offspring.

All women who might become pregnant should ensure an adequate intake of folic acid, at least around the period of conception, either through supplementation or diet. Women who have had a fetus with a neural tube defect should be counseled about the increased risk in subsequent pregnancies and offered a folic acid supplement (4 mg/day), if they intend to have another baby. Supplementation should begin before conception and continue through the first three months of pregnancy.

High-protein dietary supplements should be avoided. Balanced energy and protein nutritional supplementation, particularly in large enough amounts, reduces the incidence of small for-gestational-age birth and may reduce the perinatal mortality rate. It has no apparent effect on the mean length of gestation, only a small effect on birthweight, and no apparent effect on long-term child health. Public health programs offering nutritional supplements, dietary advice, and support for pregnant women, are intrinsically worthwhile, but should not be based on the premise that they will reduce the rate of preterm birth.

There is at present no basis for recommending supplementation with any specific nutrients for suspected impaired fetal growth. Antigen-avoidance diets have so far not shown any convincing benefit in the prevention of atopy.

Routine hematinic supplementation with iron in developed countries has not been shown to confer any benefit to either mother or baby, except to build up the woman's iron stores. Routine supplementation may be of benefit in populations in which iron deficiency is a common problem. Women who are at high risk of pre-eclampsia and have low dietary calcium intake should receive calcium supplementation during pregnancy. Vitamin D supplementation at the end of pregnancy should be considered in vulnerable groups, such as Asian women in northern Europe, and possibly others in climates with long winters. Iodine supplementation should be provided in populations with high levels of endemic cretinism. No recommendations can be made about the place, if any, for routine supplementation with zinc or magnesium, or about the role of fish oils during pregnancy.

While there is an obvious need for further research into the best means of promoting optimal nutrition in pregnancy, hungry women cannot wait for the results of such studies. They must have access to adequate amounts of food and to valid nutritional information.

Sources

Effective care in pregnancy and childbirth

Green, J., Diet and the prevention of pre-eclampsia.

Mahomed, K. and Hytten, F. Iron and folate supplementation in pregnancy.

Rush, D., Effects of changes in protein and calorie intake during pregnancy on the growth of the human fetus.

Cochrane Library

Atallah, A.N., Hofmeyr, G.J. and Duley, L., Calcium supplementation during pregnancy for preventing hypertensive disorders and related problems.

Duley, L. and Henderson-Smart, D., Reduced salt intake compared to normal dietary salt, or high intake, during pregnancy.

Gulmezoglu, A.M. and Hofmeyr, G.J., Maternal nutrient supplementation for suspected impaired fetal growth.

Kramer, M.S., Balanced protein/energy supplementation in pregnancy.

Energy/protein restriction for high weight-for-height or weight gain during pregnancy.

High protein supplementation in pregnancy.

Isocaloric balanced protein supplementation in pregnancy.

Maternal antigen avoidance during pregnancy for preventing atopic disease in infants of women at high risk.

Maternal antigen avoidance during lactation for preventing atopic disease in infants of women at high risk.

Maternal antigen avoidance during lactation for preventing atopic eczema in infants.

Nutritional advice in pregnancy.

Lumley, J., Watson, L., Watson, M. and Bower, C., Periconceptional supplementation with folate and/or multivitamins for preventing neural tube defects.

Makrides, M. and Crowther, C.A., Magnesium supplementation during pregnancy.

Mahomed, K., Folate supplementation in pregnancy.

Iron supplementation in pregnancy.

Iron and folate supplementation in pregnancy.

Zinc supplementation in pregnancy.

Mahomed, K. and Gulmezoglu, A.M., Maternal iodine supplements in areas of deficiency.

Pyridoxine (vitamin B6) supplementation in pregnancy.

Vitamin D supplementation in pregnancy.

Other sources

Kramer, M. (1998). Maternal nutrition, pregnancy outcome and public health policy. *Can. Med. Assoc. J.*, **159**, 663–5.

Olsen, S.F., Sorensen, J.D., Secher, N.J., Hedegaard, M., Henriksen, T.B., Hansen, H.S. *et al.* (1992). Randomised controlled trial of effect of fish-oil supplementation on pregnancy duration. *Lancet,* **339**, 1003–07.

Onwude, J.L., Lilford, R.J., Hjartardottir, H., Staines, A. and Tuffnell, D. (1995). A randomised double blind placebo controlled trial of fish oil in high risk pregnancy. *Br. J. Obstet. Gynaecol.* **102**, 95–100.

Salvig, J.D., Olsen, S.F. and Secher, N.J. (1996). Effects of fish oil supplementation in late pregnancy on blood pressure: a randomised controlled trial. *Br. J. Obstet. Gynaecol.*, **103**, 529–33.

Screening

Risk scoring

1 Introduction

One of the primary objectives of antenatal care is to identify factors that might put mother or baby at an increased risk of an adverse outcome, at a time when interventions can be undertaken to prevent or ameliorate the harmful consequences. Other chapters in this book address the process of screening for specific problems. In this chapter we consider a quite different aspect, the overall risk status of the woman and the pregnancy.

Caregivers have long recognized that some women are more likely than others to develop problems during their pregnancies. Factors in their family history, past medical history, past obstetrical history, or findings that are noted in their physical or laboratory examination, may increase their risk of serious sequelae. Clinicians, consciously or subconsciously, formally or informally, attempt to identify these women, and provide them with increased surveillance and care. Questions remain, however, as to whether assessing risk status in a formal, quantitative manner, is more effective than the informal methods traditionally used, and whether the labels and interventions that arise from risk assessment improve the outcome for mother or baby.

2 Theoretical considerations

The primary purpose of a risk-scoring system is to classify individual women into different categories, for which specific actions can be planned, advised, and implemented. A number of scoring systems have been proposed, in which a woman's putative risk factors are identified and summed to produce an overall 'risk score'. In some, the process has been refined (or complicated) by allotting a weighting factor to each risk, so that relatively minor risks add little to the score, while more serious risks are given greater emphasis.

In theory, a process of rationally based risk scoring should be more accurate than the rather nebulous process of clinical impression that is part of daily clinical practice. There are, however, a number of problems with this approach. First, it is difficult to make quantitative estimates of the exact risk associated with a given factor. That information is available only for certain factors, usually the most serious factors, which in themselves are enough to alert the clinician. Second, there is no evidence to suggest that assigning a number or weight to a feature allows it to be added to others to arrive at a valid overall measurement of risk status. A combination of three similar risk factors does not provide three times the risk of one of them.

There are difficulties also in the definition of risk factors. Does 'bleeding', for example, also include spotting, or bleeding from a local lesion in the vagina or cervix? The need to dichotomize continuous variables that are as different from each other as blood pressure (how high?) or smoking (how much?), imposes a rigidity that can often be counterproductive. With formalized risk scoring, a woman may be assigned to a high-risk group because of fixed definitions of the risk markers, whereas a capable clinician – or the woman herself – could have assessed the situation more sensitively with clinical judgement or common sense.

Scoring is more predictive of outcome in second or later pregnancies, than when used for women pregnant for the first time. The poor predictive value of the scoring systems for nulliparae is, at least in part, inherent in the choice of risk markers, many of which relate to characteristics of past obstetric history.

Some scoring systems require women to be scored only once, at the initial visit, while others may require reassessment at each antenatal visit. Reassessment allows the inclusion of complications appearing in the current pregnancy, and revision of the score upwards or, less typically, downwards depending on new circumstances. A useful scoring system should allow ascertainment of risk in time for appropriate action to be taken. Scoring systems correspond better to outcomes if they are implemented late in pregnancy, or allow for readjustment during pregnancy. This leads to the paradox, that the most precise predictions are made at a time when there is less need or opportunity to influence the course of events, whereas the potentially more useful early risk identification is imprecise.

3 Usefulness of scoring

In essence, risk scoring is a screening test, and should be required to conform to the criteria required for all good screening tests. The test should be able to discriminate clearly between those who are, and those who are not, at high risk, and effective management should be available for those who are identified as at high risk. Both the positive and the negative predictive values of all scoring systems are poor. Depending on the cut-off point and the test chosen, only between 10 and 30% of the women who are allocated to the high-risk groups actually experience the adverse outcome for which the scoring system declares them to be at risk. Between 20 and 50% of mothers who deliver preterm or low-birthweight infants have low risk scores. As for many other tests, the sensitivity, specificity, validity, and utility of risk-scoring systems remain to be determined.

It may be useful to the clinician to know which pregnancies under his or her care are most likely to result in an adverse outcome. To the individual woman, however, being labeled as 'high-risk' will be beneficial only if something can be done either to decrease the risk or to reduce its consequences. If, on the other hand, the label results in the use of an intervention that was not needed, it will have caused more harm than good.

Although often referred to as risk factors, most of the elements that are incorporated in the scores are merely risk markers, indicating that there is a statistical association with a particular outcome. These risk markers do not cause the outcome. The most important of them, such as parity, prepregnancy weight, height, and past reproductive performance, cannot be altered by any intervention. For the individual woman who is labeled as 'high risk', both the threat of adverse outcome and the inability to change its markers may create anxiety. As well, being labeled 'low risk' does not guarantee a good outcome. It is too easy to fall into the trap of thinking that 'risk' implies a fate, rather than a frequently incorrect prediction.

The most powerful way to test the effectiveness of formal risk-scoring systems is to mount randomized, controlled trials in which formal risk scoring is a component of the antenatal care of one group of women, while a control group receive the usual antenatal care without formal risk scoring. No such trials have been carried out.

A number of observational studies have claimed a reduction in preterm births following the introduction of systematic scoring. They attributed this improvement to better selection of those women who require treatment, and to better 'systematization of interventions'.

In many settings there was an increase in the frequency with which interventions of dubious value were performed. Although some authors expressed the belief that their prevention policy had played a part in the overall reduction of preterm birth rates, most of the improved results occurred in the women scored to be at low risk.

4 Conclusions

Formal risk scoring systems are a mixed blessing for the individual woman and her baby. They may help to provide a minimum level of care and attention in settings where these are inadequate. In other settings, however, formal risk scoring and labeling may result in a variety of unwarranted interventions. The introduction of risk scoring into clinical practice carries the danger of replacing a potential risk of adverse outcome with the certain risk of dubious treatments and interventions.

The potential benefits of risk scoring have been widely publicized, but the potential harm is rarely mentioned. Such harm can result from unwarranted intrusion in women's private lives, from superfluous interventions and treatments, from creating unnecessary stress and anxiety, and from allocating scarce resources to areas where they are not needed.

Sources

Effective care in pregnancy and childbirth

Mohide, P. and Grant, A., Evaluating diagnosis and screening during pregnancy.

Alexander, S. and Keirse, M.J.N.C., Formal risk scoring during pregnancy.

Other sources

Chard, T. and Carrol, S. (1990). A computer model of antenatal care: relationship between the distribution of obstetric risk factors in simulated cases and in a real population. *Eur. J. Obstet. Gynecol. Reprod. Biol.*, 35, 51–61

Hall, P. (1994). Rethinking risk. *Can. Fam. Physician*, 40, 1239–44

CHAPTER 8

Imaging ultrasound in pregnancy

1 Introduction

Ultrasound imaging is now firmly embedded in antenatal maternity care. Improvement in resolution and quality of ultrasound imaging equipment has been rapid; progress from the first detection of the gross abnormality of anencephaly in 1972 to the current sophisticated diagnoses of subtle fetal anomalies has been impressive.

Whether ultrasound imaging should be used routinely for prenatal screening or only used selectively for specific indications has not, as yet, been firmly established.

2 Selective use of ultrasound

There is a clear difference between selective and routine use of ultrasound. The time taken, the detail inspected, the sophistication of the equipment used, and, perhaps, the experience of the ultrasonographer, will vary with the reason for the examination. To identify fetal presentation, for example, takes seconds and can be carried out by a minimally trained technician. To thoroughly investigate a suspected fetal abnormality, may require considerable time and expertise. Routine examinations must be accomplished quickly for practical reasons;

some fetal malformations are, therefore, less likely to be detected than when there are specific reasons to anticipate their presence. The selective examination should be tailored to answer a specific question posed by the person who requests the examination.

There can be little doubt about the value of information provided by ultrasound in many specific clinical situations. Ultrasound has the ability to establish rapidly and accurately whether a fetus is alive or dead, and to predict whether a pregnancy is likely to continue after threatened miscarriage. Gestational age can be accurately estimated from early measurements of fetal size in the first or early second trimesters. In the investigation of possible fetal malformation, ultrasound can often visualize the malformation, and can facilitate other diagnostic techniques, such as amniocentesis and chorion villus sampling. It can assess fetal size and growth in the second-half of pregnancy with reasonable accuracy. It can locate placental position in cases of suspected placenta praevia. Other situations in which the selective use of ultrasound can provide valuable help include: confirmation of suspected multiple pregnancy; assessment of amniotic fluid volume in suspected polyhydramnios or oligohydramnios; confirmation of fetal position; and assistance for other procedures, such as cervical cerclage or external cephalic version.

The great value of selective ultrasound to answer specific questions does not provide information as to whether or not routine ultrasound screening of all women during pregnancy would be worthwhile. The greatest controversy surrounding obstetrical ultrasound has been whether its use should be extended from specific indications to the routine screening of all pregnant women, either early (usually 18–20 weeks, but sometimes earlier) or later in pregnancy (usually 32–36 weeks).

3 Routine early ultrasonography

The postulated benefits of routine ultrasonography in early pregnancy include: better gestational age assessment; earlier detection of multiple pregnancy; and detection of clinically unsuspected fetal malformation at a time when termination of pregnancy is possible. Data from controlled studies show that these expectations have been largely fulfilled.

When compared with selective ultrasonography in early pregnancy, routine ultrasound examination results in a reduced rate of induction of labor for apparent post-term pregnancy (probably as a result of better gestational dating) and there are fewer undiagnosed twins at 26 weeks' gestation among the screened group. Both of these effects may reduce the mother's anxiety and the costs of care, but neither has so far been shown to improve fetal outcome. Earlier evidence suggesting fewer low-birthweight babies among screened pregnancies has not been confirmed by further studies.

If the screening examination is performed early in pregnancy, some clinically unsuspected non-viable pregnancies (e.g. blighted ova and hydatidiform moles), may be detected. Some promising reports of early (first trimester) screening for anomalies have appeared, but without controlled evaluation. Satisfactory inspection of fetal anatomy to detect malformation cannot, however, be performed before 18 weeks. The usual choice of 18–20 weeks is in effect a trade-off. It is still not possible to detect all ultrasound-detectable anomalies at this period of pregnancy. If inspection of the heart is to be included, examination closer to 22 weeks may be necessary. A choice of 18–20 weeks is a balance between doing ultrasound as late as possible, in order to pick up as many anomalies as possible, but still early enough to allow women choices about whether or not to proceed with their pregnancies.

Only two of the controlled trials of routine early ultrasound included the specific aim of detecting malformed fetuses and in only one of these was effective prenatal diagnosis linked to a widespread willingness to terminate pregnancies if the fetus was malformed. In this study, the screened group had a lower perinatal mortality (but no increase in the proportion of live births) because of early detection and selective termination of pregnancies in which the baby had a malformation.

Recent studies of routine ultrasound screening at earlier stages of pregnancy suggest an association between increased nuchal translucency (measurement of a fluid filled area at the baby's neck) at 10–14 weeks, and chromosome and other abnormalities. A policy of this very early screening would permit definitive diagnostic procedures and earlier diagnosis of these abnormalities, and, if indicated, earlier termination. The inevitable false positives with such a policy would, however, result in a greater loss of normal pregnancies from these invasive diagnostic procedures. The diagnosis of a chromosomal abnormality places an additional burden on some women who would have miscarried spontaneously, but who now will have to make a difficult decision about termination. The balance of advantages and disadvantages to each woman must be carefully weighed. The financial implications of routine detailed ultrasound examinations in early pregnancy, and of more time-consuming and costly cytogenetic analyses in the laboratory, must also be considered.

4 Routine late ultrasonography

The main purpose of routine scanning in late pregnancy is to identify unsuspected growth-restricted or compromised fetuses who may benefit from elective delivery. The randomized trials of routine ultrasound measurements in late pregnancy suggest an increased incidence of antepartum hospital admissions and of induction of labor, with no improvement in perinatal outcome. There were no detectable effects on the incidence of low Apgar score, admission to the special-care nursery, or perinatal mortality. These trials provide no support for routine ultrasonography in late pregnancy for fetal measurement (see Chapter 12).

5 Placental grading

One randomized trial of reporting placental 'texture' grading was conducted in a maternity unit in which routine ultrasound examinations were performed at 30–32 and 34–36 weeks' gestation. Reports of placental appearances were made available to clinicians caring for women assigned to the experimental group, and not for those in the control group. Knowledge of the result of placental grading was associated with increased use of other fetal assessment techniques, and a tendency to increased use of elective delivery for fetal compromise. There was a better pregnancy outcome among women whose physicians knew their results, with less frequent meconium-staining of amniotic fluid, fewer babies with low Apgar scores at 5 min, and fewer deaths of normally formed babies during the perinatal period. Several unexplained intrauterine deaths in the group of women whose physicians did not know their results were associated with (unreported) placental grades that were thought to be predictive of fetal compromise.

The results of this study strongly suggest that knowledge of placental appearances can result in clinical action that may improve pregnancy outcome. Although firm recommendations cannot be made on the basis of a single study, it might be worthwhile for ultrasonographers to report the placental grade at any late pregnancy ultrasound examination. At the very least, the findings should not be ignored, and warrant confirmation or refutation by further controlled research.

6 Women's reactions to ultrasound in pregnancy

An ultrasound examination has the potential to be a fascinating and happy experience for prospective parents, but real or mistaken diagnoses of fetal abnormality on ultrasound can lead to psychological devastation. Women's reactions to ultrasonography during pregnancy have not received the systematic attention from researchers that they deserve. A majority of the women interviewed in the available studies valued ultrasonography in early pregnancy because it confirmed the reality of the baby for them, and because the examination often led to a reduction in anxiety and an increase in confidence.

Women's views on the desirability of routine ultrasonography during pregnancy, in addition to being influenced by what is actually available, are also influenced by differing perceptions of the potential benefits and concerns about the possible adverse effects of ultrasound. The only generalization that can be made on the basis of the available research is that women's views vary about the indications for ultrasonography. The obvious implication for practice is that it is important for both clinicians and ultrasonographers to take this variation into account.

Another important message is that the experience of having a scan, even if the findings are normal, can be unpleasant because of uncommunicativeness on the part of the ultrasonographer. Some ultrasonographers, technicians in particular, may be put under professional constraints not to communicate freely with the women they are examining. Whether as a result of these constraints or for other reasons, uncommunicativeness can reduce or eliminate the potential psychological benefit of the examinations. The risk of this adverse effect is likely to be increased when the human resources available for ultrasonography are stretched, as may be the case when ultrasonography is routinely performed on every pregnant woman.

7 Potential hazards of obstetric ultrasound

Any consideration of the use of diagnostic ultrasound in obstetrical practice must weigh potential benefits against potential risks. There has been surprisingly little well-organized research to evaluate possible adverse effects of ultrasound exposure on human fetuses. Based on the available follow-up of children included, as fetuses, in randomized trials, there is no evidence of a greater risk of impaired school performance at age 8–9, or of dyslexia, following routine imaging ultrasonography during the second and third trimesters of pregnancy, but there are suggestions (perhaps a chance finding) of an increased incidence of left-handedness.

Two apparently well-designed and well-conducted case-control studies have sought a relationship between ultrasound exposure and childhood malignancy. Both were reassuring, with one possible exception: neither study showed any difference in exposure between the cases and controls up to the age of 5, but in one of the studies, children dying of leukaemia or cancer over the age of five were more likely than controls to have been exposed to ultrasound as fetuses. This difference was not seen in the other, statistically more powerful study.

There has been a suggestion of more growth-restricted babies born after repeated ultrasound examinations during pregnancies in one human study, although differences were no longer evident at one year of age, and this may have been a chance finding. The randomized, controlled trials conducted to date have been far too small to have a reasonable chance of identifying an effect of ultrasound exposure on any rare adverse outcome.

8 Conclusions

The value of selective ultrasound for specific indications in pregnancy has been clearly established. The place, if any, for routine ultrasound has not been clearly determined as yet.

Many obstetric units already practice routine ultrasonography in early pregnancy. For those considering its introduction, the benefit of the demonstrated advantages need to be considered against the theoretical possibility that ultrasound during pregnancy could also be hazardous, and against the need for additional resources. At present, there is no sound evidence that ultrasound examination during pregnancy is harmful.

The available randomized trials do not support the use of routine ultrasonography in late pregnancy for fetal measurement. The only imaging ultrasound technique of late pregnancy that appears to relate to improved outcome is placental grading, and this finding requires confirmation. During ultrasound examinations at any time in pregnancy, mothers should see the monitor screen, have their baby's image pointed out, and receive as much information as they desire.

Sources

Effective care in pregnancy and childbirth

Neilson, J. and Grant, A. Ultrasound in pregnancy.

Cochrane Library

Alfirevic, Z., Early amniocentesis versus transabdominal chorion villus sampling for prenatal diagnosis.

Alfirevic, Z., Gosden, C. and Neilson, J.P., Chorion villus sampling vs amniocentesis for prenatal diagnosis.

Bricker, L. and Neilson, J.P., Routine ultrasound in late pregnancy (> 24 weeks gestation).

Neilson, J.P., Ultrasound for fetal assessment in early pregnancy.

Other sources

Kinnier Wilson, L.M. and Waterhouse, J.A.H. (1984). Obstetric ultrasound and childhood malignancies. *Lancet*, 2, 997–9.

Macdonald, W., Newnham, J., Gurrin, L. and Evans, S. (1996). Effect of frequent prenatal ultrasound on birthweight: follow up at one year of age. *Lancet*, **348**, 482.

Neilson, J.P. (1997). Assessment of fetal nuchal translucency test for Down's syndrome. *Lancet*, 350, 754–5.

Newnham, J.P., Evans, S.F., Michael, C.A., Stanley, F.J. and Landau, L.I. (1993). Effects of frequent ultrasound during pregnancy: a randomised controlled trial. *Lancet*, 342, 887–91.

Saari-Kemppainen, A., Karjalainen, O., Ylostalo, P. and Heinonen, O.P. (1990). Ultrasound screening and perinatal mortality: controlled trial of systematic one-stage screening in pregnancy. *Lancet*, 336, 387–91.

CHAPTER 9

Screening for congenital anomalies

1 Introduction

Prenatal screening for congenital abnormalities and genetic disorders has become increasingly important and increasingly complex, since the introduction of amniocentesis in 1969. A number of factors must be considered in the planning of a genetic-screening program, including the prevalence of the condition in the population to be tested, the severity of the disorder, how successfully available tests separate those with the condition from those without it (sensitivity and specificity), and the costs.

Costs are not wholly financial. It is equally important to weigh the human costs. Although screening programs may bring reassurance to some women who are tested, for others they may generate anxiety by merely raising the question of abnormality. The consequences of erroneous diagnoses, both positive and negative, warrant particularly careful consideration.

2 Genetic counseling

The prevention and treatment of genetic disease is still a new branch of medicine, but genetic counseling is becoming an increasingly important component of health care. The list of disorders that are amenable to prenatal diagnosis continues to grow, especially with advances in molecular genetics.

Counseling prior to prenatal testing is important. The central issue is, of course, one of risk. What is the risk of producing an abnormal child? What is the risk of the investigating procedure? How can that risk be most clearly explained to the woman who must make the final decision? One individual may interpret risk figures very differently from another. Parental decisions may depend, not only on the actual level of risk, but on whether or not they could imagine handling the consequences of having an abnormal child.

The decision to screen, and the action taken as a result of a screening test, should be determined by the individuals concerned, after they have been made thoroughly aware of the potential risks, adverse effects, and possible benefits. Therefore, every screening program must provide adequate time for thorough counseling when it is required. The practice, common in some centers, is for women undergoing amniocentesis to be scheduled for counseling on the same day that the procedure is carried out. It would be preferable, as a rule, for counseling to be given earlier, to allow time for couples to think carefully without feeling pressured into reaching a decision.

Personal or religious beliefs will influence whether screening is undertaken at all. There is seldom any point in carrying out prenatal diagnosis for chromosome studies when the couple would refuse a termination under any circumstances. Nevertheless, no one should be made to feel that once they have undergone screening they are bound to follow a rigid course of action. The couple should feel free to exercise whatever options they choose.

Genetic-screening tests often yield information that is relevant to other family members. Usually there is no barrier to a free exchange of information within the family but, occasionally, individuals will wish to keep the results of tests to themselves. This puts the counselor in a difficult position. He or she must preserve confidentiality, but at the same time may be concerned about relatives at risk of genetic disease who should be traced and tested. The woman's preference must be respected.

3 Methods of screening and diagnosis

3.1 Ultrasound

Ultrasound may be employed in three ways to assist the identification of fetal malformations: to directly visualize the malformation; to facilitate other diagnostic techniques, such as amniocentesis and chorion villus sampling; and to allow fetal measurement (thereby maximizing the performance of other tests that require accurate knowledge of gestational age).

A large and growing number of abnormalities can be detected by modern ultrasound imaging. Some defects, such as anencephaly, are easily identified, while others, such as certain cardiac anomalies, may be very difficult to identify. The presence of one defect may suggest the presence of others and/or a chromosomal abnormality. Sometimes features that are not malformations in themselves but identify an increased risk of genetic conditions, can be identified. Detection rates may vary with the quality of the equipment, the expertise of the ultrasonographer, and the time available for the examination. More time and expertise are likely to be available when the ultrasound examination is performed because of high-risk features (such as a previously malformed baby or raised alpha-fetoprotein levels), than when it is performed as a routine screening examination. Ultrasound can be particularly helpful in demonstrating to parents who have previously had a malformed baby that their fetus in the current pregnancy does not have the same defect.

Termination of pregnancy will be acceptable to many couples when the fetus has a lethal abnormality, such as anencephaly, or a defect likely to result in major handicap, such as spina bifida with hydrocephalus. Difficulties can arise when defects have less predictable sequelae, and also because diagnostic errors may occur. Prior consultation with surgical colleagues should help to reduce unnecessary elective early delivery (and the morbidity resulting from iatrogenic immaturity) of babies with conditions that will not benefit from early surgery.

The increasing sophistication of ultrasound technology can lead to the 'diagnosis' of many minor defects, of uncertain significance. It is vital that ultrasound does not lead to a diagnosis of abnormality in a baby that is normally formed. Such false-positive 'diagnoses' are particularly tragic if they lead to the termination of a wanted normal pregnancy.

The finding of a malformation does not mandate termination of the pregnancy. Diagnosis of a malformation may help some parents prepare for the birth of an impaired child. On the other hand, some parents may suffer a prolonged and devastating upset through such information. Skilled counseling is needed to help them plan ahead for the care of their child. Imparting information about important defects requires personal sensitivity and the availability of people who can be supportive.

The use of ultrasound during amniocentesis can probably minimize the risk of placental and fetal contact during the insertion of the needle into the amniotic cavity. In addition, the presence of a multiple pregnancy may be identified, fetal life confirmed, and gestational age estimated. Both the pregnant woman and the operator may be reassured by seeing that the fetus appears unaffected by the procedure.

3.2 Cytogenetic techniques
Studies on newborn infants show a worldwide frequency of chromosome disorders of about 6 per 1000 births. The total population load of chromosome abnormalities is far greater still, as the majority of affected embryos are spontaneously miscarried early in pregnancy. Over half of all clinically recognizable spontaneous miscarriages are chromosomally abnormal.

There has been a steady rise in demand for prenatal diagnosis for chromosome disorders. The majority of referrals for prenatal chromosome diagnosis have been of older women (aged 35 and over), who have an increased risk of carrying a fetus with Down syndrome (trisomy 21) and most other chromosomal abnormalities. Up to the age of about 29 there is little effect of maternal age on the frequency of Down syndrome (the incidence ranging from approximately 0.5 to 1.0 per 1000 live births). Between the ages of 30 and 34 the frequency begins to rise; by age 35 it is 2–3 per 1000 live births, and at the age of 40 it is 8 or 9 per 1000. Until recently, most centres used an age of 35 as the cut-off point for offering prenatal diagnosis, a decision governed partly by available resources. Policies are changing with the introduction of new tests that offer improved detection rates. Risk assessment based on measurements of one or more of serum alpha-fetoprotein, human chorionic gonadotrophin (HCG), and oestriol, together with maternal age, can further improve the selection of women for cytogenetic study.

Invasive techniques in current use for the prenatal diagnosis of chromosome disorders are amniocentesis, chorion villus sampling, and, less frequently, fetal blood sampling (cordocentesis).

3.2.1 Amniocentesis

The overall safety of early second trimester amniocentesis has been well established from several large studies, but the procedure is not without hazard. A controlled trial of genetic amniocentesis in over 4000 women at low risk of an abnormality showed that the procedure was associated with a high incidence of feto-maternal bleeding, an almost three-fold increase in the miscarriage rate, and perhaps most noteworthy, a significant increase in the incidence of very-low-birthweight babies and of respiratory distress syndrome. In absolute terms, the additional risk of miscarriage associated with the procedure is approximately 0.5–1%, and of a very-low-birthweight baby, about 0.5%.

Amniotic fluid cell chromosome studies have two major drawbacks. First, it usually takes 2–3 weeks from the time the sample is taken until the result is available. Many women find this long wait in itself distressing. Second, amniocentesis is not usually carried out before the 14th–16th week of pregnancy. Thus, if termination is requested, it has to be carried out at a relatively late stage in pregnancy. Culture failure occurs in about 2% of samples. In these cases a repeat sample becomes necessary, and the pregnancy may be distressingly far advanced by the time the result is available.

To try to obtain earlier diagnoses, amniocentesis at around 10–12 weeks has been tested in trials to assess safety and diagnostic performance. The results are not reassuring, since there are higher miscarriage rates when compared with both chorion villus sampling and mid-trimester amniocentesis.

3.2.2 Chorion villus sampling

Chorion villus sampling constitutes a theoretically attractive alternative to conventional amniocentesis, since it can be performed in the first trimester. It involves the use of a cannula (catheter) or biopsy forceps under ultrasound guidance, to take a small biopsy of villi from the developing placenta. In general, the transabdominal route results in a lower failure rate, less bleeding, and fewer miscarriages than the transcervical route. Some small trials have attempted to evaluate differences between different types of cannulas, or between cannulas and biopsy forceps, for chorion villus sampling; no clear differences have emerged. No benefit has been demonstrated from betamimetic administration prior to chorion villus sampling.

The advantages of first-trimester diagnosis are obvious, but for some women these are likely to be offset by obstetrical and cytogenetic problems. Direct comparisons of first-trimester chorion villus sampling with second-trimester amniocentesis, show that complications are uncommon with both procedures, but that chorion villus sampling is associated with significantly more need for a repeat test, more bleeding following the test, and more false-positive diagnoses. Total pregnancy loss (including miscarriage, stillbirths, and neonatal deaths) were more common among the women allocated to chorion villus sampling, and fewer of these women were able to achieve a term delivery or have a normal birthweight baby. Thus, the increased risk of the procedure has to be balanced against the advantage of earlier diagnosis. A couple with, for example, a 1 in 4 risk of having a baby with cystic fibrosis, may feel this risk justified; others, with lower risks of anomaly, may not.

The possibility has been raised that chorion villus sampling, especially when performed very early in pregnancy, may cause face or limb abnormalities on rare occasions. This risk has not been proven; there is, however, sufficient concern for some experts to recommend that chorion villus sampling should not be used before 10 weeks, thereby reducing some of its advantages. Information about the risks of early diagnostic procedures (chorion villus sampling and first-trimester amniocentesis) represent important data to inform decisions about whether first-trimester screening programs for Down syndrome by biochemical testing, or ultrasound measurement of nuchal translucency (see Chapter 8), or both, should be developed.

Apart from technical difficulties, there are other important aspects of prenatal diagnosis by chorion villus sampling that require consideration. A number of chromosomally unbalanced embryos are miscarried spontaneously in early pregnancy. Thus, a significant proportion of the chromosomally abnormal fetuses that are detected through chorion villus sampling may have been destined for spontaneous miscarriage before amniocentesis would have been carried out.

3.3 Serum alpha-fetoprotein

Serum alpha-fetoprotein determination for the detection of neural tube defects has made screening of the general population feasible. Such screening is cost-effective where the incidence of this disorder is high. When the result from a serum test shows an elevated level of alpha-fetoprotein the woman should undergo either a detailed ultrasound examination or amniocentesis to allow the more sensitive amniotic fluid alpha-fetoprotein assay to be carried out. When appropriate ultrasound expertise is available, amniocentesis is unnecessary.

4 Conclusions

Genetic screening and diagnosis now has a well-established place in modern obstetric care. It should be offered as an option to those women or couples who are deemed to be at significant risk. The potential benefits and potential adverse effects should be made known to them, so that they can make a properly informed choice.

The indications for genetic screening require further clarification, including, in particular, surveys of women's views of the desirability of the screening and of the psychological effects of both positive and negative results.

The benefits of earlier exclusion or diagnosis of some fetal disorders afforded by first-trimester chorion villus sampling, as compared with late amniocentesis, must be set against the greater risks of the former. Women considering prenatal diagnosis must be fully informed about the risks and benefits of the alternative procedures.

Sources

Effective care in pregnancy and childbirth

Daker, M. and Bobrow, M., Screening for genetic disease and fetal anomaly during pregnancy.

Cochrane Library

Alfirevic, Z., Instruments for transcervical chorionic villus sampling for prenatal diagnosis.

Early amniocentesis versus transabdominal chorion villus sampling for prenatal diagnosis.

Alfirevic, Z., Gosden, C. and Neilson, J.P., Chorion villus sampling versus amniocentesis for prenatal diagnosis.

Bastian, H., Keirse, M.J.N.C., Middleton, P. and Searle. J., Interventions to influence people's experiences of screening [protocol].

Thornton, J.G., Ways of providing information for helping parents make decisions about prenatal testing [protocol].

Other sources

Tabor, A., Philip, J., Madsen, M., Bang, J., Obel, E.B. and Norgaard-Pedersen, B. (1986). Randomised controlled trial of genetic amniocentesis in 4606 low-risk women. *Lancet*, 1, 1287–93.

Screening for pre-eclampsia

1 Introduction

Hypertensive disorders in pregnancy comprise at least two etiologically distinct entities. One is a disorder mainly, but not exclusively, of women having their first baby, which appears during the course of pregnancy and is reversed by delivery. This is referred to as 'pregnancy-induced hypertension', if there is hypertension alone, and as 'pre-eclampsia', if there is associated proteinuria. Pre-eclampsia is the more severe form, with increased risk for the woman and fetus. In contrast, the outcome following pregnancy-induced hypertension is very similar to that for women with normotensive pregnancies. The risk following pregnancy-induced hypertension is only increased if there is progression to pre-eclampsia.

The other condition is pre-existing or chronic hypertension, unrelated to, but coinciding with, pregnancy. It may be detected for the first time in pregnancy, but does not regress after delivery. Chronic hypertension is a major predisposing factor for pre-eclampsia ('superimposed pre-eclampsia'). The maternal and fetal risks of chronic hypertension in pregnancy seem to be mainly attributable to the development of superimposed pre-eclampsia; the majority of chronically hypertensive women who do not develop pre-eclampsia have a normal perinatal outcome.

Since the causes of the hypertensive disorders of pregnancy are not fully understood, definition and diagnosis are usually based on the signs that are considered to be most characteristic: hypertension and proteinuria. These are signs, not the disease itself. They constitute secondary features of an underlying circulatory disorder, thought to originate in faulty implantation of the placenta. As signs they are non-specific; they can be induced by pregnancy itself, as well as by a variety of conditions unrelated to, but coinciding with pregnancy. Hypertension and proteinuria are usually asymptomatic and must, therefore, be detected by screening.

2 Clinical history

The first step in screening is to assess the risk of pre-eclampsia by taking a careful history. Factors that increase this risk include primiparity, first pregnancy with a new partner, history of pre-eclampsia in a close relative, early onset pre-eclampsia in a previous pregnancy, chronic hypertension, diabetes, and multiple pregnancies. Although useful for helping to determine the appropriate level of antenatal care, none of these factors is very specific or sensitive. For example, women who have previously had severe early onset pre-eclampsia constitute a small group with very high risk; one in five of them will develop pre-eclampsia in a subsequent pregnancy.

3 Blood pressure

The diagnosis of hypertension is made only when blood pressure passes a predefined threshold. Many pregnancies develop normally in spite of the raised blood pressure, indicating that adequate uteroplacental and maternal organ flows are maintained. A certain degree of hypertension may well be beneficial, maintaining perfusion pressures in the face of an elevated vascular resistance.

Many factors, such as age, parity, and race, cause marked variability in blood-pressure between individuals, while others, such as time of day, level of activity, emotions, and posture, may result in variations within the same pregnant woman. Measurements by doctors or mid-wives in antenatal clinics can be higher than those obtained at home ('white coat hypertension').

Although measurement of blood pressure is the mainstay of screening, diagnosis, and decision-making in pregnant women, the inherent technical and sampling errors, whether by auscultation or by automatic devices, constitute an important limitation of the accuracy and precision of this measurement. Errors in blood-pressure measurement cannot be abolished by spending money on automated equipment. The mercury sphygmomanometer and stethoscope are still compatible with good antenatal care, and will most likely remain so in the foreseeable future. Automated devices should be used with caution for women with severe pre-eclampsia, as in this situation they may underestimate blood pressure. Continuous ambulatory monitoring of blood pressure may improve diagnosis and subsequent care, but awaits formal evaluation.

The way in which blood pressure is measured is also important, and poor or inconsistent technique will lead to errors and reduced predictive value of measurements. Either the left lateral or a sitting position, with the arm at the level of the heart, may be used. The cuff size should be appropriate for arm circumference. There is disagreement about how best to measure diastolic pressure. Until recently, the consensus favored the point of muffling of Korotkoff sounds, the fourth phase, but obstetrics is coming in line with the rest of the medical world and disappearance of the sounds, the fifth phase, is increasingly being accepted as preferable.

Hypertension in pregnancy can be defined either as a diastolic pressure above a predetermined cut-off point, or as a rise from a woman's pre-existing blood pressure level. Pregnant women with a diastolic blood pressure between 90 and 100 mmHg in the second-half of pregnancy experience an increased incidence of proteinuria and perinatal death. For that reason, a diastolic blood-pressure level somewhere between 90 and 100 mmHg may be considered to be a threshold between women at low risk and women with an increased risk of pregnancy complications. Mid-trimester blood pressure and mean arterial pressure are not useful for predicting pre-eclampsia, although they do predict pregnancy-induced hypertension.

A diagnosis of hypertension thus defined, is not a diagnosis of a disease but a marker of an increase in risk, and an indication for careful monitoring of mother and fetus. It is clinically important to realize that, in view of the physiological blood-pressure changes in pregnancy, a diastolic blood pressure of 90 mmHg in mid-pregnancy is more abnormal than such a pressure would be if it occurred for the first time at term.

Pregnancy-induced hypertensive disorders rarely occur before 20 weeks' gestation. Hypertension and/or proteinuria diagnosed before

20 weeks will usually be due to pre-existing chronic hypertension or renal disease. Hypertension may also be diagnosed for the first time during labor; such hypertension will often be transitory, due to effort and/or anxiety.

The differential diagnosis between pregnancy-induced hypertension and pregnancy associated with chronic hypertension can be difficult. In comparison with pregnancy-induced hypertension or pre-eclampsia, which usually occurs in young nulliparous women, women with chronic hypertension tend to be older and parous. Many women with chronic or renal hypertension show an even greater physiological fall in blood-pressure during the first half of pregnancy than do normotensive women, with an exaggerated rise in the third trimester. The earlier in pregnancy that hypertension is noted, the more likely it is to be chronic hypertension.

4 Proteinuria

Renal protein excretion increases in normal pregnancy, and proteinuria is not considered abnormal until it exceeds 300 mg in 24 h. An increase in protein output will usually, but not always, lead to higher concentrations in random urine samples. The volume and concentration of urine will affect protein concentration and may give rise to erroneously high or low results of tests on random urine specimens.

Proteinuria may be a temporary phenomenon due to pre-eclampsia, or it may be an expression of pre-existing renal disease coinciding with pregnancy. In the first case it should disappear at some time after delivery; in the latter it will remain present.

Proteinuria is usually a late sign in pregnancy-induced hypertensive disorders, and it is associated with an increased risk of poor fetal outcome. The overall correlation between the degree of elevation of blood-pressure and the occurrence of proteinuria is weak. On the other hand, the magnitude of protein loss correlates positively with the severity of renal lesions. Thus, urine testing is a vital part of the screening process for hypertensive disorders in pregnancy.

In practice, screening for proteinuria is usually done with reagent strips or 'dipstick' tests, which will start detecting protein (albumin) concentrations of approximately 50 mg/l. Protein concentrations depend on urine volume and specific gravity. Dipsticks may give up to 25% false-positive results with a trace reaction, and 6% false-positive results with a one + reaction on testing of random specimens from women with normal 24-h total protein excretion. Testing for micro-albuminuria before the onset of proteinuria does not appear to be helpful in predicting pre-eclampsia.

The definitive test for proteinuria in pregnancy is determination of total protein excretion in a 24-h urine collection, using a reliable quantitative method (e.g. Esbach's). This is too complicated to be used for screening, but may be considered whenever significant proteinuria is detected on screening of a random urine specimen. Alternative approaches to the measurement of 24-h protein excretion, such as determination of the protein/creatinine index in random urine specimens, have so far been disappointing.

5 Edema

Moderate edema occurs in 50–80% of healthy normotensive pregnant women. This physiological edema of pregnancy is often confined to the lower limbs, but it may also occur in other sites, such as the fingers or face, or as generalized edema. Most pregnant women note that the rings on their fingers become tight in the course of the third trimester. Physiological edema usually develops gradually and is associated with a smooth rate of weight gain. The finding that pregnant women with generalized edema, without hypertension or proteinuria, have larger babies than women without obvious edema, strongly suggests that edema is a part of the normal maternal adaptation to pregnancy.

Edema affects approximately 85% of women with pre-eclampsia. It may appear rather suddenly, and may be associated with a rapid rate of weight gain. It cannot be differentiated clinically from edema in normal pregnancy. Pregnant women without edema, and with early- or late-onset edema, all have a similar incidence of hypertension.

The combination of hypertension and edema, or hypertension and increased maternal weight gain, is associated with a lower fetal death rate than is hypertension alone. Pre-eclampsia without edema ('dry pre-eclampsia') has long been recognized as a dangerous variant of the condition, with a higher maternal and fetal mortality than pre-eclampsia with edema.

As edema in pregnancy is common and does not define a group at risk, it should not be used as a defining sign of hypertensive disorders in pregnancy.

6 Biochemical and biophysical tests

A number of tests have been devised to demonstrate the presence or absence of an abnormal vascular responsiveness before the clinical onset of pregnancy-induced hypertension. These include the cold-pressor test, the flicker-fusion test, the isometric-exercise test, the roll-over test, and infusions of catecholamines or vasopressin. Evaluation of these tests has shown them to be worthless, and they are of historical interest only. The angiotensin-sensitivity test is too complicated and time-consuming to be of clinical use, and has recently been shown to have a poor predictive value for pre-eclampsia.

There is insufficient evidence to warrant the use of uric acid levels as a screening test to predict the later development of pregnancy-induced hypertension. In women with established pre-eclampsia, however, serum uric acid levels appear to reflect fetal prognosis. For that reason, uric acid levels can be used in the care for women with pre-eclampsia to monitor the course of the disease. Determination of hematocrit values, platelet counts, and, to a lesser extent, plasma antithrombin III concentration and factor-VIII-related antigen, may also be of value in monitoring the progress of established hypertensive disorders in pregnancy.

A range of other biochemical tests, assays of placental proteins, and measures of vascular cell adhesion, have been shown to be associated with pre-eclampsia. These include kallikrein, fibronectin, alpha-feto-protein, human chorionic gonadotrophin, activin A, urinary calcium, and inhibin. So far none have proven clinically useful for the prediction of pre-eclampsia.

7 Doppler ultrasound

Doppler ultrasound is an easily learned and non-invasive way of examining the uterine circulation. Continuous-wave Doppler is cheaper than pulsed-wave Doppler systems, but has poorer reproducibility. During normal pregnancy, uterine artery blood flow changes from one of high resistance and low flow to one of high flow and low resistance. As the uterine circulation becomes one of low resistance, the diastolic notch in the flow velocity waveform disappears, and by 24 weeks is present in only 5% of women. Failure of this physiological adaptation to pregnancy is associated with an increased risk of pre-eclampsia, and other pregnancy complications such as preterm birth. The presence of bilateral notches in the uterine artery flow velocity waveform at 20–24 weeks seems to identify a group of women at particularly high risk of developing complications that will require delivery before 34 weeks. The role of this test within clinical practice remains unclear, however, and awaits further evaluation. For low-risk women, uterine artery Doppler ultrasound screening probably has little to offer, but it may be beneficial for high-risk women. An additional limitation is that routine screening will only be practical where there is access to sufficient trained staff and equipment.

8 Conclusions

Hypertension and pre-eclampsia are usually asymptomatic; screening and diagnosis depend mainly on the clinical history and careful determination of blood pressure and proteinuria.

Pregnancy-induced hypertension may occur at any time in the second half of pregnancy. It rarely occurs before 28 weeks of pregnancy, but when it does occur this early it frequently leads to pre-eclampsia with its associated high rate of perinatal morbidity and mortality. On the other hand, when pregnancy-induced hypertension occurs late in the third trimester, a much more frequent occurrence, the maternal and fetal risks are much smaller. Therefore, although routine antenatal screening for hypertensive disorders before 28 weeks' gestation may have a low productivity in terms of the number of positive diagnoses per visit, it has a high potential to prevent maternal and fetal morbidity and mortality. For that reason the number of antenatal visits of nulliparae in the second trimester should not be reduced without further evidence of safety.

Simple blood-pressure measurement remains an integral part of antenatal care; it should be performed in a standardized fashion by a skilled midwife or nurse, or by the attending physician.

The appearance of proteinuria in a previously non-proteinuric woman with pregnancy-induced or pre-existing hypertension is associated with a marked increase in maternal and fetal risk. For that reason, screening for proteinuria using a dipstick remains a valuable tool.

Of the other tests advocated for screening, prediction, and early diagnosis of pregnancy-induced hypertensive disease, only Doppler ultrasound seems promising in terms of being clinically useful, particularly for high-risk women. There is a growing interest in the use of combinations of tests, but none are yet of proven value for clinical use.

Determination of hematocrit values, serum uric acid concentrations, platelet counts, and, to a lesser extent, plasma antithrombin III concentration and factor-VIII-related antigen, may be of value in monitoring the progress of established hypertensive disorders in pregnancy.

Sources

Effective care in pregnancy and childbirth

Wallenburg, H.C.S., Detecting hypertensive disorders of pregnancy.

Cochrane Library

Bergel, E. and Carroli, G., Ambulatory versus conventional methods for monitoring blood pressure during pregnancy [protocol].

Neilson, J.P. and Alfirevic, Z., Doppler ultrasound for fetal assessment in high-risk pregnancies.

Other sources

Chien, P.F.W., Arnott, N., Gordon, A., Owen, P. and Khan, K. (2000). How useful is uterine artery Doppler flow velocimetry in the prediction of pre-eclampsia, intrauterine growth retardation and perinatal death? An overview. *Br. J. Obstet. Gynaecol.*, **107**, 196–208.

Conde-Agudelo, A., Lede, R. and Belizán, J. (1994). Evaluation of methods used in the prediction of hypertensive disorders of pregnancy. *Obstet. Gynaecol. Survey*, **49**, 210–22.

Kyle, P.M., Buckley, D., Kissane, J., de Swiet, M. and Redman, C.W. (1995). The angiotensin sensitivity test and low-dose aspirin are ineffective methods to predict and prevent hypertensive disorders in nulliparous pregnancy. *Am. J. Obstet. Gynecol.*, **173**, 865–72.

Penny, J.A., Shennan, A.H., Halligan, A.W., Taylor, D.J., de Swiet, M. and Anthony, J. (1997). Blood pressure measurement in severe pre-eclampsia. *Lancet*, **349**, 1518.

Perry, I.J., Wilkinson, L.S., Shinton, R.A. and Beevers, D.G. (1991). Conflicting views on the measurement of blood pressure in pregnancy. *Br. J. Obstet. Gynaecol.*, **98**, 241–3.

Gestational diabetes

1 Introduction

The concept of gestational diabetes evolved from the earlier concept of prediabetes, which held that much of the pathology associated with overt diabetes develops before the appearance of insulin dependency. The glucose-tolerance test became the mainstay of this diagnosis, as it was believed to uncover a defect in glucose homeostasis that could only be demonstrated after a glucose challenge. It was not until 1973 that an attempt was made to link prediabetes (an abnormal glucose-tolerance test in the absence of overt disease) to perinatal outcome. Although this link is remarkably tenuous, it gave rise to the concept of gestational diabetes as a disease entity, to be searched for and treated. Caregivers and women became anxious lest 'gestational diabetes' develop, and various forms of glucose-challenge screening were introduced and carried out to identify the condition.

2 Risks of 'gestational diabetes'

From the evidence available, the small increase in perinatal mortality associated with abnormal glucose tolerance appears to be predicted as much by the indication for glucose-tolerance testing (such as obesity, large fetus, previous stillbirth, or malformation) as by the test result. The glucose intolerance thus is simply a marker for other underlying conditions that adversely influence perinatal outcome.

Even as only a marker for increased perinatal mortality, the glucose-tolerance test could still be a useful indicator of risk. The question remains as to whether or not identification and treatment of women with gestational diabetes can prevent some of the associated adverse perinatal outcomes (see Chapter 7).

The 'adverse outcome' most frequently associated with gestational diabetes is 'fetal macrosomia' (a larger than average baby). The adverse outcomes of cesarean section, shoulder dystocia, and trauma, derive from this primary outcome. Up to 30% of mothers with an abnormal glucose-tolerance test have a baby with a birthweight of more than 4000 g. Clinical judgement, however, based on assessment of prepregnant weight, weight gain, and a pregnancy past 42 weeks, without any reference to glucose tolerance, is more predictive of fetal macrosomia than is the glucose-tolerance test. Wide application of glucose-tolerance testing to pregnant women would thus be of limited value in identifying women at increased risk of fetal macrosomia.

3 Therapy in 'gestational diabetes'

There is no convincing evidence that treatment of women with an abnormal glucose-tolerance test will reduce perinatal mortality or morbidity. Trials of dietary regulation for 'gestational diabetes' do not demonstrate a significant effect on any outcome, with the possible exception of macrosomia. Trials comparing the use of insulin plus diet with diet alone, show a decrease in macrosomia but no significant effect on other outcomes, such as use of cesarean section, the incidence of shoulder dystocia, or perinatal mortality. There is also no evidence that such treatment reduces the incidence of neonatal jaundice or hypoglycemia. One trial actually assessed the use of elective cesarean section for 'gestational diabetes'. The result was a statistically significant increase in maternal morbidity, with no benefit shown for the baby. In one trial, no significant differences were found in maternal or neonatal outcome by use of elective early induction of labor.

4 Effects of glucose-tolerance testing

The diagnosis of 'gestational diabetes', as currently defined, is based on an abnormal glucose-tolerance test. This test is not reproducible at least 50–70% of the time, and the increased risk of perinatal mortality and morbidity said to be associated with this 'condition' has been considerably overemphasized. As no clear improvement in perinatal mortality has been demonstrated with insulin treatment for gestational diabetes, screening of all pregnant women with glucose-tolerance testing is unlikely to make a significant impact on perinatal mortality or morbidity.

An abnormal glucose-tolerance test is associated with a two- or threefold increase in the incidence of macrosomia, but the majority of macrosomic infants will be born to mothers with a normal glucose-tolerance test.

There is, in addition, a great potential for doing more harm than good by performing a glucose-tolerance test. A positive test labels the woman as having a form of diabetes. Her pregnancy is likely to be considered as 'high-risk', invoking an extensive and expensive program of tests and interventions of unproven benefit. A negative glucose-tolerance test, on the other hand, also has a potential for harm by falsely reassuring the physician and the woman that the risk, engendered by the indication for the test, has been removed.

As no benefit has yet been established for glucose screening during pregnancy, the method used for this screening is irrelevant. However, for those who use this test of unproven value, it should be noted that a glucose polymer has been shown to be more acceptable than glucose to women undergoing such screening, and is associated with less nausea and headache. If any value for screening for minor degrees of glucose intolerance during pregnancy should ever be demonstrated, the possible advantages of using a glucose polymer rather than glucose for this screening should be reviewed.

5 Conclusions

All forms of glucose-tolerance testing should be reviewed. Women in whom overt diabetes is suspected should be followed with fasting or blood glucose estimations 2 h after meals, throughout pregnancy.

The available data provide no evidence to support the wide recommendation that all pregnant women should be screened for 'gestational diabetes', let alone that they should be treated with insulin. Until the risk of minor elevations of glucose during pregnancy have been established in appropriately conducted trials, therapy based on this diagnosis must be critically reviewed. The use of injectable therapy on the basis of the available data is highly contentious and in many other fields of medical practice, such aggressive therapy without proven benefit would be considered unethical.

Sources

Effective care in pregnancy and childbirth

Hunter, D.J.S. and Keirse, M.J.N.C., Gestational diabetes.

Cochrane Library

Walkinshaw, S.A., Dietary regulation for 'gestational diabetes'.

Pre-Cochrane reviews

Walkinshaw, S.A., Glucose polymer vs glucose for screening/diagnosing 'gestational diabetes'. Review no. 06652.

Elective caesarean for 'gestational diabetes'. Review no. 06648.

CHAPTER 12

Assessment of fetal growth, size, and well-being

1 Introduction

A wide range of tests of fetal well-being have been introduced during the last thirty years, and have enjoyed waves of popularity. Both biochemical tests (which monitor the endocrine function of the placenta or the fetoplacental unit) and biophysical methods of monitoring (which provide different information about fetal growth and physiological function) have the theoretical ability to detect changes in fetal well-being that may occur over hours, days, or weeks. No known method of assessment can predict sudden events, such as cord prolapse or placental abruption, which may also cause fetal damage or death.

Two general assumptions underlie the contention that antenatal monitoring is clinically useful: first, that these methods can detect or predict fetal compromise; and second, that with appropriate interpretation and action, they can reduce the frequency or severity of adverse perinatal events or prevent needless interventions.

Tests of fetal well-being have been used both as screening tests with the purpose of preventing those otherwise unpredictable fetal problems that occur from time to time, and in specific clinical situations with a high estimated fetal risk. 'High-risk' circumstances include diabetes or pre-eclampsia, multiple and post-term pregnancy and, most of all, when the fetus is thought to grow poorly. Because of the frequency with which such babies are monitored, and because of the controversy over what constitutes 'growth restriction', it is worthwhile to re-examine the definitions and underlying pathophysiological concepts.

2 Size and growth

Fetal size and fetal growth are often confused in clinical practice. It is common to see 'birthweight-for-gestational age' standards described as 'fetal growth charts', and a weight-for-gestation below some arbitrary centile referred to as 'intrauterine growth restriction'. There are two main reasons why this may lead to false conclusions. First, the weights of babies born at a given length of gestation are not a good reflection of fetal weights at the same gestation. Second, some authors have made inferences about fetal growth by comparisons with cross-sectionally derived mean or median birthweights at consecutive weeks of gestation. This approach is misleading because it ignores the important distinction between size and growth. Infants below a particular centile are 'light-for-gestational age' without necessarily being 'growth restricted'. Growth cannot be estimated without two or more measurements of size. What the clinician would like to know is whether fetal growth has deviated from its normal progression.

The term 'intrauterine growth restriction' should be used only for fetuses with definite evidence that growth has faltered. Such infants may not necessarily be 'light-for-gestational age'; a fetus whose weight falls from the 90th centile to the 30th in a short period of time is almost certainly in greater peril than a fetus who has maintained a position on the 5th centile.

Genuine fetal growth restriction is attributed to an inadequate supply of nutrition to the fetus by a malfunctioning placenta (or, more accurately, insufficient blood supply to the placenta). The fetus responds to this unfavorable environment by making adjustments that maximize the chances of survival. These include redistribution of blood flow (more to brain and heart, less to liver and kidneys) and limiting unnecessary movements. These adaptive phenomena provide the basis of some tests of fetal well-being.

3 Abdominal examination

The simplest clinical method of estimating fetal size – abdominal palpation – is so inaccurate as to be little better than a blind guess: 20% of such assessments just before birth are not within 450 g of the actual birthweight, and the errors are worse at the extremes of the range, where the information is most needed. A more quantitative approach is to measure the increase in size of the maternal abdomen, which must, to some extent, reflect uterine growth. The two most widely practised techniques are the measurement of fundal height (the distance between the upper border of the pubic symphysis and the uterine fundus) and the measurement of abdominal girth at the level of the umbilicus.

There have been several studies of fundal height as an indicator of fetal size, but little investigation of the potential of this measurement for assessing growth. This is understandable, given the considerable inter- and intra-observer variation in measuring fundal height. Nevertheless, several studies have shown quite good sensitivity and specificity of fundal height for predicting low birthweight for gestation. The ability to predict low birthweight is not the same as the ability to detect growth restriction, but fundal height may be useful as a screening test for further investigation – albeit that only very limited trial information is available. Abdominal girth measurement has not been adequately evaluated at all.

4 Fetal movement counting

Reduction or cessation of fetal movements may precede fetal death by a day or more. In theory, recognition of this reduction, followed by appropriate action to confirm fetal jeopardy and expedite delivery, could prevent fetal death. This is the basis for using counts of fetal movements as a test of fetal well-being. The most commonly used method is to ask the mother to record on a chart each day, the time at which she has noticed 10 kicks.

Not all late fetal deaths are even theoretically preventable in this way. Some are not preceded by a reduction in fetal movements. For others, there may be insufficient time between the reduction and fetal death to allow clinical action. Still others may be preceded by conditions that are recognizable in their own right, such as pre-eclampsia or intra-uterine growth restriction. In the latter circumstances, fetal movement counting might still be theoretically useful as a supplement to other tests of fetal well-being.

The cause of most antepartum late fetal deaths, however, is unknown. These deaths are unpredictable and the extent to which they can be prevented by current forms of antenatal care is, therefore, limited. Screening by fetal movement counting, because it can be performed each day, has theoretical advantages over other tests of fetal well-being, all of which are either difficult or impossible to perform daily for practical reasons.

Two randomized, controlled trials have addressed the question of whether clinical actions taken on the basis of fetal movement counting improve fetal outcome, the largest involving over 68 000 women. These trials collectively provide no evidence that routine formal fetal movement counting reduces the incidence of fetal death in late pregnancy. Routine counting results in more frequent reports of diminished fetal activity, greater use of other techniques of fetal assessment, more frequent antepartum admission to hospital, and an increased use of elective delivery for decreased movement, hence an increase in the use of resources without compensating benefit. The practice does not appear to result in either a significant increase or decrease in feelings of anxiety among mothers.

There is a marginal possibility that an occasional late fetal death might be prevented by fetal movement counting. The wider social, psychological, and economic implications of recommending routine fetal movement counting, however, must be taken into account as they affect all women.

5 Biophysical tests

5.1 Ultrasound measurements
Ultrasound imaging has the potential to assist assessment of fetal growth and well-being in a number of ways: by assessing fetal size at a single point in time to confirm or refute the clinical impression that a fetus is small for gestational age; by measuring fetal growth over a period of time by repeated measurements; by assessing amniotic fluid volume (and therefore indirectly fetal urine production); by investigating the appearance of the placenta; and by examining the movement and behavior of the fetus.

The use of fetal measurements to assess whether or not the fetus is growing satisfactorily may be considered in the general framework of diagnostic tests, and appraised from the standpoints of their test properties: sensitivity, specificity, and predictive values. It is not clear, however, precisely what one is trying to predict. There is no absolute postnatal criterion of growth restriction that can be used to assess the validity of the 'test'. In the absence of an appropriate outcome measure, authors frequently use some measure of 'relatively low' birthweight, such as being below the 10th centile for gestational age.

There has been very little research aimed at producing true growth curves based on repeated measurements over time of the same fetus. Such information would provide a far sounder basis for assessing fetal growth, and is arguably the only valid approach for detecting growth restriction. This approach is particularly useful when gestational age is unknown or uncertain. Ultrasonography, rather than 'birthweight-for-gestational-age', should be considered as the 'gold standard' for measuring fetal growth. Despite this, controlled trials show that routine ultrasound measurement of fetal size in late pregnancy results in an increased rate of antenatal hospital admission, and possibly of induction of labor, with no evidence of any substantive benefit to the baby. No adequately controlled trial data are available from specifically high-risk pregnancies.

'Light-for-dates' fetuses form a heterogeneous group within which individual risk varies greatly. Attempts have been made to analyze patterns of growth in the hope of uncovering the underlying pathogenesis and of providing an estimate of the risk to the individual fetus. 'Light-for-dates' fetuses can be divided into two groups: the first showing arrest of previously normal growth; the second showing early departure from normal limits of growth that continues until delivery. The first of these patterns has been attributed to 'utero-placental insufficiency', and the second to low growth potential. This latter group includes infants that are inherently abnormal (especially chromosomally abnormal), some that have suffered a major insult (e.g. from rubella) during the critical period of organogenesis, and some that are small because of their genetic endowment. Comparative measurements of the fetal head and abdomen have been suggested as a means to further differentiate these two groups. While there is a higher incidence of intrapartum fetal distress and operative delivery in the asymmetrical-growth group, the perinatal mortality and incidence of low Apgar scores are similar and high in both groups.

The significance of ultrasonically detected patterns of fetal growth requires further study, and seeking correlations with the results of Doppler studies would be of interest. Thus far, the evidence indicates that abdominal measurements are superior to head measurements in predicting 'light-for-dates' babies, but little is known about serial measurements, and particularly about their relationship to neonatal outcome.

A single trial reported in 1987 has examined the value of ultrasound placental appearances. Reporting placental 'texture' to clinicians providing antenatal care resulted in less meconium stained amniotic fluid in labor, fewer babies with low 5-min Apgar scores, and, most importantly, fewer deaths of normally formed babies, than occurred for women whose clinicians were not provided with the report of placental grading. It appears that knowledge of placental grading can lead to appropriate clinical action that can improve pregnancy outcome. This study deserves to be repeated. In the meantime, it seems advisable to report the placental grade following ultrasound examinations for specific clinical indications during the third trimester.

The only information available from randomized trials on the use of amniotic fluid volume estimation by ultrasound is in the clinical context of post-term pregnancy assessment, or as part of the biophysical-profile test (see below).

5.2 Doppler ultrasound

Doppler ultrasound has been used for a number of years to identify and record fetal heart pulsation, and, in adults, to assess blood flow in compromised vessels. The use of the technique to demonstrate blood velocity wave forms in the fetal umbilical artery was first described in 1977. Alterations in fetal umbilical blood flow may occur as an early event in conditions of fetal compromise. For this reason, Doppler studies could provide important information on the pathophysiology of compromised pregnancies (especially of fetal growth restriction), and be a useful technique for evaluating fetal well-being in high-risk pregnancies.

Information from trials supports this hypothesis. Combined evidence from several trials in high-risk pregnancies (complicated mainly by fetal growth restriction or maternal high blood pressure) shows that there are fewer stillbirths and neonatal deaths among normally formed babies when the results of Doppler velocimetry are made available to the clinicians. A number of the deaths in the control groups in these studies seem to have resulted from uteroplacental insufficiency, and these might well have been avoided by Doppler study and the clinical action prompted by it. The use of Doppler ultrasound in high-risk pregnancies so far appears also to lead to fewer admissions to hospital during pregnancy and fewer elective deliveries. There has been no demonstrated effect on the incidence of cesarean section or on the condition of the newborn baby, other than a greater likelihood of being born alive.

In contrast to its effectiveness in decreasing perinatal mortality among women at identified high risk, Doppler ultrasound appears to have little, if any effect on pregnancy outcome when used as a screening test in unselected pregnancies. This should not be surprising; when used in a low-risk population, the predictive power of any test is low, and the benefits from adequately responding to the few true positive tests can be more than counterbalanced by the harm done in response to the inevitable high proportion of false-positive tests.

5.3 Contraction stress testing

Continuous recording of fetal heart rate and uterine activity was first developed for use in labor, in an attempt to identify the fetus at risk of death or morbidity due to intrapartum asphyxia. Because many fetal deaths occur prior to the onset of labor, the stimulation of contractions with oxytocin for short periods of time was proposed to allow observation of the fetal heart rate under labor-like conditions in pregnancies at risk.

This technique, which subsequently became known as the 'oxytocin-challenge test' or 'contraction stress test', has no demonstrated benefits and suffers from a number of disadvantages. It is time-consuming, requires an intravenous infusion, and has the potential to harm the fetus. Its use is contra-indicated in some pregnancies at risk, for example, when there is antepartum bleeding, placenta praevia, a history of preterm labor, or preterm rupture of membranes.

The nipple-stimulation stress test is similar in purpose to, and has been directly compared with, the oxytocin-challenge test. The pregnant woman is encouraged to stimulate her nipples with her fingers, palms, a warm, moist face cloth, or a heating pad, either directly or through her clothing. Contractions can be stimulated effectively, but the mechanism, previously assumed to be oxytocin release, remains unknown. The nipple-stimulation stress test has some of the same disadvantages as the oxytocin-challenge test with the additional problem that, while stimulation is easily discontinued, there is a time-lag of more than three minutes between stimulation and peak uterine response. Excessive uterine activity occurs in over half the women who undergo this test, and this will result in fetal bradycardia in 7–14%. Cases of severe uterine tetany associated with fetal heart rate abnormalities have also been reported. Because of these concerns, and because it offers no clear advantages over other techniques, the nipple-stimulation stress test should be relegated to the history books.

5.4 Non-stress cardiotocography

The evaluation of fetal heart rate patterns, without the added stress of induced contractions, was first proposed in 1969. This 'non-stress test' has been widely incorporated into antenatal care for both screening and diagnosis.

There is no universally accepted technique for performing non-stress antepartum cardiotocography. Various durations and frequencies of monitoring are used, and these can have a powerful influence on the predictive properties of the test. Additional manoeuvres, such as abdominal stimulation, sound stimulation, glucose infusions, post-prandial repeat tests, and follow-up oxytocin-challenge tests for suspected abnormal records, have been suggested or used. None of these have been shown to improve the predictive value of the test.

Many factors may interfere with the interpretation of the non-stress test. Like the contraction stress test, the non-stress test requires sophisticated equipment, which may occasionally malfunction. Fetal and maternal movements may produce artefacts, since ultrasound monitoring detects movement rather than sound. During fetal rest periods, which not uncommonly last for more than thirty minutes, normal physiological reduction in heart rate variability may be confused with pathological change. Medications taken by the mother are often transferred to the fetus, and, particularly in the case of drugs with a sedative effect on the central nervous system, may in themselves produce heart-rate patterns that can be interpreted as abnormal. Likewise, the gestational age of the fetus has a strong influence on the frequency of false-positive non-reactive tests, with 'abnormal' patterns being more frequently described in the preterm fetus. When all these factors are taken into consideration, as many as 10–15% of all records may be unsatisfactory for interpretation.

A variety of methods for interpreting non-stress cardiotocograms have been described, all of which include evaluation of some or all of the following characteristics: baseline fetal heart rate; various interpretations of fetal heart-rate variability; accelerations of fetal heart rate associated with spontaneous and/or stimulated movements of the fetus; and decelerations associated with spontaneous uterine contractions. The more complicated systems assign scores to some or all of these parameters, sometimes subsequently grouping the scores. The most commonly used method is to divide traces into reactive (normal) and non-reactive (abnormal), based on the presence or absence of adequate baseline heart-rate variability and heart-rate accelerations with fetal movement. It is now well documented that even when a standardized method is used, interpretation of a trace may vary when an individual observer reads the same trace at different times, or when the same trace is read by different observers.

In addition to the difficulties with test interpretation, there is a danger inherent in any form of screening when the likelihood of the fetus being in difficulty is small. A higher proportion of positive tests will be false-positive when the probability of an adverse outcome is small. Intervention based on the results of a 'positive' non-stress test in a low-risk group of women will often do more harm than good.

This risk is real, rather than only theoretical. In each of the four trials of non-stress testing that have been reported, perinatal deaths from causes other than malformations were more common in the groups in which clinicians had access to the test results. Collectively, the increase in perinatal deaths among the women tested was importantly (more than threefold) and statistically significantly higher. There was no demonstrable effect on cesarean section rates, incidence of low Apgar scores, abnormal neonatal neurological signs, or admission to special-care nurseries. These analyses provide no support at all for the use of antepartum non-stress cardiotocography, as used in these studies, as a supplementary test of fetal well-being in 'high-risk' pregnancies. One can only speculate as to why cardiotocography continues to be used in such an extensive way, and why the results from the only four randomized trials that have been published are so widely disregarded by many obstetricians.

Antepartum cardiotocography is essentially an assessment of immediate fetal condition. Unless evidence emerges to the contrary its clinical use would seem best restricted to situations in which acute fetal hypoxemia may be present e.g. sudden reduction of fetal movement, or antepartum hemorrhage.

5.5 Fetal biophysical profile

The 'biophysical profile' was derived from a study of serial ultrasound examinations and antenatal cardiotocography (non-stress test) in high-risk pregnancies. Combining five biophysical 'variables' considered to be of prognostic significance (fetal movement, tone, reactivity, breathing, and amniotic fluid volume) into a score, reduced the frequency of false-positive and false-negative results compared to the non-stress test alone. An additional advantage of the biophysical profile over the non-stress test is that it permits assessment of the possibility of major congenital anomalies. This may be important, as detection of a serious anomaly may on occasion help to avoid a cesarean section when the baby is clearly abnormal.

Only two controlled trials of biophysical-profile testing have been performed. Both were conducted in women referred to units specializing in fetal biophysical assessment. They compared care based on biophysical score results with that based on non-stress test results, following a management protocol. In both studies, the biophysical profile score was a better predictor of low 5-min Apgar scores than the non-stress test. The biophysical profile was both more sensitive and more specific in predicting overall abnormal outcome than the non-stress test.

Despite the better predictive value of the biophysical score than the non-stress test, its use did not result in any improvements in outcome for the baby. Outcomes measured included perinatal death, fetal distress in labor, low Apgar score, and low birthweight-for-gestational-age. Compared with cardiotocography alone, biophysical-profile testing showed no obvious effect (either beneficial or deleterious) on these outcome measures. The available evidence provides no support at all for the use of biophysical profile as a test of fetal well-being in high-risk pregnancies. However, the number of women included in these studies is so small that any estimates of effect are extremely imprecise.

6 Biochemical tests

Biochemical testing in late pregnancy is now only of historical interest. The enthusiasm for estrogen assays that prevailed in the 1960s and 1970s was based on the observation that perinatal mortality rates were twice as high in women with low estriol excretion than in the general population. However, the usefulness of the tests was marred by the facts that they were not sensitive enough to detect the majority of pregnancies destined to have an adverse outcome, and that a great many women with normal pregnancies falsely appeared to be at risk.

Among the many studies reported, there has been only one randomized, controlled trial. In this trial, knowledge of estriol levels had no detectable effect on either perinatal mortality or the rate of elective delivery. Similar conclusions were reached from comparison of pregnancy outcomes within the same institution in two consecutive periods with and without the use of estriol assays. Thus, there is no evidence to suggest any benefit from estriol assays.

Similarly, there was only one randomized intervention study of human placental lactogen measurement. The results of this trial suggest, on first inspection, that revealing the results of human placental lactogen measurements to a clinician armed with a predetermined intervention program, statistically significantly reduced fetal and perinatal mortality. Although the data of this trial have been cited to indicate that human placental lactogen measurements are beneficial for the surveillance of high-risk pregnancy, they relate only to the 8% (4% in each group) of pregnancies that had abnormal human placental lactogen values. Data on the large majority of pregnancies (92%) that did not belong to that category were not reported, and are no longer available. One cannot exclude the possibility that the apparent benefit in the small minority with abnormal placental lactogen values was offset by negative effects in the majority of pregnancies with normal tests.

7 Conclusions

Tape measurement of symphysis–fundal height is simple, inexpensive, and widely used during antenatal care. Fundal height could be used as a screening device for referral of women to an obstetrician for further assessment, but many small fetuses will be missed, and many perfectly well-grown fetuses will be considered worryingly small. Nevertheless, in our present state of knowledge it would be unwise to abandon the practice.

Ultrasound techniques have the capacity to detect abnormalities of fetal growth, but have not been effectively exploited. There is a need for prospective studies to examine the differential growth of fetal parts, in large populations, to see whether patterns of growth that are associated with fetal compromise and later infant morbidity can be defined. Such studies should be carried out with scheduled repeated measurements. It is particularly crucial that better measures of outcome should be defined. Intervention based on assessments of size or growth should be evaluated in randomized trials before they are accepted into general obstetrical practice. For the present, the evidence provides no support for routine ultrasonography for fetal measurement in late pregnancy.

Biochemical tests of fetal well-being are expensive and have a low predictive value for adverse outcome. While they have added immensely to knowledge of placental and fetal physiology, none of them have been shown to be clinically useful. Their use should be restricted to research, and they should not be employed in clinical practice.

Monitoring of fetal movements by the mother is a simple and inexpensive test of fetal well-being that can be performed daily. There is no evidence, however, that a policy of routine fetal movement counting will have beneficial results. If used at all, it should be used in individual circumstances, for example, where a woman perceives diminished fetal movements. The results should prompt other diagnostic tests rather than more definitive obstetric intervention. The possibility of congenital malformation should be considered before delivery is expedited.

Biophysical tests are employed today with the same enthusiasm that characterized biochemical testing in the past. These tests have greatly increased our understanding of fetal behavior and development, but with the exception of Doppler studies of umbilical artery wave form in high-risk pregnancies, and possibly placental grading, their use has not been demonstrated to confer benefits in the care of an individual woman and her baby. For this reason, and despite their widespread clinical use, most biophysical tests of fetal well-being should be considered of experimental value only, rather than as validated clinical tools. They should be acknowledged as such and, at the very least, further extension of their clinical use should be curtailed until or unless they can be demonstrated to be of benefit in improving the outcome for mother or baby.

The role of non-stress cardiotocography as either a screening or a diagnostic test seems questionable, because of its poor predictive properties. The biophysical profile may have greater potential as a diagnostic test for women in whom there is a high risk of fetal problems, but the usefulness of this approach is still not established.

Doppler ultrasound has been evaluated more rigorously and extensively than any other test of fetal health or fetoplacental function. The encouraging results justify the use of Doppler ultrasound during high-risk pregnancy to guide clinical care, but there is no evidence that any benefit is derived from routine Doppler screening in unselected pregnancies.

Sources

Effective care in pregnancy and childbirth

Alexander, S., Stanwell-Smith, R., Buekens, P. and Keirse, M.J.N.C., Biochemical assessment of fetal well-being.

Altman, D. and Hytten, F., Assessment of fetal size and fetal growth.

Grant, A. and Elbourne, D., Fetal movement counting to assess fetal well-being.

Mohide, P. and Keirse, M.J.N.C., Biophysical assessment of fetal well-being.

Neilson, J. and Grant, A., Ultrasound in pregnancy.

Cochrane Library

Alfirevic, Z. and Neilson, J.P., Biophysical profile for fetal assessment in high-risk pregnancies.

Bricker, L. and Neilson, J.P., Routine ultrasound in late pregnancy (> 24 weeks gestation).

Routine Doppler ultrasound in pregnancy.

Cloherty, L.J. and Neilson, J.P., Hormonal placental function tests for fetal assessment in high-risk pregnancies.

Neilson, J.P., Symphysis-fundal height measurement during pregnancy.

Neilson, J.P. and Alfirevic, Z., Doppler ultrasound for fetal assessment in high-risk pregnancies.

Pattison, N. and McCowan, L., Cardiotocography for antepartum fetal assessment.

Tan, K.H., Fetal manipulation for facilitating tests of fetal well-being [protocol].

Maternal glucose administration for facilitating tests of fetal well-being [protocol].

Tan, K.H. and Smyth, R., Fetal vibroacoustic stimulation for facilitating tests of fetal well-being [protocol].

Pre-Cochrane reviews

Neilson, J.P., Routine formal fetal movement (FM) counting.

Other sources

Alfirevic, Z. and Walkinshaw, S.A. (1995). A randomised controlled trial of simple compared with complex antenatal fetal monitoring after 42 weeks of gestation. *Br. J. Obstet. Gynaecol.*, 102, 638–43.

Proud, J. and Grant, A. (1987). Third trimester placental grading by ultrasonography as a test of fetal wellbeing. *Br. Med. J.*, 294, 1641–44.

Pregnancy problems

CHAPTER 13

Unpleasant symptoms in pregnancy

1 Introduction

Although an uncomplicated pregnancy is generally considered to be a state of health rather than a disease, it is frequently accompanied by symptoms that, at other times or in other circumstances, might be thought to be signs of illness. The so-called 'minor symptoms' of pregnancy, such as nausea and vomiting, tiredness, backache, heartburn, constipation, hemorrhoids, vaginal discharge, leg cramps, varicose veins, and edema, are unpleasant and can cause significant discomfort. The many women who suffer from them may have to make major changes in their lifestyle and behavior. Preventing or alleviating those symptoms is an important aspect of antenatal care.

2 Nausea and vomiting

Nausea and vomiting are among the most frequent, the most characteristic, and perhaps the most troublesome symptoms of early pregnancy. Almost three-quarters of all pregnant women suffer from nausea, and for 1 in 10 the condition persists beyond the first trimester. Despite the popular name 'morning sickness', many women experience the symptom throughout the whole day. For women with a multiple pregnancy it is often more severe and longer lasting.

The most severe form of nausea and vomiting (hyperemesis gravidarum), with dehydration and electrolyte disturbance, is fortunately rare today. Although women who suffer from hyperemesis may require admission to hospital and active treatment, the associated morbidity and mortality have declined dramatically.

The causes of nausea in pregnancy are still largely unknown, and the variety of treatments that have been recommended reflect the many theories about underlying causes. As might be expected for a self-limiting condition, uncontrolled studies of these 'treatments' have yielded rather spectacular, if spurious, results. In contrast, the results of controlled trials have been less impressive.

In recent years, the use of anti-emetic drugs has declined because of possibly justified fears of the effects of medication on the fetus. Non-pharmaceutical approaches to relieve nausea and vomiting are often preferred, particularly during the first few weeks when the developing fetus is most vulnerable. Common-sense suggestions about rest and diet for women with nausea or vomiting during pregnancy have not been evaluated in randomized trials, but are likely to be harmless, and may be helpful. Small amounts of carbohydrate, such as biscuits or bananas, may relieve some women, and if retained will provide needed nutrition. Rest may be impractical when women have other responsibilities, such as employment or small children, but may help when it is possible.

An unconventional approach, using acupressure at the Neiguan (P6) point on the wrist has been evaluated in several placebo-controlled randomized trials. The trials were small, but suggest that the acupressure may reduce the frequency of persistent nausea. The commonly available wrist bands used for travel sickness may help some women, and are unlikely to be harmful. The role of acupressure deserves further evaluation.

Vitamin B6 (pyridoxine) has been tested in two trials. Their results suggest that B6 may be effective in reducing the severity of nausea, but it is unclear by how much. The evidence for any effect on vomiting is inconclusive. For hyperemesis, powdered ginger root and ACTH have been compared with placebo but these trials were too small for any reliable conclusions.

Several trials, mostly conducted in the 1950s and 1960s, have demonstrated a variety of antihistamines to be better than placebos. A trial of dramamine showed it to be less effective alone than when combined with benzylamine. Simple antihistamines are generally considered to be safe during pregnancy, although they sometimes cause troublesome side-effects, such as drowsiness and blurring of vision. There have been no major epidemiological studies to look for possible adverse effects on the fetus.

The drug at one time most widely used to treat nausea and vomiting of pregnancy was a compound containing the antihistamine doxylamine succinate and pyridoxine (marketed as Debendox in the UK, as Bendectin in the United States and Canada, and as Lenotan in some other countries). The three small placebo-controlled trials that have been published provide reasonable evidence that Debendox relieved nausea during pregnancy. It was withdrawn from the market in 1983 as a direct result of litigation brought against the manufacturers. There were claims that the drug had caused congenital malformations when used in pregnancy. At the time of its recall, Debendox had been used by over 30 million women worldwide. In many countries between a quarter and a third of all pregnant women used Debendox. If congenital malformations occur in 3.5% of all babies, by chance alone Debendox would have been used by the mothers of over a million babies born with a congenital malformation. In the inevitable search for what may have produced the children's malformations, it is not surprising that many mothers implicated Debendox, and, perhaps prompted by over-eager lawyers, some chose to sue.

The litigation was brought despite overwhelming evidence *against* Debendox being a teratogen. From the 19 epidemiologic studies of Debendox, there is widespread agreement that the drug is *not* associated with an increased risk of congenital malformations. Despite the abrupt withdrawal of Debendox, there has been no correlated reduction in the reported incidence of any group of malformations. The removal of Debendox has probably led to an increased use of other medications for treating nausea and vomiting, about which, for any single product, much less human research has been conducted.

If an anti-emetic is used during pregnancy, the choice now is often an antihistamine. These agents appear to be efficacious, as shown by the early trials, but their safety has not been as extensively studied.

3 Tiredness

Many women report feelings of extreme tiredness, especially in the early months and again during the last few weeks of pregnancy. In spite of the adverse effect that this has on women's lives, there has been little research into the causes or treatment of this symptom. Interesting questions relate to the relationship between tiredness and nausea, and into factors that might help, such as taking time off work outside the home. In the absence of controlled research, it seems sensible to reassure women that tiredness is a common symptom that is likely to lessen during the second trimester, to advise those who are excessively tired to rest whenever they can, and to seek help with home and work commitments whenever this is feasible.

4 Backache

Backache is common in the general population, and even more common among pregnant women. Up to three-quarters of women report having backache at some time during pregnancy, and a third find it a severe problem. Potential causes of backache in pregnancy include altered posture with an increased lumbar lordosis (curve in the spine), and hormonal changes leading to a loosening of the ligaments and greater water retention within the tissues. Symptoms are often worse at night and contribute to difficulties with sleeping, especially during the last three months of pregnancy. Women should be reassured that the problem usually resolves spontaneously soon after the birth, particularly for those who did not have backache before pregnancy.

There is little information from controlled trials about how to prevent or treat backache during pregnancy. Common-sense advice about lifestyle, such as using chairs with good back support and avoiding heavy lifting, has not been evaluated in controlled trials, but seems worth trying. One study has evaluated a program of exercises and education, delivered either as two small group sessions with written material, or as five individual sessions with a tape and written material. Pain-related problems were reduced in both treatment groups compared to the group with normal antenatal care, and women who had the individualized program needed less time off work. These results must be interpreted with caution, however, because of methodological weaknesses in the study.

A single trial of the Ozzlo pillow, a special pillow developed in Australia for backache, suggested that it was somewhat better than a standard pillow in alleviating backache in late pregnancy. This treatment may be worth considering in places where the pillow is available.

5 Heartburn

Heartburn affects about two-thirds of all women at some stage of pregnancy. It is another so-called 'minor' disorder of pregnancy, but it causes more discomfort and distress than do many more serious conditions. It is commonly associated with eating, stooping, or lying down. The most clear-cut precipitating factor is posture.

Initial advice to women with heartburn should include sensible measures such as avoiding fatty or spicy foods, and minimizing bending over or lying flat after eating. If this is insufficient, self-medication with proprietary antacids is the most commonly employed treatment, and often provides adequate relief. There is little evidence of differences in efficacy between the various preparations available.

Acid-suppressing drugs, such as cimetidine or ranitidine, and omeprazole, a proton-pump inhibitor, have been shown to be highly effective in the treatment of severe or persistent heartburn or gastroesophageal reflux. All H_2-blockers cross the human placenta, but neither animal or human epidemiologic studies have shown them to be teratogenic. There is little information on the fetal or neonatal effects of taking H_2-blockers late in pregnancy, but studies have shown no differences in any aspects of pregnancy outcomes or neonatal health from their use. More studies are needed, however, to confirm the safety of these agents during late pregnancy. One small trial has evaluated ranitidine in pregnant women, and the results are promising.

In situations where simple and sensible dietary and lifestyle measures have failed to provide adequate relief from heartburn, the evidence suggests that antacids should be prescribed initially, and the use of acid-suppressing agents reserved for persistent symptoms. Individuals should choose their preferred product among different preparations, since therapeutic compliance will be increased when the product is found to be palatable as well as effective.

6 Constipation

Constipation is a troublesome problem for many women during pregnancy, particularly during the last trimester. Women who are habitually constipated usually become more so during pregnancy. The frequency of constipation among pregnant women will reflect their dietary habits, fluid intake, and pattern of physical exercise.

Alteration in diet, fluid intake, and exercise, have been found, in observational studies, to bring relief to many women. More recently, interest has focused on using modest supplemental intake of dietary fibre to reduce constipation. In a small randomized trial comparing two forms of dietary bran supplement with no supplementation, pregnant women with constipation in the fibre-supplemented groups increased their number of bowel movements compared to the untreated women.

Nevertheless, many women with troublesome constipation may require laxatives if physiological approaches afford no relief. Laxatives are usually classified by their mode of action. Bulking agents (polysaccharide and/or cellulose derivatives) and detergent stool-softeners (the dioctylsulphosuccinates) are safe to use during pregnancy, because they are inert and not absorbed. Some laxatives, such as the diphenylmethanes (e.g. bisacodyl and phenolphthalein), the anthraquinones (aloe, cascara, and senna), and castor oil, operate by their irritant action on the intestine. The most common maternal side-effects include cramping or griping, increased mucus secretion, and excessive catharsis with resultant fluid loss. Chronic use of irritant laxatives can result in loss of normal bowel function and laxative dependence. These irritant laxatives are all absorbed systemically to some extent. Most of them probably cross the placenta, but there is little information about possible effects on the fetus.

Saline cathartics (magnesium, sodium, and potassium salts) and lubricants (such as mineral oils) should not be used during pregnancy; the former because of the danger of inducing electrolyte disturbances and the latter because they interfere with absorption of fat-soluble vitamins.

The initial advice for women with constipation should be to use physiological measures and to increase their dietary fibre. Both bulking agents and stool softeners are safe for long-term use during pregnancy and lactation. If these preparations fail to relieve symptoms, irritant laxatives, such as standardized senna or bisocodyl, should be used on a short-term basis. Saline cathartics and lubricant oils should not be used at all.

7 Hemorrhoids

Effective prevention or treatment of constipation will help to reduce the severity of hemorrhoids, another common and painful symptom of pregnancy. In the absence of sound research about the best means of preventing or treating this condition, advice similar to that given to non-pregnant sufferers may be appropriate, such as rest, elevation of the legs, and avoiding constipation. Women can also be reassured that hemorrhoids usually improve or disappear after the birth. One small placebo controlled trial has compared a rutoside with placebo. Although this study suggested some relief of symptoms, there is little evidence about the safety of rutosides during pregnancy.

8 Vaginitis

8.1 Candidiasis

Vaginal candidiasis (thrush or yeast infection) is a frequent problem during pregnancy, and causes an intensely irritating, itchy vaginal discharge. The infection is found between two and ten times more frequently in pregnant women than in non-pregnant women, and it is more difficult to eradicate during pregnancy. It usually clears spontaneously soon after delivery.

The clinical diagnosis of vaginal candidiasis is neither specific nor sensitive. For some women, it may be difficult to distinguish between symptoms of candida and the increase and changes in normal vaginal secretion in pregnancy. Typical symptoms include an irritating vaginal discharge and pruritus (itch). Examination reveals reddened mucosa of the labia minora, introitus, and lower third of the vagina, with white patches and a thin discharge containing white flakes. Definitive diagnosis can be made by laboratory examination.

Candida infections can affect infants of very low birthweight and cause pneumonia and skin infections. These infections in the newborn, however, are rare considering the high frequency of vaginal candidal carriage in pregnant women, and for this reason screening of pregnant women without symptoms for candida is not indicated.

A variety of different local antifungal agents, as well as different dosages and frequencies of administration, have been studied. Imidazoles are more effective than nystatin. There is no evidence that a 14-day course of antifungal therapy is more effective in curing candidiasis than a 7-day course, but a 7-day course is more effective than a 4-day course. Cure rates for a 7-day course are up to 90%. Recently, single-dose vaginal treatments have been used, but no comparative trials in pregnancy have been reported.

The initial treatment of symptomatic vaginal candidiasis should consist of a 7-day course of a topical imidazole, such as clotrimazole, because of their proven superior efficacy over nystatin. Repeat courses may be required, given the tendency of the infection to recur. No treatment is indicated in asymptomatic infection.

Oral drugs, such as fluconazole, are now also being prescribed. In theory, they may be more effective than vaginal treatments, as they are effective against bowel, as well as vaginal, organisms. However, this form of treatment has not been tested during pregnancy, and it cannot be assumed to be safe.

8.2 Trichomoniasis

The protozoan *Trichomonas vaginalis* is frequently isolated from vaginal secretions during pregnancy. Infection with *Trichomonas vaginalis* in pregnancy may cause severe symptomatic vaginitis in some women, with vaginal discharge, severe irritation and soreness, and painful urination. Whether or not it can have adverse effects on the course of pregnancy or on the newborn is uncertain. Unsubstantiated reports have suggested that failure to treat trichomonas vaginitis leads to preterm birth, but one randomized, controlled trial reported no statistically significant difference in birthweight or gestational age at birth, whether asymptomatic *Trichomonas vaginalis* infection was treated with a single dose of metronidazole or left untreated. Colonization of the baby following vaginal delivery appears to be rare.

As *Trichomonas vaginalis* is often associated with other sexually transmitted infections in pregnancy, these should be specifically sought when *Trichomonas vaginalis* is identified.

Up to half the women carrying the organism are asymptomatic. Vaginal discharge is the most common complaint, but the classically described green frothy discharge is found in only a small proportion of women. Microscopic examination of a wet preparation of vaginal secretions is simple to perform and highly specific, but its sensitivity compared to culture may be as low as 50%. To maximize the sensitivity of a wet preparation, a drop of vaginal discharge diluted in saline should be examined under the microscope immediately. The characteristic jerky movements of the organism are lost if the secretions are allowed to cool before examination.

Culture is the best method to diagnose *Trichomonas vaginalis*, but the methodology is time-consuming and not generally available. Papanicolaou smears have been used to diagnose the disease, but the sensitivity of this method compared to culture is only 40%.

Metronidazole is a highly effective treatment of infection with *Trichomonas vaginalis*. A single 2-g dose has cure rates of more than 90% for up to one month. This single-dose therapy will also maximize compliance. The sexual partner should be treated at the same time as the woman.

Metronidazole readily crosses the placenta. Although it has been found to be carcinogenic in rodents and mutagenic for certain bacteria, there is no evidence for teratogenicity in humans after its administration to pregnant women. Most obstetricians, however, refrain from its use during the first trimester of pregnancy. Imidazoles, which have been shown to be effective *in vitro* against *Trichomonas vaginalis*, may provide symptomatic relief during early pregnancy.

8.3 Bacterial vaginosis

Bacterial vaginosis is caused by large numbers of a mixed group of organisms, including *Gardnerella vaginalis*, *Mycoplasma hominis*, and various anaerobes. It is common, but often asymptomatic. When symptoms do occur, they include vaginal discharge and vulval itch. Infection will usually resolve spontaneously. There is evidence that bacterial vaginosis is associated with preterm birth, however, and several trials have evaluated antibiotic treatment for both symptomatic and asymptomatic women. Although these studies show antibiotics have good cure rates, they are too small to establish whether there is any associated benefit in terms of reducing perinatal morbidity and mortality (see Chapter 19).

9 Leg cramps

Leg cramps (painful spasms of the calf muscles) are experienced to some extent by almost half of all pregnant women, particularly in the later months of pregnancy. The symptom tends to occur at night, and may recur repeatedly for weeks or months, causing considerable distress. The cause and mechanism of these cramps are still not clear. Sometimes based on rather astonishing analogies and unsupported hypotheses, a number of drugs have been widely prescribed for treatment and prophylaxis. Quinine, Benadryl, vitamin D, and dietary calcium were acclaimed to be of benefit on the basis of uncontrolled studies.

Sodium chloride tablets were demonstrated to be more effective than placebo, no treatment, or calcium lactate, in one controlled trial, but this study had methodological problems and the results have not been confirmed. A placebo-controlled trial of calcium failed to show any improvement in symptoms among women who took 1 g of calcium twice daily for 3 weeks. Another trial suggested that 5 mmol magnesium in the morning and 10 mmol at night for 3 weeks might prevent cramps, but this study was too small for any firm conclusions.

Calcium salts are still widely prescribed for the syndrome of nocturnal calf cramps in pregnancy, despite the lack of evidence from controlled trials that they have any benefit beyond that of a placebo. Unfortunately, no further trials of the efficacy of increased sodium or magnesium intake appear to have been conducted. It is probable that the observed benefits may be restricted to women who are sodium or magnesium deficient.

Massage, and stretching the affected muscles, often afford relief during an attack, and these innocuous measures are surely worth trying.

10 Varicose veins and leg edema

Varicose veins of the legs and vulva, are very common during pregnancy. Leg edema (swelling) can affect up to 80% of pregnant women, and should not be considered to be a sign of pregnancy-induced hypertension or pre-eclampsia (see Chapter 10). Symptoms can include pain, feelings of heaviness, night cramps, numbness, and tingling. The standard treatment for symptoms of varicose veins during pregnancy is support stockings. These seem to provide relief, although they have not been tested in randomized trials. They can be very uncomfortable during hot weather.

Two small trials provide some evidence that rutosides are associated with better relief than placebo for symptoms of varicosities, including cramps, tiredness, and edema. Further trials are required to confirm these findings, and to provide reassurance that rutoside use in pregnancy has no harmful effects on the fetus. Trials should also be designed to evaluate physical remedies, such as elastic support hosiery and exercises such as swimming, and to compare them with drugs.

Other methods of providing symptomatic relief of edema, such as intermittent external pneumatic compression, and immersion in a bath for almost an hour, can result in short-term reduction in leg volume or increased urine output, but they are of little practical help. The main importance of edema is the discomfort experienced by women, and there is no evidence that these measures provide symptomatic relief.

11 Other symptoms

Small trials have attempted to assess the effectiveness of a cream to prevent stretch marks (striae gravidarum), of sunscreen cream for melasma (dark skin patches), of antihistamines compared to aspirin for itching in late pregnancy, and of vitamin B to prevent tooth decay. None had adequate methodology or sample size to clearly establish whether or not the treatments provided any benefit or relief.

12 Conclusions

Some of the symptoms commonly experienced during pregnancy can be relieved by simple and physiological approaches. Others persist and cause significant discomfort.

Acupressure has shown promise for the relief of nausea and vomiting of pregnancy, and should be further investigated. Where medication is deemed to be necessary, antihistamines appear to be the drugs of choice, although no single product has been satisfactorily tested for efficacy in enough trials, and few studies are available to inform us about possible teratogenic risks.

No information is available to help in the alleviation of tiredness. Where possible, women should be encouraged to rest, and to seek help with home and work responsibilities.

When symptoms of heartburn fail to respond to postural and diet measures, antacids or acid-suppressing agents should be taken. For constipation in pregnancy, modification of the diet, including increasing dietary fibre and fluid intake, should be considered before resorting to laxatives. Bulking agents, if necessary combined with stool-softeners, should be used if dietary measures do not provide sufficient relief. Irritant laxatives (such as standardized senna) should be reserved for short-term use in refractory cases.

Symptoms of candidal vaginitis respond well to short courses of clotrimazole, which will often give relief from the symptoms of trichomonas vaginitis as well. No treatment is indicated in asymptomatic infection. Metronidazole, which is most effective for *Trichomonas vaginalis*, readily crosses the placenta, and probably should be withheld during the first trimester.

No pharmaceutical treatment for leg cramps has yet been firmly based on scientific evidence. At present, there is little evidence to recommend any treatment for edema which is either effective or acceptable. Despite the lack of objective evidence, support stockings remain the standard treatment for troublesome varicose veins and edema.

Prevention and treatment of the so-called 'minor', often extremely unpleasant symptoms of pregnancy have received little systematic study in clinical trials. Because of their wide prevalence, and the significant discomfort that they cause, such systematic study is urgently required.

Sources

Effective care in pregnancy and chilbirth

Bracken, M., Enkin, M., Campbell, H. and Chalmers, I., Symptoms in pregnancy: nausea and vomiting, heartburn, constipation, and leg cramps.

Cochrane Library

Brocklehurst, P. and Rooney, G., Interventions for treating genital chlamydia trachomatis infection in pregnancy.

Brocklehurst, P., Hannah, M. and McDonald, H., Interventions for treating bacterial vaginosis in pregnancy.

Gulmezoglu, A.M., Interventions for trichomoniasis in pregnancy.

Jewell, M.D. and Young, G., Interventions for nausea and vomiting in early pregnancy.

Interventions for preventing and treating backache in pregnancy.

Interventions for treating constipation in pregnancy.

Mahomed, K. and Gulmezoglu, A.M., Pyridoxine (vitamin B6) supplementation in pregnancy.

Young, G.L. and Jewell, M.D., Interventions for varicosities and leg edema in pregnancy.
Antihistamines versus aspirin for itching in late pregnancy.
Creams for preventing stretch marks in pregnancy.
Interventions for leg cramps in pregnancy.
Topical treatment for vaginal candidiasis in pregnancy.

Pre-Cochrane reviews

Jewell, M.D., Antacid therapy for heartburn in pregnancy.
Compound antacid preparations for heartburn in pregnancy.
Young, G.L., Sunscreen cream for melasma in pregnancy.

Other Sources

Bardhan, K.D., Müller-Lissner, S., Bigard, M.A., Bianchi Porro, G., Ponce, J., Hosie, J. *et al.* (1999). Symptomatic gastro-oesophageal reflux disease: double blind controlled study of intermittent treatment with omeprazole or ranitidine. *BMJ*, 318, 502–7.

Magee, L.A., Inocencion, G., Kamboj, L., Rosetti, F. and Koren, G. (1996). Safety of first trimester exposure to histamine H_2 blockers. *Dig. Dis. Sci.*, 41, 1145–9.

Östgaard, H.C., Zetherström, G., Roos-Hansson, E. and Svanberg, B. (1994). Reduction of back and posterior pelvic pain in pregnancy. *Spine*, 19, 894–900.

Wijayanegara, H., Mose, J.C., Achmad, L., Sobarna, R. and Permadi, W. (1992). A clinical trial of hydroxyethylrutosides in the treatment of hemorrhoids of pregnancy. *J. Int. Med. Res.*, 20, 54–60.

Miscarriage

1 Introduction

Miscarriage is the spontaneous loss of a pregnancy before the fetus is viable. Caregivers and family may sometimes not consider this to be as tragic a loss as fetal demise later in pregnancy, but it often results in a similar degree of mental suffering and anguish for the woman and her partner. Miscarriage is common. One in seven clinically recognized pregnancies will miscarry, usually during the first 14 weeks of pregnancy. Over half the babies who are miscarried during this period have a chromosomal abnormality. Other factors that influence the risk of miscarriage include maternal age over 35 years, multiple pregnancy, polycystic ovaries, autoimmune disorders, poorly controlled diabetes, and having had two or more previous miscarriages. Recurrent early pregnancy loss is suffered by 1–2% of couples. A number of interventions have been proposed and used in efforts to prevent miscarriage, particularly for women perceived to be at greater than average risk. Chief among these have been the prescription of bed-rest, either at home or in hospital, and the use of various hormones. For each woman, the choice of care should depend on evidence of effectiveness and on her personal preferences.

Psychological support for women who are at high risk of early pregnancy loss has not been formally evaluated in randomized trials. However, non-randomized comparisons suggest that such support alone may be associated with an improved pregnancy outcome. Proper evaluation of additional interventions is, therefore, of particular importance for the care of these women.

2 Confirmation of fetal life

Ultrasound has the ability to establish rapidly and accurately whether a fetus is alive or dead, and to predict whether a pregnancy is likely to continue when there is bleeding (threatened miscarriage). This ability has rationalized the care of women with threatened miscarriage in early pregnancy. The gestational sac can be visualized by 6 weeks menstrual age, and the fetus by 7 weeks. As soon as the fetus can be demonstrated with ultrasound, it can be measured and its viability confirmed by detection of heart movement. Fetal life is confirmed by observation of heart pulsation, and fetal death by its absence. Except in very early pregnancy, there should be no doubt about the diagnosis. Blighted ova, which constitute the largest group of early pregnancy failures, are diagnosed by the inability to detect a fetus on careful examination. When the sac is small, the pregnancy without an embryo has to be differentiated from the normal, very early pregnancy by a repeat ultrasound examination. Missed abortion can be diagnosed by absence of heart movement. The small group of pregnancies in which the embryo is alive but destined to miscarry cannot be predicted with certainty by ultrasound. These constitute less than 15% of the total number of miscarriages. Although a reduction in amniotic fluid volume, diminished fetal activity, or the presence of large intra-uterine hematomas may suggest a poor prognosis, there are no specific ultrasound features.

3 Prevention of miscarriage

3.1 Bed-rest and hospitalization

Bed-rest is often recommended for women whose pregnancies are complicated by a number of conditions, including a history of recurrent miscarriage or early bleeding in the present pregnancy. Women with these problems may be advised to rest in bed at home and in some cases may be admitted to hospital, to facilitate bed-rest and to permit closer investigation and surveillance of their pregnancy.

The extent to which women are advised to rest in bed varies considerably, but such advice is very common in some places. The intervention is not innocuous. Bed-rest and immobilization can increase the risk of thromboembolic disease. Both confinement to bed at home and hospitalization during pregnancy may result in great financial and social costs for pregnant women and their families, especially those with children. Antenatal hospitalization is often a disruptive and stressful experience involving separation of women from their families at a time of great anxiety. In addition, adoption of this policy has brought substantial costs to the health services.

The only reported attempt to undertake any form of controlled evaluation of the effectiveness of bed-rest in the management of threatened miscarriage was made over 45 years ago. The results of this study give no support to the view that a policy of recommending bed-rest reduces the risk of miscarriage after bleeding occurs in early pregnancy.

Bed-rest is sometimes advised for many days if spotting or bleeding is persistent, and this may cause considerable family disruption. Yet, in a substantial proportion of these pregnancies, the fetus is already dead. The presence of a non-viable pregnancy can now be demonstrated by ultrasound and no form of care can preserve these pregnancies.

Even with a viable embryo, there is no valid basis for advising bed-rest. The preferences of individual women should, therefore, be the deciding factor in whether or not they should rest, and this need not be in bed. Some women may feel they wish to rest. Women should be encouraged to do whatever feels best for them, although it would seem prudent to advise against prolonged immobilization.

3.2 Hormones

Over the last fifty years, various hormones have been given to pregnant women in attempts to prevent miscarriage, as well as fetal death, preterm delivery, and other adverse outcomes of pregnancy. Studies in the mid-1930s suggested a link between abnormal hormone levels and complications of pregnancy. The conclusion that inadequate hormone secretion meant that additional hormones should be administered is a classic example of the danger of applying pathophysiological reasoning to clinical practice without appropriate evaluation.

3.2.1 Diethylstilbestrol

The synthetic hormone, diethylstilbestrol, was administered to pregnant women on a wide scale for over thirty years. Based on animal studies and uncontrolled observations in humans, it was thought that it would be effective in preventing a variety of adverse outcomes. This hypothesis appeared to be supported by studies using observational data, but studies with contemporary controls did not substantiate the postulated beneficial effects. By the mid-1950s these controlled trials, individually and collectively, indicated that diethylstilbestrol did not reduce the risk of miscarriage, pre-eclampsia, low birthweight, preterm birth, stillbirth, neonatal death, nor increase the likelihood of a woman's pregnancy resulting in a surviving infant.

Thus, strong evidence was available by the mid-1950s to challenge the claims made on behalf of diethylstilbestrol. The drug should have been abandoned at that time, or prescribed only in the context of further trials. Despite this lack of evidence of benefit, obstetricians continued to use diethylstilbestrol until the 1970s, when several cases of vaginal adenocarcinoma (a very rare form of cancer in women less than 50 years old) were reported in young women whose mothers had received diethylstilbestrol while pregnant with them.

The randomized cohorts of women and their children generated by three of the trials have been studied for between 20 and 40 years after receiving diethylstilbestrol or placebo. The data suggest that there may be an increased risk of breast cancer in the women, and they clearly demonstrate an increased incidence of psychiatric illness and urogenital abnormalities in the children of both sexes. These abnormalities include benign tumours, vaginal adenosis, vaginal/cervical ridges, abnormal cervical smears, amenorrhoea/oligomenorrhoea, and infertility among the daughters, and low sperm density and other urogenital abnormalities among the men. The long-term adverse effects of the use of diethylstilbestrol in pregnancy that later became evident could have been minimized if more attention had been paid to the results of the controlled trials showing the drug to be ineffective.

3.2.2 Progestogens

Pregnancy loss in the first 3 months is associated with low serum progesterone. One possible explanation for this is that low progesterone causes miscarriage; another is that a failing pregnancy leads to reduced progesterone levels. Several randomized trials have evaluated the use of progestogens in early pregnancy. There is no evidence to suggest that they reduce the risk of miscarriage, stillbirth, or neonatal death, in women either with bleeding (threatened miscarriage) or with a history of recurrent miscarriage. The trials, however, have not been large enough to exclude an important effect, in either direction (increase or decrease in the risk of miscarriage), and in many of the studies ultrasound examinations were not done. These could have shown the fetus to be already dead, so that there may have been few pregnancies in which the progestogens could have been effective.

One small trial evaluated combined progesterone and estrogen for women having *in vitro* fertilization, started at the time of embryo transfer. This study has only reported outcome during the first 3 months of pregnancy, however.

Although the progestogen follow-up studies have been largely anecdotal and uncontrolled, there have been suggestions from some studies that fetal exposure to the drugs may increase the risk of esophageal atresia, cardiac, neurological, neural tube and other major malformations, and female masculinization, or 'tom-boyishness' in girls. Other studies, however, have failed to detect these adverse effects, and so the safety of progestogens, like their postulated benefits, remains an open question.

3.2.3 Human chorionic gonadotrophin

Data from the several controlled trials that have examined the effects of human chorionic gonadotrophin on the risk of miscarriage in women with a past history of repeated early pregnancy loss suggest that this treatment may be effective in preventing recurrent miscarriage.

The results of these trials must be interpreted with great caution because of methodological weaknesses in the studies. They need to be replicated in good quality randomized trials before any recommendation can be made about the use of human chorionic gonadotrophin in practice.

3.2.4 Luteinizing hormone releasing hormone agonists

High levels of luteinizing hormone are associated with early miscarriage. For women who have had repeated early pregnancy loss, it is therefore plausible that suppressing secretion of luteinizing hormone with a luteinizing hormone-releasing hormone agonist may reduce the risk of miscarriage. One trial has compared suppression of luteinizing hormone secretion, combined with low-dose ovulation induction, with spontaneous ovulation. This study was too small for any reliable conclusions about the effect on pregnancy loss.

3.3 Immunotherapy

During pregnancy, a woman's immune system is modified to allow her body to accept the growing fetus, and not to reject it as foreign tissue. Failure of this response, for whatever reason, is one possible but unproven cause of early pregnancy loss. Immunologic laboratory tests have no predictive value for pregnancy success, and should be abandoned. Immunotherapy has been suggested as a possible treatment for some women with an unexplained history of recurrent miscarriage: those with no identifiable cause and the same partner for each pregnancy. The most commonly used form of immunotherapy is injection of the women with her partners white blood cells. White cells from a third party, trophoblast membrane, and immune globulin have also been used.

Initial uncontrolled studies of immunotherapy for recurrent miscarriage suggested a beneficial effect. To date, however, these benefits have not been confirmed in trials with proper controls. Although the use of paternal white cells may lead to a small reduction in the risk of miscarriage, this needs to be balanced against the possible serious adverse effects, which have not been adequately quantified. These potential hazards include anaphylactic shock, transfusion reactions, and hepatitis. In addition, immunotherapy is expensive and so, even if further trials do confirm a worthwhile benefit, its usefulness will be limited by the high cost.

3.4 Interventions for women with autoimmune conditions

Around 15% of women with recurrent early pregnancy loss have antibodies to some of their own cells, autoimmune factors. These include antiphospholipid antibodies, lupus anticoagulant, and anticardiolipin antibodies. In contrast, autoimmune factors are present in 2% of women with a normal obstetric history. Women with autoantibodies have a very high risk of further miscarriage, and various interventions have been tried in the hope of improving their chance of having a healthy baby.

In theory, corticosteroids might improve the chance of these women having a healthy baby. The two trials that have evaluated steroid therapy, with or without aspirin, were too small for firm conclusions about the effect on having a liveborn baby, but they do suggest an increase in the risk of preterm delivery and of complications for the mother.

Two trials have evaluated low-dose heparin, injected subcutaneously (under the skin) and aspirin for women with autoantibodies and a history of recurrent pregnancy losses. The results of these studies are promising in terms of improving the chances of having a liveborn baby, although the risk of pregnancy complications, particularly preterm birth, remained high. Confirmation in larger trials is needed before any recommendation can be made about the overall effectiveness and safety of heparin treatment for women with recurrent pregnancy loss.

3.5 Other medications

The use of indomethacin for threatened miscarriage has been tested in one small trial, and no effect on the rate of miscarriage was demonstrated. Small trials evaluating tocolytic and antispasmodic medications suggest a reduction in the rate of miscarriage, but methodological flaws in these studies mean that these results should be interpreted with caution.

4 Care following spontaneous miscarriage or missed abortion

If miscarriage occurs within the first few weeks of pregnancy, it is usually complete, with the gestational sac expelled intact, and rarely requires admission to hospital or any intervention. After 6 weeks there is an increasing risk that some products of conception will be retained within the uterus, leading to an increased risk of continued bleeding and infection. Ultrasound scanning is widely used to confirm or refute the presence of retained products. Although this has not been evaluated in trials, the overall impression is that ultrasound will help reduce the need for intervention.

For many decades women with suspected retained products of conception, including missed abortion, have routinely been admitted to hospital for surgical evacuation of the uterus. This approach has recently been challenged and there are now three options for women with retained products of conception during the first trimester: a 'wait and see' approach; medical evacuation; or surgical curettage. Some women have strong preferences for one or other of these options.

4.1 'Wait and see' versus surgical evacuation

For women with an estimated gestational age of below 12–13 weeks and clinical evidence of retained products, the conservative 'wait and see' approach has been compared with surgical evacuation. In these trials, overall, around 20% of women managed with the expectant approach needed a surgical evacuation. There was insufficient evidence for reliable conclusions about any differential effect on pelvic infection but following the 'wait and see' approach, there did seem to be fewer complications. In the two studies reporting subsequent fertility, there was no evidence of any difference. Where women's views have been sought, they seem to prefer the 'wait and see' approach.

No trials have evaluated a 'wait and see' approach for women with a missed abortion (see Chapter 27).

4.2 Medical versus surgical evacuation

Following the successful introduction of hormonal methods for terminating pregnancy early in the first trimester, these agents are now being used for the care of women with spontaneous miscarriage. The drugs most widely used are prostaglandins and antiprogesterones, often in combination. These have been compared to surgical evacuation in a few trials. In one small study evaluating a single dose of a prostaglandin, most women with a medical evacuation went on to have a surgical evacuation, usually because of continued bleeding. This trend has not been confirmed in other studies.

One study in the UK has suggested that medical evacuation is cheaper if the theatre time freed up is put to good use. If the extra theatre time is not used, medical treatment will be more expensive than surgical evacuation. This study also suggests that about half the women with spontaneous miscarriage will have a strong preference for either medical or surgical evacuation.

Two large ongoing three-arm trials are comparing the 'wait and see' approach with medical and surgical evacuation.

4.3 Surgical evacuation

Surgical evacuation has been the standard treatment for incomplete miscarriage and first-trimester missed abortion for most of this century. It is, therefore, surprising that very few aspects of this procedure have been evaluated in adequately controlled trials.

4.3.1 Analgesia versus general anesthetic

One trial has compared systemic analgesia on the ward with a general anesthetic in theatre. Women having a systemic analgesic were less likely to need a blood transfusion, and had their operation more quickly.

4.3.2 Suction versus conventional curettage

Another trial has compared suction evacuation with conventional curettage. Women who had a suction evacuation had less blood loss. This procedure was also faster and less painful.

4.3.3 Prophylactic antibiotics

One trial has evaluated the use of prophylactic doxycycline during surgical evacuation in a hospital where the risk of infection following incomplete miscarriage was low. There was no apparent effect on postoperative pelvic infection. Another trial in Zimbabwe evaluated 1 week of oral tetracycline postoperatively. The risk of infection was high, but again there was no effect. However, in this study poor compliance was thought to have been a factor.

5 Conclusions

Hospitalization during pregnancy is costly and disruptive for many families. Discussion with individual women will make it clear that a prescription for rest, either at home or in hospital, would sometimes be welcome. As there is no strong evidence that this is likely to have harmful effects, women's views should be taken into account. By the same token, women with bleeding in early pregnancy should not be coerced into resting at home or in a hospital against their better judgement.

In the present state of knowledge, hormone administration of any type during pregnancy should be used only within randomized trials until the ratio of benefits to hazards has been more clearly established. Future trials should involve only those women who have had ultrasonography to confirm that the fetus is alive. A similar caution must be made in regard to indomethacin, tocolytics, and antispasmodics.

The use of immunotherapy for women with an unexplained history of recurrent miscarriage should also be restricted to those participating in randomized trials. Maternal injection of paternal white blood cells appears to show most promise, but it may also be associated with serious hazards. A greater understanding of the theoretical basis for immunotherapy may help guide further research in this field.

For women with autoantibodies, combined heparin and aspirin treatment appears promising, but further evaluation of the possible hazards and the long-term effects is needed before this can be recommended for clinical use.

Following spontaneous miscarriage with retained products of conception, surgical evacuation is probably necessary if the uterine size is more than 12–13 weeks. If the uterine size is less than this and there is clinical and ultrasound evidence of retained products, the options are 'wait and see', medical evacuation, or surgical curettage. Women may have strong preferences, and these should be taken into account in the decision about what form of care is given. A 'wait and see' approach will mean that 80% of women avoid the need for surgery. The role of medical evacuation remains unclear and awaits further evidence about the optimal agents and their effects at different gestations. Prophylactic antibiotics following surgical evacuation may have a role in areas were the risk of postoperative infection is high.

Sources

Effective care in pregnancy and childbirth

Crowther, C. and Chalmers, I., Bed-rest and hospitalization during pregnancy.

Goldstein, P.A., Sachs, H. and Chalmers, T.C., Hormone administration for the maintenance of pregnancy.

Neilson, J. and Grant, A., Ultrasound in pregnancy.

Cochrane Library

Scott, J.R., Human chorionic gonadotrophin for recurrent miscarriage.

Immunotherapy for recurrent miscarriage

Pre-Cochrane reviews

Prendiville, W.J., Progestogens to prevent miscarriage and preterm birth.

Tocolytics/antispasmodics for threatened miscarriage.

17alpha-hydroxyprogesterone caproate in pregnancy.

Progestogens in pregnancy.

Progestogens for threatened miscarriage.

Indomethacin for threatened miscarriage.

Progestogen/estrogen prophylaxis in early normal pregnancy.

Other sources

Clifford, K., Rai, R., Watson, H., Franks, S. and Regan L. (1996). Does suppressing luteinising hormone secretion reduce the miscarriage rate? Results of a randomised controlled trial. *BMJ*, 312, 1508–11.

de Jonge, E.T., Makin, J.D., Manefeldt, E., De Wet, G.H. and Pattinson, R.C. (1995). Randomised clinical trial of medical evacuation and surgical curettage for incomplete miscarriage. *BMJ*, 311, 662.

Laskin, C.A., Bombardier, C., Hannah, M.E., Mandel, F.P., Ritchie, J.W., Farewell, V. *et al.* (1997). Prednisone and aspirin in women with autoantibodies and unexplained recurrent fetal loss. *N. Eng. J. Med.*, 337, 148–53.

Nielson, S. and Hahlin, M. (1995). Expectant management of first trimester spontaneous abortion. *Lancet*, 345, 84–6.

Prieto, J.A., Eriksen, N.L. and Blanco, J.D. (1995). A randomised trial of prophylactic doxycycline for curettage in incomplete abortion. *Obstet. Gynecol.*, 85, 692–6.

Rai, R., Cohen, H., Dave, M. and Regan, L. (1997). Randomised controlled trial of aspirin and aspirin plus heparin in pregnant women with recurrent miscarriage associated with phospholipid antibodies (or antiphospholipid antibodies). *BMJ*, 314, 253–7.

Silver, R.K., MacGregor, S.N., Sholl, J.S., Hobart, J.M., Neerhof, M.G. and Ragin, A. (1993). Comparative trial of prednisone plus aspirin versus aspirin alone in the treatment of anticardiolipin antibody-positive obstetric patients. *Am. J. Obstet. Gynecol.*, 169, 1411–7.

Verkuyl, D.A. and Crowther, C. (1993). Suction v conventional curettage in incomplete abortion. A randomised controlled trial. *S. Afr. Med. J.*, 83, 13–5.

Hypertension in pregnancy

1 Introduction

Two etiologically distinct entities account for most hypertensive disorders in pregnancy. One is a disorder induced by pregnancy, which, in this chapter, we refer to as 'pregnancy-induced hypertension', if not accompanied by proteinuria, as 'pre-eclampsia' if there is associated proteinuria, and as 'eclampsia' if it leads to convulsions and/or coma. The other is chronic hypertension that precedes or coincides with pregnancy, and is sometimes associated with a known underlying condition, such as renal disease. In addition, a combination of the two conditions may occur; this is referred to as 'superimposed pre-eclampsia'.

The outcome for pregnancies complicated by hypertensive disorders is often good, but sometimes these conditions may have devastating consequences for mother and baby. For example, the woman may develop renal or hepatic failure, disseminated intravascular coagulation, or a cerebrovascular hemorrhage. The baby may have intrauterine growth restriction, suffer the consequences of being born too early, or die *in utero*.

The risk of adverse effects has been recognized for a long time, and a bewildering array of medical and surgical regimens have been proposed or used for the prevention and treatment of pre-eclampsia and eclampsia. One author reports that women with eclampsia have been 'blistered, bled, purged, packed, lavaged, irrigated, punctured, starved, sedated, anesthetized, paralyzed, tranquillized, rendered hypotensive, drowned, given diuretics, had mastectomies, been dehydrated, forcibly delivered, and neglected'. Thankfully, most of these 'remedies' are now obsolete. In this chapter we assess the available evidence about current approaches to either preventing or treating pregnancy-induced hypertension, pre-eclampsia, and eclampsia.

2 Prophylaxis

2.1 Dietary measures

As discussed in the chapter on dietary modification, there is no evidence that any modification of protein or calorie intake can protect against pregnancy-induced hypertension. Two trials from the Netherlands have compared advice to restrict dietary salt with continuing a normal diet. These were not large studies, and there is little suggestion of any effect on the development of pregnancy-induced hypertension or pre-eclampsia. Salt intake during pregnancy should, therefore, be a matter of taste and personal preference.

Certain long-chain fatty acids, contained in fish oils, have shown an antiplatelet and antithrombotic effect similar to that of aspirin. Observational studies, as well as the results of a supplementation trial carried out over fifty years ago, suggested the possibility of a prophylactic effect of fish oil, and prompted more rigorous controlled trials These more recently carried out trials show a promising reduction in the incidence of hypertension, proteinuric pre-eclampsia, and preterm birth, but there are insufficient data to show a decrease in any measure of perinatal mortality or morbidity. Oil of evening primrose, another source of fatty acids, has also been suggested for prevention of pre-eclampsia. It has been tested in a few trials, but these were too small to provide any guidance for clinical practice.

Calcium supplementation during pregnancy appears to reduce the risk of women developing pre-eclampsia, particularly if they were at high risk and had low-calcium intake early in pregnancy. There is little evidence of any effect on other important outcomes, such as cesarean section, intra-uterine growth restriction, or perinatal death, although the studies were not large enough to exclude a small but clinically worthwhile benefit. Calcium supplementation may be well worth considering, particularly for high-risk women with low dietary calcium.

Supplementation with magnesium, zinc, and selenium also have been suggested to reduce the risk of pre-eclampsia, but the trials that have evaluated these minerals have all been too small to provide a reliable basis for clinical practice.

The search for something that will prevent pre-eclampsia, and is also cheap and easy for women to take, continues.

2.2 Diuretics
There is no evidence that excessive water retention or even frank edema either causes pre-eclampsia, or defines a group of women at particular risk of developing the condition. Nevertheless, many attempts have been made and, indeed, are still being made by some obstetricians and midwives to prevent retention of salt and water in pregnancy by prescribing diuretics or a rigidly sodium-free diet in the belief that this will prevent pre-eclampsia.

The effects of the prophylactic use of diuretics in pregnant women with normal blood pressure (with or without edema or excessive weight gain), and of their therapeutic use in women with moderate hypertension, have been studied in a number of randomized trials carried out many years ago. The results reflect the ability of diuretics to reduce blood pressure, but fail to show any improvement in substantive outcomes. There is no clear evidence of benefit with respect to the prevention of pre-eclampsia or the risk of perinatal death. This could mean either that the treatment was ineffective, or that the numbers studied were too small to detect some modest but worthwhile benefit. None of the serious side-effects of diuretic treatment in pregnancy that have been described in occasional case reports, were observed in these trials. These findings suggest that both the benefits and the risks of diuretic administration may have been overstated.

2.3 Antithrombotic and antiplatelet agents
Changes in the blood-clotting system are well documented in established pregnancy-induced hypertension. The extent of the clotting

disorders appears to be related to the severity of the disease and early activation of the clotting system may contribute to the pathology of pre-eclampsia. Aspirin has been shown to prevent thrombotic occlusion of arteriovenous shunts and coronary artery bypass grafts, and to reduce death and reinfarction in unstable angina, and after myocardial infarction and cerebral ischemic attacks. For these reasons, the use of anticoagulant or antiplatelet agents, and aspirin in particular, has been considered for the prevention of pre-eclampsia and associated intra-uterine growth restriction.

Several small trials of antiplatelet prophylaxis for pre-eclampsia and intra-uterine growth restriction suggested that the incidence of both these conditions might be substantially reduced. Unfortunately, this early promise was not confirmed in larger studies. There are now nearly 40 studies, which include among them over 30 000 women. Overall, these trials confirm that there is a small (15%) reduction in pre-eclampsia. This is reflected in a similar reduction (14%) in the risk of a stillbirth or neonatal death, and an 8% reduction in the risk of a preterm birth. Remaining questions include whether aspirin might be more helpful for women at very high risk of developing pre-eclampsia, such as those with a history of severe early onset disease, and whether treatment needs to be started in the first half of pregnancy. Current research into the inherited thrombophilias and their possible link to early-onset pre-eclampsia may help identify a sub-group of women in whom the role of aspirin may be worthy of re-exploration in the future.

Low dose aspirin does seem to be reasonably safe. More is now known about the short- and medium-term safety of aspirin than for most other drugs used during pregnancy, and early fears that it might be associated with an increased risk of bleeding have not been confirmed. Although the routine widespread use of prophylactic aspirin is not supported by the results of the trials, it would appear that low dose aspirin does have some limited clinical value. Further research is required to determine which women are most likely to benefit.

Heparin requires subcutaneous (or intravenous) administration, making it an inconvenient form of treatment, and its use may be associated with dangerous side-effects. It has been tested in a few trials, but these were too small to provide a reliable guide to clinical practice. Warfarin has also been used prophylactically in an attempt to prevent recurrent pre-eclampsia in multiparous women. Anecdotal reports of its use do not provide any evidence of benefit for either the mother or the baby, and there is some suggestion that it may have serious side-effects.

2.4 Antioxidant vitamins

One small trial has evaluated high doses of vitamins C and E as antioxidant agents for prevention of pre-eclampsia. The results were very promising, but require confirmation in larger studies before these vitamins can be recommended for clinical practice. Two such trials are being planned.

3 Mild or moderate pregnancy-induced hypertension and pre-eclampsia

Chronic hypertension and mild or moderate pregnancy-induced hypertension carry little risk to the mother or the fetus, unless severe hypertension, pre-eclampsia, or eclampsia ensue. For this reason, the aim of treatment of mild to moderate hypertensive disease in pregnancy has been to defer or prevent the development of severe hypertensive disease. Rest in bed, and a variety of medications have been used.

3.1 Bed rest

Women with hypertension or mild or moderate pre-eclampsia are often advised to rest in bed at home, or they may be admitted to hospital to facilitate bed-rest and to permit closer investigation and surveillance of their pregnancies. The extent to which women are advised to rest in bed at home or in hospital varies considerably, but such advice is very common in some places. The intervention is not innocuous. Both confinement to bed at home and hospitalization during pregnancy may result in financial and social costs for pregnant women and their families, and carry an additional risk of thromboembolic disease. Antenatal hospitalization is often a disruptive and stressful experience, and adoption of this policy has brought substantial costs to the health services. It would only be justified if there were clear health benefits from the practice.

The effectiveness of bed-rest for non-proteinuric hypertension has been evaluated in three controlled trials. Unfortunately, no clear picture emerges from these trials on the value of this practice. One trial suggests that hospitalization may have a beneficial effect on the evolution of pre-eclampsia, while another tends to suggest the opposite. There are also contrasting patterns in the frequency of preterm birth among the trials.

When proteinuria develops in addition to hypertension in pregnancy, the risks for both mother and fetus are substantially increased.

Admission to hospital is then considered necessary for evaluation and increased surveillance, to detect any deterioration in maternal or fetal condition as soon as possible. Whether the hospitalization should be linked to strict rest in bed is less clear. The two small trials that have addressed this question have not provided clear answers. To date, there is no good evidence to support a policy of strict bed-rest in hospital for a woman with mild or moderate pre-eclampsia.

3.2 Antihypertensive agents

Antihypertensive medication for either mild to moderate pregnancy-induced hypertension or for chronic hypertension in pregnancy reduces blood pressure, but the effects on other important outcomes are less clear. It may possibly reduce the risk of perinatal death and preterm birth, but the evidence for this remains weak. There is no evidence that antihypertensive treatment with any of the drugs available prevents proteinuria, and there is insufficient evidence for reliable conclusions about the effects of antihypertensive treatment on other important endpoints, such as cesarean section or neonatal morbidity. Few children exposed to antihypertensive drugs *in utero* have been followed up beyond the perinatal period.

Methyldopa is the most widely used drug in women with mild to moderate pregnancy-induced hypertension. A proportion of the children in one study have been followed to age seven. These data provide a degree of reassurance about the safety of methyldopa that is not available for the other drugs. The use of methyldopa for women with moderate hypertension does reduce their risk of developing severe hypertension. There is also a strong suggestion that it may reduce the risk of perinatal death, although the results marginally fail to reach statistical significance. In the same way as for diuretics, there is no evidence of an effect on the incidence of proteinuria, intra-uterine growth restriction, preterm birth, or cesarean section. Clonidine is similar to methyldopa in most respects, except for a more rapid onset of action (about 30 min compared with 4 h for methyldopa).

The beta-blockers, including labetalol, are also well established in clinical practice. Although there are several trials in women with mild to moderate hypertensive disease in pregnancy, even when taken together there is not enough information to allow reliable assessment of their effects on clinically important outcomes or on deterioration of the disease. Administration of beta-blockers will reduce the incidence of severe hypertension, but there is a suggestion that it may increase the risk of intra-uterine growth restriction. Beta-blockers are effective antihypertensive agents that reduce cardiac output, and it is possible that this effect would be unfavorable in pregnancy, since adequate perfusion of the maternal and uteroplacental circulation depends on maintenance of the elevated cardiac output of pregnancy.

Direct comparisons of beta-blockers with methyldopa, hydralazine, and nifedipine, do not indicate any significant differential effects, but the trials have been far too small to provide reliable information on the relative safety and efficacy of these agents.

Randomized trials of calcium-channel blockers in pregnancy-induced hypertension, compared either with placebo or with beta-blockers, have been too small to provide useful estimates of their effects.

Another question about the use of antihypertensive agents is whether there is any advantage to starting treatment early. In a recent study ketanserin, a selective serotonin-2-receptor antagonist, was given to women with mild hypertension during the first half of pregnancy. Although the study was small, there was a trend towards less pre-eclampsia among the women receiving early treatment.

The small numbers of women studied in adequately controlled trials of antihypertensive medication for both the prevention and treatment of moderate hypertensive disease preclude definitive conclusions about their effects, even when the results of all trials are considered together. It seems likely that antihypertensive treatment prevents the development of severe hypertension in pregnancy, and for that reason may reduce the number of hospital admissions and emergency deliveries. If true, this may in itself reduce the risk of preterm birth and thereby improve outcome for the baby. There is no clear evidence that antihypertensive treatment with any of the drugs available may defer or prevent the occurrence of proteinuric pre-eclampsia or of associated problems, such as fetal growth restriction and neonatal morbidity. Nor is there good evidence about the safety of such treatments, in particular with respect to child development. Methyldopa has been the most studied agent. If an antihypertensive agent is to be used, it is probably the agent of choice, except in the context of randomized comparisons with other agents.

3.3 Other treatments

Small trials have attempted to assess the efficacy of magnesium, prostaglandin precursors, and antioxidants, such as vitamins C and E, in the treatment of pre-eclampsia. The trials are too small to provide reliable information about either the effectiveness or the safety of these approaches.

4 Severe pre-eclampsia and eclampsia

Although treatment of hypertension does not strike at the basic disorder, it may still benefit the mother and fetus. One of the important objectives in severe hypertension in pregnancy is to reduce blood pressure in order to avoid hypertensive encephalopathy and cerebral hemorrhage in the mother. For this reason, the aim in treating severely hypertensive pregnant women is to keep the blood pressure below dangerous levels (less than 170/110 mmHg) and to maintain adequate circulating blood volume.

4.1 Antihypertensive agents

Hydralazine is the antihypertensive drug most commonly used for women with severe pregnancy-induced hypertension and pre-eclampsia, followed by labetalol and nifedipine. Methyldopa is also used, although it has the disadvantage of a relatively slow onset of action (about four hours). Agents that have been evaluated in trials comparing one drug with another include hydralazine, labetalol, calcium antagonists (nifedipine, nimodipine, and isradipine), diazoxide, prostacyclin, ketanserin, and magnesium sulphate. Ketanserin was more often associated with persistent maternal hypertension than hydralazine. These studies are all small, however, and there is currently no evidence to justify a strong preference for any one of the various drugs available for treating severe hypertension in pregnancy over another.

In clinical practice, therefore, the choice of drug should probably depend on the familiarity of an individual clinician with a particular drug. In general, maternal side-effects are not different from those in the non-pregnant state, and are listed in pharmacology texts. All drugs used to treat hypertension in pregnancy cross the placenta, and so may affect the fetus directly, by means of their action within the fetal circulation, or indirectly, by their effect on uteroplacental perfusion.

From what is known about direct and indirect adverse effects on the fetus and neonate, hydralazine appears to be relatively safe. Labetalol may cause severe and long-lasting fetal and neonatal bradycardia, particularly after high doses. These effects may be clinically important in the presence of fetal and neonatal hypoxia. In one small trial comparing diazoxide with labetalol, diazoxide appeared to provoke a precipitous fall in maternal arterial pressure and was associated with an increased risk of cesarean section. In addition, hyperglycemia has been reported in the newborn after maternal treatment with diazoxide.

Although this study was small, it would seem prudent to avoid this drug and use one of the other available options.

There is, as yet, little clinical information on the fetal or neonatal effects of maternal use of calcium antagonists. Various problems have been observed in the neonatal period following their use in uncontrolled studies, but these effects could not definitely be attributed to maternal drug treatment.

4.2 Plasma volume expansion

Women with severe pre-eclampsia often have a reduced circulating plasma volume. This has led to a recommendation that plasma volume should be expanded with either colloid or crystalloid solutions, in an attempt to improve the maternal systemic and uteroplacental circulation. Some uncontrolled studies suggested that rapid replenishment of intravascular volume may result in decreased arterial blood pressure in pregnant women with moderate third-trimester hypertension or preeclampsia. Although blood pressure was not restored to normal by volume expansion, these uncontrolled studies suggest that such treatment may be an effective adjunct to the administration of antihypertensive drugs and by reducing the drug doses needed, might minimize the risks of maternal and neonatal side-effects.

It should be borne in mind, however, that intravascular volume expansion carries a serious risk of volume overload, which may lead to pulmonary and perhaps cerebral edema in pre-eclamptic women in whom colloid osmotic pressure is usually low. Plasma volume expansion may be particularly dangerous after birth, when venous volume tends to rise. It should not be applied without careful monitoring. Also, the choice of agent may have a major impact on outcome. Recently it has become clear that for critically ill people plasma expansion with colloid is associated with a higher mortality than either not using any plasma expander or expansion with crystalloid. Although none of these studies included pregnant women, it would seem prudent to avoid colloid solutions until data from randomized trials involving women with pre-eclampsia become available.

There is insufficient evidence from controlled trials to provide reliable guidelines for the use of plasma volume expansion for hypertension in pregnancy. Further studies are clearly needed to define the place of plasma volume expansion, with or without additional antihypertensive treatment, in the care for women with severe pregnancy-induced hypertension.

4.3 Anticonvulsant agents

Anticonvulsant drugs are widely used in the management of eclampsia, as well as in severe hypertensive disease and pre-eclampsia, in an attempt to prevent the occurrence of eclamptic seizures.

For eclampsia, there is now good evidence from randomized trials that magnesium sulphate is considerably better than either diazepam or phenytoin for the prevention of further seizures. The trends in maternal mortality are also in favor of magnesium sulphate, although these are not statistically significant. In comparison with diazepam, the use of magnesium sulphate does not appear to be associated with any other effects for either the woman or her baby. In comparison with phenytoin, women who had magnesium sulphate also did better in terms of needing fewer admissions to intensive care, requiring ventilation less often, and having a lower risk of pneumonia. Their babies were less likely to need intubation at the place of delivery or admission to a special care nursery.

Uncertainty remains about whether anticonvulsants are useful therapy for women with pre-eclampsia. In the United States, parenteral magnesium sulphate is given to women with severe pre-eclampsia, and it may also be used for relatively mild or moderate pre-eclampsia, usually during labor and delivery. In contrast, a quarter of obstetricians in the UK and Ireland never use prophylactic anticonvulsants, and those who do usually reserve such agents for severe or fulminating pre-eclampsia. When anticonvulsants are felt to be necessary, magnesium sulphate is now a popular choice of agent in the UK, but diazepam is also widely used.

Four controlled trials with a total of 1200 women have compared magnesium sulphate with placebo or no anticonvulsant for women with pre-eclampsia, and one small study compared oral diazepam with no treatment. Although there is promising evidence that magnesium sulphate does reduce the risk of eclampsia, the studies are too small to indicate whether this effect is big enough to be clinically worthwhile. Also, little is known about whether magnesium sulphate has any other important effects and whether it is safe for the woman and her child. As for any prophylaxis, most women who receive this treatment would not develop eclampsia anyway, and so it is particularly important to be sure that it does more good than harm. A large international trial is currently comparing magnesium sulphate with placebo for women with pre-eclampsia.

Magnesium sulphate is not an innocuous drug. It can reach life-threatening levels as a result of excessive dosage or diminished excretion (e.g. due to renal failure). Since an overdose can cause death by cardiorespiratory arrest, women receiving magnesium sulphate must be closely monitored at all times, and calcium should be readily available as an antidote. Clinical monitoring of urine output, tendon reflexes, and respiratory rate will usually be adequate, and it is not normally necessary to measure serum levels.

Only a small amount of magnesium appears to cross the blood–brain barrier after intravenous administration of magnesium sulphate and it has virtually no sedative effect. Magnesium readily crosses the placenta, and high magnesium concentrations in cord blood have been shown to be associated with respiratory depression of the baby.

There is conflicting evidence about the possible long-term effects of *in utero* exposure to magnesium sulphate. Case control studies have suggested this may reduce the risk of cerebral palsy for very low-birthweight babies, a hypothesis now being tested in randomized trials. However, there is also concern that *in utero* exposure to magnesium sulphate may be harmful, particularly in high doses. In addition to evaluation of the effects of magnesium sulphate on the women, more information is required about the effects on long-term growth and development for the children.

4.4 Interventionist versus expectant management

For women who have severe pre-eclampsia before 34 weeks, the decision about the best time to deliver the baby is often difficult. The hazards to the baby of being born too early need to be balanced against the risks to both the woman and the baby if the pregnancy is allowed to continue for too long. Two trials have compared an interventionist policy (early resort to elective delivery) with a more expectant approach between 28 and 32 or 34 weeks. The trends in these studies were towards beneficial effects for the babies of an expectant policy, but with possibly greater risks to the woman. The trials were too small to provide a reliable guide to clinical practice.

5 Conclusions

Preliminary results with antiplatelet agents were promising, but the evidence from recent large trials does not support their use for routine prophylaxis against pre-eclampsia. Calcium supplementation may be useful for high-risk women with low dietary calcium.

Discussion with individual women will make it clear that a prescription of rest, either at home or in hospital, would sometimes be welcome. But hospitalization and bed-rest is an expensive and intrusive intervention, with as yet no clear evidence of value. Thus, women with non-albuminuric hypertension, or with mild to moderate pre-eclampsia, should not be coerced into either resting in bed at home, or into being hospitalized against their better judgement.

Antihypertensive medication for mild to moderate hypertension in pregnancy prevents further increases in blood pressure. This in turn may reduce the number of hospital admissions, inductions, and emergency deliveries, although these effects have not been studied systematically. Trials to date have been too small to provide reliable information about other important outcomes. At present, there is insufficient evidence to assess at what level of hypertension the benefits of antihypertensive therapy outweigh the disadvantages.

For treatment of severe hypertensive disease, most agents seem equally effective in lowering blood pressure, although there is little information about other possible effects. The exceptions are diazoxide, which should be avoided due to the risk of hypotension and cesarean section, and ketanserin, which was more often associated with persistent hypertension than hydralazine.

Magnesium sulphate is the anticonvulsant of choice for treatment of eclampsia. For pre-eclampsia there is insufficient evidence to assess whether, overall, prophylactic anticonvulsants do more good than harm. If an anticonvulsant is to be used, magnesium sulphate is the best choice and is now being evaluated in a large trial.

In view of the promising effects of antihypertensive agents in preventing the development of severe hypertension, and their widespread use by many doctors, there is an urgent need for evaluation in large-scale trials.

There is little reliable information about the value of plasma volume expansion. Until further data are available, if plasma expansion is to be done this should be with crystalloid rather than colloid.

Current treatment of hypertensive disorders in pregnancy appears to be largely based on clinical experience fed by anecdotal reports, rather than on reliable evidence from properly controlled trials of sufficient size. Given the large number of women who develop hypertensive disease in pregnancy, multicenter collaborative studies involving much larger numbers of women than have so far been studied should be mounted. These could assess the effects of the various treatments that are used more reliably than has been done so far.

Sources

Effective care in pregnancy and childbirth

Collins, R. and Wallenburg, H.C.S., Pharmacological prevention and treatment of hypertensive disorders in pregnancy.

Cochrane Library

The Albumin Reviewers (Alderson, P., Bunn, F., Lefebvre, C., Li Wan Po, A., Li, L., Roberts, I., Schierhout, G.), Human albumin solution for resuscitation and volume expansion in critically ill patients.

Atallah, A.N., Hofmyr, J.G. and Duley, L., Calcium supplementation during pregnancy to prevent hypertensive disorders and related problems.

Duley, L. and Henderson-Smart, D., Magnesium sulphate versus diazepam for eclampsia.

Magnesium sulphate versus phenytoin for eclampsia.

Drugs for rapid treatment of very high blood pressure during pregnancy.

Reduced salt intake compared to normal dietary salt, or high intake, during pregnancy.

Duley, L., Gulmezoglu, M. and Henderson-Smart, D., Anticonvulsants for pre-eclampsia.

Gulmezoglu, A.M. and Hofmeyr, G.J., Plasma volume expansion for suspected impaired fetal growth.

Knight, M., Duley, L., Henderson-Smart, D. and King, J., Antiplatelet agents for preventing and treating pre-eclampsia.

Mahomed, K., Zinc supplementation in pregnancy.

Makrides, M. and Crowther, C.A., Magnesium supplementation during pregnancy.

Schierhout, G., Roberts, I. and Alderson, P., Colloids compared to crystalloids in fluid rescusitation of critically ill patients.

Pre-Cochrane reviews

Duley, L., Aggressive vs expectant management of pre-eclampsia.

Diuretics for prevention of pre-eclampsia.

Diuretics for treatment of pre-eclampsia.

Diuretics for prevention/treatment of pre-eclampsia.

Strict bed rest for proteinuric hypertension in pregnancy.

Hospitalization for non-proteinuric pregnancy hypertension.

Other sources

Broughton Pipkin, F., Crowther, C., de Swiet, M., Duley, L., Judd, A., Lilford, R.J. *et al.* (1996). Where next for prophylaxis against pre-eclampsia? *Br. J. Obstet. Gynaecol.*, 103, 603–7.

Chappell, L.C., Seed, P.T., Briley, A.L., Kelly, F.J., Lee, R., Hunt, B.J., Parmar, K., Bewley, S.J., Shennan, A.H., Steer, P.J., and Poston, L. (1999). Effect of antioxidants on the occurrence of pre-eclampsia in women at increased risk: a randomised trial. *Lancet*, 354, 810–16.

Duley, L. and Neilson, J.P. (1999). Magnesium sulphate and pre-eclampsia. *BMJ*, 319, 3–4.

Hutton, J.D., James, D.K., Stirrat, G.M., Douglas, K.A. and Redman, C.W. (1992). Management of severe pre-eclampsia and eclampsia by UK consultants. *Br. J. Obstet. Gynaecol.*, 99, 554–6.

Nelson, K. (1996). Magnesium sulfate and risk of cerebral palsy in very low-birth-weight infants. *JAMA*, 276, 1843–4.

Fetal compromise

1 Introduction

In general, the care of women whose fetus is diagnosed or suspected of being in jeopardy involves a choice between pre-emptive delivery and conservative care in order to avoid potentially serious consequences for the baby. A number of conservative measures have been considered in controlled trials.

2 Impaired fetal growth

Suboptimal maternal blood flow to the placenta is thought to be an important cause of both impaired fetal growth and pre-eclampsia. There are, however, no well-validated methods for increasing utero-placental circulation (except change from a supine position).

2.1 Bed-rest

In theory, uteroplacental perfusion may improve with bed-rest. On the other hand, bed-rest may increase the likelihood of thrombosis. It may be stressful for women with children or other responsibilities. If in hospital, it will be costly for the health services.

Despite the fact that it is commonly advised, only one trial to assess the effects of bed-rest in hospital for women with a small-for-gestational age fetus has been reported. This trial failed to show any effect of hospitalization for bed-rest on any clinical outcome. Thus, there is no good evidence that bed-rest in hospital promotes fetal growth, although the trial was too small to exclude that possibility. No controlled studies have been mounted to assess the effects, good or bad, of bed-rest at home.

2.2 Abdominal decompression

Abdominal decompression was developed initially as a method of enhancing the forward movement of the uterus during labor contractions, with a view to relieving pain. Apparent beneficial effects on the condition of the infant at birth, which were not anticipated, led to the hypothesis that repeated brief decompression of the abdominal region may increase the flow of blood to the placenta. The concept has intrigued a number of enthusiasts, but has not found acceptance in mainstream obstetrical practice.

A rigid dome is placed about the abdomen and covered with an airtight suit. The space around the abdomen is decompressed to −50–100 mmHg for 15–30 seconds out of each minute for 30 minutes once to thrice daily, or continuously during labor. This is thought to 'pump' blood through the intervillous space. Physiological data suggest that the technique may reduce intra-uterine pressure, increase maternal placental blood flow, increase fetal movements, and increase fetal heart-rate acceleration and variability. Not surprisingly, some thought that this might foster fetal well-being, and the modality was tried both prophylactically and therapeutically.

2.2.1 Prophylaxis in normal pregnancy

Abdominal decompression came into clinical use in normal pregnancies in the early 1960s on the basis of the results of several poorly controlled studies, which appeared to show that it improved fetal well-being and subsequent intellectual development. Two prospective studies followed, in which attempts were made to compare the outcome in women subjected to abdominal decompression with comparable control groups. None of the available data suggest that prophylactic abdominal decompression affects duration of pregnancies or infant birthweight. They give no support to suggestions that prophylactic abdominal decompression has a beneficial effect on the condition of the infant at birth. One carefully controlled trial studied the effects of abdominal decompression on child development. Although the developmental scores were slightly higher in the study group at 28 days and at 3 years of age, the differences were neither clinically nor statistically significant.

These studies provide convincing evidence that antenatal abdominal decompression used in uncomplicated pregnancies does not improve any of the outcomes measured. There is thus no support for the use of antenatal abdominal decompression as a prophylactic procedure.

2.2.2 Treatment of the compromised fetus

There is some evidence to suggest that abdominal decompression may have a place in the management of pregnancies in which the fetus is likely to be compromised.

Abdominal decompression appears to slow the progression of pre-eclampsia. In addition, one trial showed abdominal decompression to be associated with a statistically significantly larger weekly growth in the fetal biparietal diameter. These differences between experimental and control groups were reflected in somewhat fewer inductions of labor for 'placental insufficiency' and less non-reassuring fetal status during labor in the women who had received decompression.

Observer bias and possibly reporting bias may account for some or all of the putative effects of abdominal decompression noted above. The assessment of birthweight is less subject to large observer biases. Abdominal decompression was associated with a substantial reduction in the incidence of low birthweight, and an increase in mean birthweight (2800 g versus 2296 g) . The available data suggest a reduction in the incidence both of depressed Apgar scores and of perinatal mortality.

The studies thus suggest a beneficial effect of abdominal decompression on fetuses with impaired growth, although their methodological shortcomings limit the confidence that one can place in these conclusions. It may be important to assess whether or not abdominal decompression affects uteroplacental blood flow. The advent of Doppler flow measurements offers an opportunity to assess this more rigorously than has been done in the past.

2.3 Betamimetics

Small trials mounted to assess the effects of betamimetics for women whose fetus does not appear to be growing adequately have not provided sufficient data to determine the clinical effects. There were no significant differences found for any of the outcomes measured between groups of women who received or did not receive betamimetics but, because of the small numbers studied, clinically important differences may have been missed. While there is a possibility that betamimetic therapy may promote fetal growth, either by improving uteroplacental circulation or by increasing blood sugar and plasma insulin levels, there is insufficient evidence to support their use except in the context of randomized clinical trials.

2.4 Maternal oxygen administration

Two small trials of maternal oxygen administration for suspicion of inadequate fetal growth have shown a reduction in perinatal mortality in the oxygenation group. Methodological shortcomings in these trials, a preponderance of extremely preterm babies in the control group, and small sample sizes preclude reliance on this finding.

Biochemical data available suggest that oxygen treatment for impaired fetal growth may have both beneficial and harmful effects. In view of the suggestion from some studies that oxygen administration may decrease uterine blood flow, the effectiveness of oxygen administration would need to be demonstrated in larger, well-controlled clinical trials before its use in clinical practice could be recommended.

2.5 Hormone treatment

No clinically relevant outcomes are available from the trials of various types of hormone treatment for suspected impairment of fetal growth. Thus, we have no evidence to support the use of hormones for this purpose.

2.6 Calcium channel blockers

The only controlled trial to assess the clinical effect of calcium channel blockers for suspected impairment of fetal growth showed the mean birthweight to be higher in babies of the women in the actively treated group than in those in the placebo group. There was also a non-significant trend towards lower perinatal mortality.

The evidence from this trial is not strong enough to support the use of calcium channel blockers in pregnancies with an increased risk of impaired fetal growth. The results are, however, sufficiently encouraging to justify further trials with adequate numbers to assess the effects on substantive outcomes.

2.7 Energy/protein supplementation

Observational studies have reported that gestational weight gain is associated with fetal growth. Evidence from the quasi-experimental Dutch Famine Study suggests that energy/protein restriction is associated with impairment in fetal growth. Randomized trials of balanced protein/energy supplementation show a modest increase in maternal weight gain and fetal growth, but no long-term effects on the child.

The available evidence provides no justification for prescribing high-protein or isocaloric balanced protein nutritional supplements to pregnant women. Not only do such supplements appear to lack beneficial effects; the evidence suggests that they may even be harmful (see Chapter 6).

2.8 Other measures

Plasma volume expansion with hydroxyethyl starch, transcutaneous electrostimulation, and nutrients such as intravenous calf blood extract, have been tried as conservative treatments for suspected placental insufficiency or impaired uterine growth. There is insufficient evidence to justify the clinical use of any of these measures.

Oral hydration has been shown to increase amniotic fluid volume in the short-term, but substantive clinical outcomes have not been studied.

3 Acute 'fetal distress'

3.1 Tocolytics

The use of acute tocolysis with betamimetic and other agents as a treatment for acute non-reassuring fetal status has become widespread in clinical practice. This is based on the presumption that uterine relaxation improves uteroplacental blood flow and, therefore, fetal oxygenation, and that this advantage outweighs the adverse cardiovascular effects of the treatment on the mother. Surprisingly, few well-controlled studies have addressed this question.

In two small studies, persistent fetal heart rate abnormalities were significantly reduced with tocolysis, but the improvements found in perinatal outcome are compatible with the effect of chance.

The limited evidence available suggests that intravenous beta-mimetics are a useful treatment for 'buying time' when non-reassuring fetal status is diagnosed during labor. Such time may be useful for preparing for cesarean section or operative delivery, setting up regional analgesia, transferring a woman from home or from a unit without the necessary surgical or neonatal facilities to an appropriate hospital, or reviewing the need for urgent delivery. Whether poor outcomes or the need for operative delivery can in fact be reduced by this treatment remains to be demonstrated.

On the basis of the one trial comparing magnesium sulphate with terbutaline as a tocolytic, it appears that terbutaline (and presumably other betamimetics) is more likely to be effective in this respect than magnesium sulphate.

3.2 Maternal oxygen administration

Oxygen is frequently given to the mother in the management of suspected 'fetal distress'. Several non-randomized studies have suggested a beneficial effect, while others have disputed this. To our knowledge, no randomized clinical trials have assessed the effectiveness of maternal oxygen administration for non-reassuring fetal status. In one randomized trial of maternal oxygen administration in the absence of non-reassuring fetal heart rate patterns, cord blood pH values were significantly reduced in those receiving oxygen administration. Whether or not a similar adverse effect might occur in the presence of 'fetal distress' is not yet known. There is thus a need for trials to evaluate the beneficial or adverse effects of oxygen administration for non-reassuring fetal status.

4 Conclusions

The effectiveness of bed-rest in hospital for impaired fetal growth has not been demonstrated, but it has not been adequately evaluated. Because of the enormous financial and personal costs of prolonged hospitalization, this form of care should be used only in the context of well-designed controlled trials to test its effectiveness. Bed-rest at home may also be seriously disruptive for the woman, and should not be strongly recommended without proper evaluation.

There is some evidence that abdominal decompression may be of value in certain abnormal states of pregnancy, but the studies reported to date are not sufficiently strong to support its use outside the context of methodologically sound controlled trials. Because there are so few options for managing the compromised fetus other than elective delivery, it is important to subject abdominal decompression to further evaluation.

There is a reasonable theoretical basis for investigating the usefulness of tocolytic treatment for suspected impaired fetal growth, but as yet no evidence to support its clinical use.

Preliminary evidence suggests an effect of calcium channel blockers on fetal growth, but further research is needed to evaluate their effectiveness in terms of substantive pregnancy outcomes.

The effectiveness of maternal oxygen administration for both impaired fetal growth and non-reassuring fetal status is unproven. Tocolytic therapy for acute non-reassuring fetal status improves fetal heart rate patterns. Further studies are needed to evaluate substantive outcomes.

Sources

Effective care in pregnancy and childbirth

Crowther, C. and Chalmers, I. Bed-rest and hospitalization during pregnancy.

Hofmeyr, G.J., Abdominal decompression during pregnancy.

Rush, D., Effects of changes in protein and calorie intake during pregnancy on the growth of the human fetus.

Cochrane Library

Gulmezoglu, A.M. and Hofmeyr, G.J., Bed-rest in hospital for suspected impaired fetal growth.

Betamimetics for suspected impaired fetal growth.

Calcium channel blockers for potential impaired fetal growth.

Transcutaneous electrostimulation for suspected placental insufficiency (diagnosed by Doppler studies).

Hormones for suspected impaired fetal growth.

Maternal oxygen administration for suspected impaired fetal growth.

Maternal nutrient supplementation for suspected impaired fetal growth.

Plasma volume expansion for suspected impaired fetal growth.

Hofmeyr, G.J., Abdominal decompression in normal pregnancy.

Abdominal decompression for suspected fetal compromise/pre-eclampsia.

Maternal hydration for increasing amniotic fluid volume in oligohydramnios and normal amniotic fluid volumes.

Kramer, M.S., Balanced protein/energy supplementation in pregnancy.

High protein supplementation in pregnancy.

Isocaloric balanced protein supplementation in pregnancy.

Kulier, R. and Hofmeyr, G.J., Tocolytics for suspected intrapartum fetal distress.

Other sources

Crowther, C.A. (1995). Commentary: bed-rest for women with pregnancy problems: evidence for efficacy is lacking. *Birth*, 22, 13–4.

Kramer, M.S. (1993). Effects of energy and protein intakes on pregnancy outcome: an overview of the research evidence from controlled clinical trials. *Am. J. Clin. Nutr.*,58, 627–35.

Multiple pregnancy

1 Introduction

Multiple pregnancy poses particular problems for women, their infants, and for their caregivers. Women are likely to experience the common, unpleasant symptoms of pregnancy, such as heartburn, backache, hemorrhoids, difficulty walking, and tiredness to a greater degree than women with a singleton pregnancy. They are more likely to suffer from anemia, hypertension, pre-eclampsia, preterm labor, and operative delivery. The increased risks to the babies include congenital malformations, monochorionicity (both babies sharing one placenta), poor fetal growth, preterm birth, and perinatal death. For the survivors, in the long term there is a greater risk of cerebral palsy.

2 Prenatal care

A wide range of options for regular antenatal attendance are practised, ranging from modified shared care between obstetrician and general practitioner to weekly visits from the 20th week of gestation onwards. There is no evidence to suggest that one pattern of prenatal care is better than another, because this important research question has never been properly addressed. Regular prenatal visits permit screening for hypertension and pre-eclampsia by careful determination of blood pressure, and, if elevated, checking for proteinuria. Care for women with a multiple pregnancy who develop hypertension may be particularly important, and should follow current treatment recommendations (see Chapter 15).

2.1 Advice and support

Women with a multiple pregnancy need advice and support from caregivers to help them deal with the particular problems of multiple pregnancy and with the common, unpleasant symptoms of pregnancy, such as hemorrhoids, heartburn, and backache (see Chapter 13). They may be especially anxious about the pregnancy, the birth, and their ability to cope with the practical and financial demands of more than one new baby. Assisting women to find support, such as a special antenatal class for women with a multiple pregnancy or referring them to a multiple-birth support group, may help.

2.2 Nutrition

Fetal demands for iron and folate are increased in multiple pregnancy and anemia is reported more frequently than in singleton pregnancies. Routine iron and folate supplementation is often advised from the beginning of the second trimester, although this has not been shown to improve the clinical outcome of the pregnancy (see Chapter 6).

2.3 Ultrasound

If routine ultrasonography is not carried out, an ultrasound examination is indicated when multiple pregnancy is suspected. Routine early ultrasonography results in earlier detection of multiple pregnancies, the detection of mono-amniotic pregnancies (with greater risk), and the detection of some unsuspected congenital abnormalities. Earlier detection of multiple pregnancy has not been shown to improve fetal outcome.

The risk of neural tube defects, cardiac anomalies, and bowel atresias, have all been reported to be increased in twin pregnancies. Conjoined twins and twin reversed arterial perfusion sequence are rare anomalies that are found exclusively in multiple pregnancies. Early diagnosis of fetal anomaly enables appropriate counseling as to the care options available.

The prediction of amnionicity (number of amniotic sacs) and chorionicity (separate or joined placentas) by first-trimester ultrasound is possible, though its accuracy and the relevance to pregnancy outcome remains to be determined. In theory at least, knowledge of amnionicity and chorionicity may be helpful in a number of ways, such as in the differentiation of twin-to-twin transfusion syndrome from a twin pregnancy complicated by intra-uterine growth restriction, in management after a single fetal death, or where one of the twins has a major congenital malformation and selective termination is considered.

If twin-to-twin transfusion syndrome develops, several therapeutic options have been advocated. These include: non-steroidal anti-inflammatory drugs, repeated therapeutic amniocenteses, and techniques that interrupt the pathological placental circulation. The results of controlled trials of these therapies are awaited, although there has been minimal evidence to date that any of these improve infant outcome.

Poor fetal growth of one or more babies is a risk in a multiple pregnancy. No adequately controlled data are available on the value of regular ultrasound or umbilical artery Doppler for assessing fetal growth and well-being in multiple pregnancy.

3 Preterm birth

Preterm birth presents the greatest threat to infant survival. Counseling as to the signs and symptoms of preterm labor with advice to present to the hospital if they occur, together with a written information sheet, may be of value, although this approach has not been subjected to a controlled evaluation.

Prediction of preterm birth is difficult. Cervical assessment by digital examination or by ultrasonography has been reported to provide useful prediction of the risk of preterm birth. How frequent these assessments should be made is uncertain, and whether they are more beneficial than harmful is unknown.

Cervical fibronectin may prove to be useful in predicting which women will give birth preterm, although the main strength lies in its negative predictive value. Whether the measurement of fibronectin will be useful clinically to improve pregnancy outcome remains to be established by controlled trials.

Several prenatal treatments have been used in attempts to reduce the risk of preterm birth and its sequelae in women with multiple pregnancy. These include cervical cerclage, beta-mimetic agents, home uterine-activity monitoring, and hospitalization for bed rest. All have been evaluated by controlled trials but, to date, none have proven to be of value in reducing the risk of preterm birth.

3.1 Cervical cerclage

In normal pregnancy, the uterine cervix is thought to assume a sphincter-like function to retain the contents of the uterus. A congenital or traumatically-acquired weakness of the cervix, or the unusual physiological circumstance of multiple pregnancy, are factors that may render the cervix incapable of performing this function as efficiently as usual. Belief in such 'incompetence' of the cervix is the basis for performing the operation of cervical cerclage.

The data available from controlled trials of cervical cerclage in twin pregnancy are too few to be clinically useful. They are compatible with both a large beneficial effect and with a large adverse effect of the operation. Cervical cerclage does affect other aspects of clinical care and carries some specific risks. It should not be adopted specifically for twin pregnancy outside the context of further controlled trials of sufficient size and quality.

3.2 Prophylactic betamimetic agents

Trials have been conducted with a number of oral betamimetic agents, including isoxuprine, ritodrine, salbutamol, and terbutaline, in various doses, for the prevention of preterm labor in women with multiple pregnancy. In spite of the diversity of agents and the varying doses used, the results are consistent. No beneficial effect of prophylactic betamimetic administration has been detected on preterm birth, low birthweight, or perinatal mortality. Although prophylactic betamimetic agents have not succeeded in postponing delivery or in improving fetal growth, the four trials that provide information on the incidence of respiratory distress syndrome suggest that the frequency of this adverse outcome may be significantly reduced. No such effect has been found with prophylactic betamimetics in singleton pregnancies, and it might be a chance finding.

In the light of the theoretical dangers of chronic fetal exposure to betamimetic agents, prophylactic administration of these drugs should only be considered in the context of well-controlled clinical trials.

3.3 Home uterine-activity monitoring

Trials of home uterine-activity monitoring in multiple pregnancy have been small, and not enough detail is available to evaluate the potential sources of bias. There are suggestions that babies born to mothers using home uterine-activity monitoring for twin pregnancy may be less likely to weigh less than 1500 g, or to be admitted to a special care nursery. Because of the high potential for bias, these data must be viewed with caution. Home uterine-activity monitoring, if adopted at all, should not be adopted outside the context of adequately controlled trials.

3.4 Hospitalization in multiple pregnancy

Prolonged bed rest in multiple pregnancy, with the aim of increasing the duration of gestation, improving fetal growth, and decreasing perinatal mortality, has been advocated for many years. The general considerations about the use of bed rest (see Chapter 14), apply equally strongly to its use in multiple pregnancy, as the practice is not innocuous.

Hospitalization and bed-rest in multiple pregnancy was introduced into clinical practice without adequate evaluation and the policy has still not been fully evaluated. Only recently have a few trials been conducted and further controlled evaluations are necessary to clarify the effects of this intervention. More information is available from twin than from higher multiple pregnancies.

There is some suggestion from these trials that routine hospitalization of women with twin pregnancies may result in a decreased risk of maternal hypertension, but a positive impact on more relevant outcomes has been negligible. Indeed the data suggest that routine hospitalization may have adverse effects. The risk of very preterm birth (less than 34 weeks gestation) and very low-birthweight babies was *increased* by routine hospitalization in these trials. No differences have been detected in the incidence of depressed Apgar score, admission to special care nurseries, or perinatal mortality.

Some obstetricians have suggested that hospitalization for bed rest in twin pregnancies should be applied only for women deemed to be at higher than average risk of preterm birth. Although this more conservative advice is possibly justified, there is remarkably little good evidence to support it. Only one such selective policy has been evaluated in a randomized trial. Comparison between the hospitalized and control groups of women with early cervical dilatation failed to show any benefits on the risk of preterm birth, perinatal mortality, fetal growth, or other neonatal outcomes. There is no basis for widespread adoption of the policy.

Only one trial of bed-rest in triplet pregnancies has been published. The results of this trial suggest that a number of adverse outcomes, including preterm birth, perinatal death, and low birthweight, can be reduced by routine hospitalization of women with a triplet pregnancy. The trial was small; the findings were compatible with chance; and further research is required.

4 Delivery

Virtually no data from controlled trials are available to help determine the choice between vaginal birth and cesarean section for women with multiple pregnancy. A single trial has assessed the effect of cesarean section for delivery when the second twin was in a non-vertex presentation. As would be expected, maternal febrile morbidity and need for general anesthesia was increased with cesarean section. No offsetting advantages in terms of decreased fetal or neonatal morbidity or mortality were found.

5 Conclusions

Additional support may be needed to help women with the emotional, practical, and financial demands of pregnancy and planning for more than one baby.

Routine early ultrasonography results in early diagnosis, detection of fetal abnormalities, and can determine amnionicity and chorionicity. Whether this improves the outcome for the mother or infant is unknown. Regular antenatal attendance permits screening for hypertension. Iron or folate supplementation may help to prevent anemia.

Prediction of preterm birth is difficult and the role of cervical assessment and clinical use of fibronectin remains to be evaluated by controlled trials. Therapies that aim to reduce the risk of preterm birth have not been shown to be effective.

There is currently no sound evidence to support the practice of routine bed-rest in hospital for women with a twin pregnancy; indeed the evidence suggests that this may be harmful. Whether or not such a policy would be justified in women at higher risk of preterm labor, such as those with triplet pregnancy or with early cervical dilatation, remains to be established.

The use of cervical cerclage, oral betamimetics, or home uterine-monitoring, for women with multiple pregnancy cannot be justified outside the context of adequately controlled trials. The indications for cesarean delivery with multiple pregnancy have not been established.

Sources

Effective care in pregnancy and childbirth

Crowther, C. and Chalmers, I., Bed-rest and hospitalization during pregnancy.

Grant, A., Cervical cerclage to prolong pregnancy.

Cochrane Library

Crowther, C.A., Hospitalization for bed-rest in multiple pregnancy.

Cesarean delivery for the second twin.

Neilson, J.P., Ultrasound for fetal assessment in early pregnancy.

Pre-Cochrane reviews

Grant, A.M., Cervical cerclage in twin pregnancy. Review no. 03280.

Keirse, M.J.N.C., Prophylactic oral betamimetics in twin pregnancies. Review no. 03462.

Home uterine-activity monitoring in twin pregnancies. Review no. 06661.

Other sources

Crowther, C.A. (1997) Multiple pregnancy. In *High-risk pregnancy management options* (ed. D. James). WB Saunders, London.

Rhesus iso-immunization

1 Introduction

Iso-immunization against rhesus antigens, which may result in hemolytic disease of the fetus and newborn, was a major cause of perinatal mortality, morbidity, and long-term disability until the 1970s. With the development of RhD immunoglobulin, and its evaluation and utilization in clinical practice since the early 1970s, severe rhesus iso-immunization is rarely seen today. A reduction in average family size may have also contributed to this welcome reduction.

The dramatic reduction in deaths from rhesus hemolytic disease has been one of the major obstetrical achievements of the past quarter-century. Despite this, rhesus hemolytic disease is unlikely to disappear, and remains a problem for women and their babies who are affected.

2 Prevention of iso-immunization

The effectiveness of anti-D immunoglobulin in the prevention of rhesus iso-immunization has been demonstrated in a number of trials conducted in different countries. The question is not whether or not women at risk of rhesus immunization should receive anti-D immunoglobulin, but which women should receive such prophylaxis, at what times, and in what doses.

There is a risk of iso-immunization in any situation in which Rh-positive red blood cells enter the circulation of a Rh-negative woman.

The degree of this risk will vary with the amount of rhesus antigen to which she is exposed.

2.1 After delivery

The most common time for Rh-positive fetal cells to enter the mother's circulation is at the birth of a Rh-positive baby. Without the administration of anti-D immunoglobulin, Rh-negative women who give birth to a Rh-positive baby have a 7.2% risk of developing rhesus antibodies within 6 months of delivery, and a much larger risk (15%) of showing evidence of sensitization in a subsequent pregnancy. With postpartum administration of anti-D immunoglobulin, these risks are reduced to 0.2 and 1.6%, respectively.

ABO incompatibility, commonly believed to confer significant protection against the development of rhesus antibody formation, does not confer sufficient protection to be useful in clinical practice.

Evidence on the optimal amount of anti-D immunoglobulin to recommend for routine prophylaxis is limited. In the UK, postnatal administration of 100 mg (500 IU) is generally used; in Australia 125 mg (750 IU); and in the USA and parts of Europe 200–300 mg (1000–1500 IU).

It is reasonably well established that 20 mg (100 IU) of anti-D will neutralize the antigenicity of 1 ml of Rh-positive red cells, or 2 ml of whole blood. Hence, the dose of 300 mg (1500 IU), applied in some countries, is sufficient to protect against a fetomaternal bleed of 30 ml. When smaller doses are given in the interests of economy, the amount of fetomaternal transfusion must be assessed. The relative cost-effectiveness of giving a smaller dose of anti-D immunoglobulin along with assessment of the amount of fetomaternal transfusion, compared with routine administration of a higher dose, will depend on local circumstances and the relative costs of anti-D immunoglobulin and of laboratory tests.

In some countries, the availability of anti-D immunoglobulin is limited. Establishing the cost-effectiveness of a smaller dose of anti-D immunoglobulin combined with screening for the degree of feto-maternal hemorrhage, compared with routine use of a larger dose of anti-D, would seem advisable.

A fetomaternal hemorrhage of 30 ml or more is uncommon but does occur in up to 0.6% of deliveries. In this case, larger doses of anti-D immunoglobulin are required to prevent immunization. Counts of fetal cells in maternal blood have become routine after birth in some centers, to determine whether a larger dose of anti-D immunoglobulin should be given. The risk of a large fetomaternal hemorrhage is increased after traumatic births, cesarean section, manual removal of the placenta, and in some cases of fetal death.

The best time to administer the anti-D immunoglobulin would be as soon as possible after birth, but immediate administration is not practical in view of the time required to determine the blood group of the baby. From the trials that have been conducted, it would appear that an interval of up to 72 hours is compatible with effective prophylaxis.

No adverse effects of treatment with anti-D immunoglobulin have been reported from the trials, although the risk of rare adverse effects of sensitivity reactions and transmission of infectious agents remains.

2.2 During pregnancy

A small proportion of women (1.5%) develop rhesus antibodies during their first pregnancy; most such immunizations take place after 28 weeks of gestation. Antenatal administration of 100 mg (500 IU) anti-D immunoglobulin at 28 and 34 weeks to RhD-negative mothers has been shown to reduce the number of women with a positive Kleihauer test (evidence of fetal blood cells entering the mother's circulation) at both 32–35 weeks and at delivery, as well as the incidence of iso-immunization. A trial using a smaller 20-mg (100 IU) dose failed to show these beneficial effects.

The combination of antenatal administration of 100 mg anti-D immunoglobulin to all unsensitized Rh-negative women, and a further dose administered after birth to all such women who give birth to a Rh-positive child, would reduce the remaining incidence of rhesus iso-immunization from 0.2 to 0.06%. The costs of such a program may be high, but must be considered against the costs of antenatal detection and treatment of the affected infant, whose mother develops immunization. Further studies are required to determine the cost-effectiveness.

Administration of anti-D immunoglobulin to unsensitized RhD-negative women is required after procedures known to carry a risk of fetomaternal transfusion. Bleeding from the fetal to the mother's circulation has been documented as a consequence of chorion villus sampling, amniocentesis, fetal blood sampling, placental biopsy, and external version of a breech presentation.

Fetomaternal transfusion may occur with either spontaneous or induced abortion, and may result in iso-immunization, if anti-D immunoglobulin is not administered. The incidence of fetomaternal transfusion in spontaneous abortion has been estimated at about 6–7% during the first trimester of pregnancy, and 20% or more in the second trimester. Up to 13 weeks of pregnancy, a dose of 50–75 mg of anti-D gamma globulin after termination of pregnancy or miscarriage is sufficient to ensure adequate protection. In the second trimester, the standard postpartum dose should be administered.

Abdominal trauma, placenta praevia, placental abruption, or any form of uterine bleeding, may occasionally cause fetomaternal transfusion. Massive fetomaternal transfusion may sometimes be suspected on the basis of the findings at cardiotocography prompted by these conditions. Fetomaternal transfusion may also occur without any obvious cause. Unexplained fetal or intrapartum death, or the birth of a pale, distressed baby, should raise the possibility that a significant fetomaternal transfusion has occurred.

3 Diagnosis of iso-immunization

All women should have routine assessment of their rhesus status in early pregnancy. Women who are RhD-negative should be further screened for the presence of antibodies. The other rhesus antigens (C and E) are far less immunogenic but occasionally can cause serious clinical problems. Anti-Kell, anti-Kidd, anti-Duffy, and some of the more rare antigens, can also, on occasion, cause hemolytic disease in the fetus and newborn. For this reason, many centers screen all pregnant women for other blood group antibodies, in addition to the RhD status.

The presence of antibodies indicates that the fetus may become affected if it carries the antigen to which the antibodies were formed; it does not indicate whether the fetus carries the antigen. For this reason, it is helpful to determine whether the woman's partner is homozygous or heterozygous for the antigen. If the father is homozygous, the fetus will always carry the antigen; if the father is heterozygous, there is a 50% risk that the fetus will carry the antigen. Zygosity of RhD cannot be determined with certainty, but it can be estimated with a probability ranging between 80 and 96%.

The level of an antibody titre does not predict the presence or severity of disease, although in a first affected pregnancy there is a reasonable correlation between the antibody titre and the severity of disease. In subsequent pregnancies, the extent to which the fetus was affected in previous pregnancies is the most powerful predictor of the severity of disease in the present one. The obstetric history, in combination with serial antibody levels, will usually allow a reasonably accurate prediction of the severity of the hemolytic disease in the current pregnancy. This information is not, however, sufficiently precise to determine the need, or the optimal time, for intervention. For this, ultrasound, amniocentesis with spectrophotometric analysis of hemoglobin degradation products (bilirubin) in the amniotic fluid, or fetal blood sampling to determine fetal blood group and fetal hematocrit, are required. This may need to be repeated at regular intervals, depending upon the severity and progression of the findings.

4 Treatment of iso-immunization

Early delivery, before the baby is too severely affected to be effectively treated by postnatal therapy, remains the mainstay of treatment for established iso-immunization.

When the hemolytic disease is sufficiently severe that it would not be safe to continue the pregnancy until the fetus is sufficiently mature, intra-uterine transfusion is the treatment of choice. RhD-negative packed cells transfused into the fetus can correct the fetal anemia and allow birth to be postponed to a more advanced stage in the pregnancy, when the baby can be successfully treated with currently available methods of intensive neonatal care. The procedure can be started as early as 16 weeks of gestation, and can be repeated as necessary.

Other treatments that have been used include plasmapheresis from early pregnancy onward, immunosuppression with promethazine, and desensitization by oral administration of RhD-positive red blood cells. These methods for treatment have not been evaluated in controlled trials.

5 Conclusions

Rhesus hemolytic disease of the fetus and newborn, while by no means the frequent condition that it once was, remains a problem that requires constant vigilance and attention. Although effective prophylaxis is available it must be properly used.

Postpartum prophylaxis with anti-D immunoglobulin should be given within 72 hours of birth to all RhD-negative women who give birth to a RhD-positive baby, or a baby whose RhD status cannot be determined, irrespective of their ABO status.

Anti-D immunoglobulin should be administered also to all RhD-negative women during pregnancy when there is an increased risk of fetomaternal bleeding.

Routine use of anti-D immunoglobulin at 28 or 34 weeks of pregnancy for all Rh-negative women is of value as well, but the costs of such a programme are high and together with the limited supplies of anti-D immunoglobulin may preclude this in some countries.

Rhesus iso-immunization has become sufficiently rare, and the treatment sufficiently complex, to warrant regionalization of care for these women and babies. Hopefully, this may facilitate adequate evaluation of the methods used for diagnosis and treatment, none of which have been as yet subjected to controlled trials.

Sources

Effective care in pregnancy and childbirth

Bennebroek Gravenhorst, J., Rhesus iso-immunization.

Cochrane Library

Crowther, C.A. and Keirse, M.J.N.C., Anti-D administration during pregnancy for preventing rhesus allo-immunization.

Crowther, C.A. and Middleton, P., Anti-D administration after childbirth for preventing rhesus allo-immunization.

Neilson, J.P., Interventions for suspected placenta praevia during pregnancy [protocol].

Infection in pregnancy

1 Introduction

In the past, bacterial infection during pregnancy was a major cause of both maternal and perinatal death. These deaths are now rare in most parts of the developed world, although maternal infection and colonization with pathogenic organisms continue to cause problems for both mothers and babies. Various infections are more prevalent among socio-economically disadvantaged pregnant women, and this may in part explain the greater frequency of adverse outcomes of pregnancy among these women.

Other organisms, such as fungi, viruses, and protozoa, may lead to serious disease during pregnancy and the perinatal period. In the last decade, infections with the human immunodeficiency virus (HIV) have become epidemic in many countries, particularly in the developing world. In many developing countries, HIV is now a major cause of maternal and infant mortality. Other organisms such as *Chlamydia trachomatis* and the genital mycoplasmas, have also been linked with disease in pregnancy and childbirth. Finally, pregnant women are subject to the same range of acute and chronic infections as non-pregnant women.

2 HIV infection

Asymptomatic HIV infection and acquired immunodeficiency syndrome (AIDS) are now major health problems. AIDS is characterized by defects in the immune system with attendant susceptibility to infections by opportunistic micro-organisms and specific tumours. Asymptomatic HIV infection is important because of the risk of transmission from the mother to the fetus or neonate. Despite improvements in survival associated with the introduction of combinations of more potent antiretroviral therapies, for many HIV-infected individuals, complications still occur.

Pediatric-acquired immunodeficiency syndrome was first recognized in 1982 and numerous case series have been reported since. HIV infection is usually not recognized at birth, but can present months to years later with recurrent bacterial infections and sepsis, persistent or recurrent thrush, and failure to thrive.

The organism in adults is usually transmitted sexually, and is frequently associated with the presence of other sexually transmitted disease. It is also transmitted through infected blood and blood products, or the sharing of infected needles among drug users. Intra-uterine transmission from mother to infant may occur during pregnancy, at birth (when most transmission occurs), or through breast milk. While the advantages of breastfeeding may outweigh the risk of transmission through breast milk, communities in less-developed countries need to identify ways to reduce the not insignificant incidence of postnatal transmission through breastfeeding.

There is now good evidence of reduced transmission of HIV infection from mother to baby by prenatal zidovudine treatment. Unfortunately, the cost of this drug is prohibitive in countries with the greatest burden of need. There may be a further reduction in vertical transmission when pregnant women are treated with the now standard, more potent antiretroviral combinations. There is also emerging evidence of reduced transmission through delivery by cesarean section.

Both symptomatic and asymptomatic women may transmit the infection to their infants. Offering screening only to women who are considered to be at high risk will only detect a small proportion of infected women. Universal screening for HIV in pregnancy is being widely advocated.

Globally, the major issue is the high prevalence of HIV infection in the poorest countries, where facilities for prevention and treatment are least available. HIV infection has become a massive problem in developing countries. In some it is the single most important cause of maternal death.

3 Syphilis

The incidence of syphilis has declined dramatically in the developed world following the widespread introduction of penicillin in the 1950s. More recently, the incidence has increased again, largely in association with HIV infection. In the developing world, syphilis remains a major public health problem.

Syphilis during pregnancy is particularly important because transmission of *Treponema pallidum* from mother to baby may result in congenital syphilis, with its tragic sequelae. Such transmission may cause abortion, preterm birth, or perinatal death (20%). Subclinical congenital infection with resulting handicap is not uncommon. Congenital syphilis can be largely prevented by identification and treatment of the infected mother during pregnancy. Transmission to the fetus occurs particularly during the second trimester, although it may occur during the first trimester as well.

Most infected women are free of symptoms, and can only be identified by blood testing. A program of screening and treating those women found to be seropositive is cost-effective, even in places where syphilis in pregnancy is rare, because effective treatment is simple and readily available, while the consequences of untreated infection are so serious.

Treatment of mothers should consist of efficacious antibiotics, preferably a penicillin. Infants and women's sexual partners should be followed up, and treated if found to be infected.

The clinical diagnosis of congenital syphilis is difficult because the presentation is variable, and many babies are free of symptoms. Treatment of infants is recommended when the adequacy of treatment of the mother is unknown or if the mother received treatment for the first time during the pregnancy with a drug other than penicillin.

4 Gonorrhoea

In some parts of the world, routine screening for gonorrhoea during pregnancy is deemed worthwhile because of the severe effects of infection on both the mother and her baby. This can be accomplished by obtaining cervical swabs for culture at the first antenatal visit. In women considered to be at particular risk, either on demographic grounds or because of a history of sexually transmitted disease, repeat cultures can be taken. Culture remains the 'gold standard' for diagnosis of gonorrhoea. The Gram stain is not sensitive enough for specimens obtained from the female genital tract. Although the infection may be asymptomatic, pregnancy appears to increase the likelihood of both arthritis and systemic disease. Where the prevalence of penicillin-resistant gonorrhoea is high, certain third-generation cephalosporins are recommended for treatment.

The most common gonococcal infection in neonates is conjunctivitis. Gonococcal ophthalmia characteristically manifests itself early, 2–5 days after birth. If left untreated, this infection may lead to permanent corneal damage and even perforation of the eye. The ideal method of preventing neonatal ophthalmia is detection and early treatment of maternal disease.

There is no evidence that routine prophylactic medication is better than careful observation and prompt treatment of ophthalmia in the newborn in most populations. Prophylaxis is required when mandated by law (as is the case in some countries or states) or in populations with a high prevalence of gonorrhoea. When such prophylaxis is necessary, antibiotic regimens that are active against both gonorrhoea and chlamydia should be used. Cohort studies of tetracycline, erythromycin, and penicillin suggest that these agents are both less irritating and more effective prophylactic agents than silver nitrate, and they are also effective against chlamydia infection.

5 Chlamydia trachomatis

Maternal infection with *Chlamydia trachomatis* is important primarily because of the potential adverse effects of infection on the newborn infant. The condition is often asymptomatic in the mother, and may not be detected clinically, although some infected women may have a mucopurulent cervicitis, salpingitis, or a urethral syndrome.

The prevalence of *Chlamydia trachomatis* in pregnant women varies widely; estimates ranging from 2% to nearly 40% have been reported. In the United States, high rates are found in young women, unmarried women, and black women, as well as in women from lower socio-economic groups and those attending inner-city ante-natal clinics.

The newborn infant can acquire chlamydial infection through contact with infected maternal genital secretions at birth. Inclusion conjunctivitis will develop in 18–50% of infants born to infected mothers, making *Chlamydia trachomatis* the most common cause of neonatal conjunctivitis. The estimated risk that an infant born to an infected mother will develop chlamydial pneumonia ranges from 3 to 18%.

The diagnosis of maternal *Chlamydia trachomatis* infection is best made by using one of the new amplified nucleic acid tests. Tissue culture and antigen detection kits are less sensitive than the amplified methods and, where available, an amplification method should be used to test cervical specimens from pregnant women. There are no data using the newer diagnostic tests to estimate the cost-effectiveness of screening for chlamydia at different prevalence rates.

Randomized, controlled trials of antibiotic treatment suggest that amoxicillin is as effective as erythromycin in eradicating colonization by *Chlamydia trachomatis* during pregnancy; a single dose of azithromycin is an alternative. Tetracycline is contra-indicated in pregnancy because of its hepatotoxicity and its effect on the development of bone and teeth in the fetus.

The natural history of *Chlamydia trachomatis* infections in pregnancy is inadequately known and the role of the organism in the adverse outcomes of pregnancy remains to be resolved. Well-designed trials are still required to clarify the usefulness of screening for and treating this condition.

6 Bacterial vaginosis

Bacterial vaginosis is a vaginal infection typified by large numbers of organisms, such as *Gardnerella vaginalis*, *Mycoplasma hominis*, and various anaerobes, and by decreased numbers of the normal population of lactobacilli. Bacterial vaginosis is not thought to be sexually transmitted, but may be associated with sexual activity. It has been postulated as a cause of adverse pregnancy outcome, notably due to preterm birth. However, bacterial vaginosis may be present in up to 20% of pregnant women and, before screening and treatment are advocated, it is important to determine whether the infection is, in fact, pathogenic.

The suggestion that bacterial vaginosis might be a cause of pregnancy wastage is largely based on case-control studies in which a higher rate of colonization was found among women with adverse pregnancy outcomes than among those without abnormal outcomes. As is true of all such studies, other factors, both known and unknown, may have caused the adverse outcomes, irrespective of the presence or absence of bacterial vaginosis. For example, if such infections are simply markers for sexually transmitted disease in general, other organisms might be the actual causes.

Trials have shown that bacterial vaginosis may be treated effectively by antibiotics. However, this did not result in any improvement in pregnancy outcome, except in women with a past history of preterm birth, who were less likely to deliver preterm after treatment. It may, therefore, be worthwhile screening such women in subsequent pregnancies (see Chapter 13).

7 Herpes simplex

Herpes simplex infection of the newborn, acquired from the mother, is a rare but potentially serious condition, occurring in between 1 in 2500 and 1 in 10 000 births. Its clinical presentation varies widely, from asymptomatic, through involvement of only the skin, to involvement of the eye or nervous system, or widespread dissemination.

The risk of transmission from mother to baby at the time of birth is high in primary herpes infection, but the risk of infection from a mother with recurrent genital herpes is very low. Viral shedding is rare in the absence of a lesion. 'Prophylactic' cesarean section should not be offered to a woman with a history of herpes simplex infection who does not have clinically active herpes at the time of birth.

Clinical assessment remains the best criterion for identifying women who are shedding virus at the time of delivery. Asymptomatic shedding at delivery cannot be predicted on the basis of cultures during the pregnancy, and repeated cultures in asymptomatic women will not identify those women who are shedding asymptomatically at the time of delivery.

One controlled trial has studied the effects of acyclovir given to women with a history of recurrent genital herpes. In this study, pregnant women with recurrent genital herpes (mean of three symptomatic recurrences in previous 6 months) received acyclovir 200 mg four times daily, beginning one week before the expected date of delivery. This treatment resulted in significant reductions in maternal viral shedding at the time of delivery, symptomatic recurrences within 10 days of delivery, and use of cesarean section for herpes. There were no cases of neonatal herpes in either the treatment or the control group, and no maternal or neonatal side-effects were seen. Although these results indicate that acyclovir can be effective in reducing maternal viral shedding and symptomatic recurrences, further confirmation is required before a firm conclusion about the role of antenatal acyclovir in recurrent genital herpes can be drawn.

There have been no randomized trials to evaluate care policies for women with herpes in pregnancy, and the evidence on which these are based is weak indeed. Current recommendations are that cesarean section should be carried out if there is clinical evidence of active disease, viral shedding cannot be ruled out, and the membranes have not been ruptured for more than 4–6 h. The infant born to a woman with a history of genital herpes should be carefully monitored.

8 Bacteriuria

Significant numbers of bacteria are harbored in the urine (bacteriuria) of 3–8% of pregnant women, usually without exhibiting any symptoms, and 15–45% of untreated women with symptomless bacteriuria will develop symptomatic infections of bladder or kidney (acute cystitis or pyelonephritis). Acute cystitis and acute pyelonephritis are found in approximately 1% of pregnancies. Urinary tract infection is thus a common medical complication of pregnancy.

Culture and colony count of a single voided specimen is the best currently available form of screening for bacteriuria. Other more economical methods to screen for infection, such as the detection of urinary nitrites or microscopic analysis of a clean catch spun urine, have been suggested. These may have a role in identifying which urines should be cultured in the interests of cost-saving, but their sensitivity in pregnant women is not high enough to replace urine culture as an adequate screening test.

Recognition and treatment of asymptomatic bacteriuria in pregnancy will result in a substantially decreased risk of acute pyelonephritis and its short-term consequences to both mother and fetus. It appears to reduce the incidence of preterm birth or low birthweight as well. The mechanism through which treatment of bacteriuria leads to a reduction in preterm birth is not clear. Prevention of pyelonephritis may be a factor. Treatment of bacteriuria with antibiotics may also eradicate organisms colonizing the cervix and vagina. Antibiotic treatment of bacteriuria in pregnancy has not been shown to reduce the risk of subsequent infection in the long term, but the only trial with any follow-up is small.

The available evidence from controlled trials suggests that sulphonamides, including co-trimoxazole, nitrofurantoin, ampicillin, and the first-generation cephalosporins, are equally effective in the treatment of asymptomatic bacteriuria when the bacteria are known to be susceptible.

The traditional approach to therapy for asymptomatic bacteriuria in pregnancy was continuous antibiotic treatment for the duration of pregnancy. Single-dose therapy for uncomplicated urinary tract infection in women who are not pregnant is well-established, however, and trials suggest that this may be effective for pregnant women as well. It has obvious advantages in terms of compliance, minimization of adverse effects, and financial savings. No trials of other regimens have been reported.

Symptomatic lower-tract infection in pregnancy may also respond to single-dose treatment, but there are insufficient data for this treatment to be recommended. Regular follow-up urine cultures should be obtained. Failures, relapses, and recurrences must be treated appropriately, and when infection recurs, consideration must be given to continuous treatment for the remainder of pregnancy. Recurrent infection during pregnancy may signify an underlying abnormality of the urinary tract, and these women should be further investigated after pregnancy.

9 Pyelonephritis

Pyelonephritis is diagnosed clinically by the presence of fever, flank pain, and dysuria, together with a positive urine culture. Women should be hospitalized and started on adequate antibiotic therapy after blood and urine cultures have been taken. In the absence of frank septicemia, oral therapy and intravenous therapy are associated with a similar duration of maternal fever, and the same incidences of systemic complications of sepsis and of re-admission for urinary tract infection. An aminoglycoside (with or without ampicillin) or a cephalosporin is appropriate initial treatment, as infection is probably due to *Escherichia coli*. Therapy should be adjusted when the results of susceptibility testing are available. The use of the quinolone class of drugs should be avoided in pregnancy. Where there is concern about maternal renal function, monitoring of serum aminoglycoside levels may be warranted to minimize fetal exposure to the drug, as high levels may be associated with hearing loss in the child.

Following an episode of acute pyelonephritis, women are at risk of relapse and recurrence of infection, but the only reported randomized trial of suppressive therapy for the remainder of pregnancy failed to detect any advantage over close surveillance with cultures.

10 Rubella

Rubella (German measles) is typically a mild childhood illness. Maternal infection, occurring early in pregnancy, can lead to fetal death, low birthweight-for-gestational-age, deafness, cataracts, jaundice, purpura, hepatosplenomegaly, congenital heart disease, and mental retardation in the infant. The objective of rubella vaccination programs is to prevent fetal infection and its consequences: the congenital rubella syndrome.

The risk to the fetus of maternal infection decreases with increasing duration of pregnancy. In a prospective study, infants whose mothers had confirmed rubella at successive stages of pregnancy were followed for 2 years. No defects attributed to rubella were found in children infected after 16 weeks' gestation, while infants infected before the 11th week had significant cardiac disease and deafness.

Two approaches to rubella vaccination have been used: universal vaccination and selective vaccination. Universal vaccination of young children to interrupt transmission has led to a significant decline in reported cases of rubella and the congenital rubella syndrome. A vaccination rate of close to 100% will be needed if congenital infection is to be eliminated.

Following a rubella infection with viremia, lifelong protection against the disease usually develops. Re-infections can occur, but the majority of these are asymptomatic and detected only by a booster response in rubella-specific antibodies. Vaccination produces an overall lower antibody response than natural infection, but protection against infection can be expected in almost all vaccinated women.

The diagnosis of rubella in a pregnant woman who has been exposed to, or develops, a rubella-like infection, is often difficult. The laboratory must be provided with a detailed history, as routine screening tests are inadequate and additional testing to detect IgM antibody is required. False-negative results can occur if the specimen is drawn too soon after exposure. The pattern of antibody response to acute infection and re-infection will vary according to the test method used, and expert consultation may be required for interpretation of data.

Pregnant women should not be given rubella vaccine, but there should be little concern if a pregnant woman is vaccinated unknowingly or if she becomes pregnant within 3 months after immunization. As rubella vaccine virus has been isolated from fetal tissue following induced abortion, the risk cannot be assumed to be zero, but receipt of rubella vaccine in pregnancy is not ordinarily an indication for termination of pregnancy. Available data suggest that the risk of teratogenicity from live rubella vaccine is virtually non-existent.

The most significant cost factors associated with rubella are related to the long-term consequences of congenital rubella. The costs of the congenital rubella syndrome far outweigh that of routine vaccination of all infants of both sexes, as well as teenage girls and postpartum rubella seronegative women.

High immunization frequency must be achieved and maintained, and all susceptible women of childbearing age should be identified and vaccinated. Prenatal screening should be carried out on all pregnant women without documented immunity, and vaccination given following childbirth, miscarriage, or termination of pregnancy, when the probability of pregnancy occurring within the next 30 days is low. Almost all vaccinated women show seroconversion, and side-effects are mild. Where follow-up cannot be assured, rubella vaccination without prior serological testing may be preferable. One-third to one-half of current cases of the congenital rubella syndrome could be prevented if postpartum vaccination programs were fully implemented.

Termination should be offered when maternal infection is diagnosed in the first 16 weeks of pregnancy. Routine use of immunoglobulins for post-exposure prophylaxis against rubella is not recommended, although it may have a role where maternal rubella occurs and termination of pregnancy is not an option.

11 Toxoplasmosis

Maternal infection with the protozoan parasite *Toxoplasma gondii* acquired during pregnancy may result in congenital infection of the infant, sometimes with serious sequelae. Individuals can be infected only once, so a woman who is immune prior to pregnancy is not at risk of transmitting the organism to her infant.

Clinical manifestations of congenital toxoplasmosis, which consist of chorioretinitis, recurrent seizures, hydrocephalus, and intracranial calcifications, may be present at birth or appear later. The vast majority of infections are asymptomatic in the mother, although lymphadenopathy may occur. Although asymptomatic infection can be confirmed by detection of specific IgM antibody to *Toxoplasma gondii* in serum, this test should only be performed by a reference laboratory and requires careful interpretation. Seroconversion or a fourfold rise in specific IgG antibody suggests recent infection, but a single high IgG antibody level cannot be used to confirm recent toxoplasmosis infection.

Studies on congenital toxoplasmosis have relied on serological results to identify maternal infection. Both the prevalence of seropositivity (indicative of past exposure and immunity) and the risk of acquisition during pregnancy vary among countries and even among different regions within the same country. This has been ascribed, at least in part, to different habits with respect to the handling and consumption of raw meat and the disposal of cat litter, both of which can be reservoirs of the organism. Routine screening for the condition is conducted in some countries (e.g. France and Austria) but not in many others, such as the United Kingdom, the Netherlands, New Zealand, and Australia.

The risk of transmission of toxoplasmosis from mother to baby is dependent on the stage of pregnancy at which maternal infection occurs. In one major study, the frequency of infection rose from 17%, in infants whose mothers were infected during the first trimester, to 65%, in infants whose mothers acquired the infection in the third trimester. Although the incidence of transmission from mother to fetus, based on serology, was highest in third-trimester infections, transmission in the first trimester was associated with more severe symptoms in the newborn. Severe disease occurred in 14% of first-trimester transmissions and in none of third-trimester transmissions. Some of the early infections may result in spontaneous abortions. The high frequency of neonatal clinical disease after infections early in gestation has led French investigators to recommend termination of pregnancy where feasible, and an antiprotozoan drug, spiramycin, when termination is not possible. There is no trial evidence that screening, or treatment by spiramycin alone or other combinations of drugs, does more good than harm.

When the incidence of new toxoplasmosis infection is low, the low pick-up would not justify the expense of a universal screening program. A health education program, advising pregnant woman against eating raw or undercooked meat, to wash their hands after its preparation, and to wear gloves when gardening or cleaning cat litter, might be more cost-effective. Although there is some evidence that knowledge of toxoplasmosis is increased following an educational session, there is no evidence that this knowledge is associated with changes in behavior and a reduced incidence of congenital toxoplasmosis.

Much work is still necessary to determine the true frequency of infection and the sequelae of congenital toxoplasmosis. Neither spiramycin nor pyrimethamine-sulpha are very efficacious against this parasite, and the latter agent is associated with a high frequency of side-effects in pregnant women. Trials of new antiprotozoan drugs, with potentially better efficacy and safety, are needed. Such studies will require prolonged follow-up, as some of the sequelae of fetal infections may only occur some time after birth.

12 Group B streptococcus

Group B streptococcus has become the most frequent cause of overwhelming sepsis in neonates. The early, and most serious, form of infection is characterized by rapid onset of respiratory distress, sepsis, and shock. The likelihood of disease, (approximately 2 per 1000 live births) is directly related to the density of maternal colonization and the immaturity of the infant. Infants with birthweights of less than 2500 g have a much higher overall infection rate than infants weighing 2500 g or more. Prelabor rupture of the membranes and maternal fever are also associated with a higher incidence of infection.

Attempts to prevent disease by giving antibiotics, to either all babies or those considered to be at high risk, have proved disappointing. Although the available data suggest that infant sepsis with group B streptococcus can be reduced with antibiotic prophylaxis given to the baby, such prophylaxis may be accompanied by an increase in sepsis with penicillin-resistant organisms, which may result in a higher rate of deaths from infection in the babies given antibiotic prophylaxis.

Since attempts at prophylaxis after the baby has been born may be too late, attention has focused on studies of the effectiveness of antepartum and intrapartum antibiotics. The available data show that a course of antibiotics given during pregnancy results in only a temporary eradication of group B streptococcal carriage, with no detectable effects on infant colonization or sepsis with group B streptococcus. Treatment during pregnancy, unless continued into labor, has only a transient effect on the vaginal flora, and will not influence the rate of sepsis in the newborn.

There is no doubt that the use of intrapartum antibiotics reduces the transmission of group B streptococcus. The studies reviewed show a beneficial effect of treatment for women who are receiving comprehensive obstetrical care and are known to be colonized with group B streptococcus; but these results are not generalizable to all pregnant women. The optimal method of detecting colonization with group B streptococcus, whether by routine prenatal cultures or a rapid test at the onset of labor in high-risk patients, has not been determined. There is clear evidence that treatment should be given to high-risk colonized women, but insufficient evidence to recommend routine screening of all women for group B streptococcus during pregnancy.

It seems reasonable that a pregnant woman in preterm labor, or a woman with either intrapartum fever or prolonged rupture of membranes, should receive intrapartum antibiotics if either a rapid diagnostic test is positive or not available, although there is no evidence from controlled trials to support these recommendations. An alternative option would be a screening culture for all women at or before 35 weeks, with treatment of women with a positive culture during labor if there are other risk factors, such as preterm labor, prelabor rupture of membranes, or fever. In high-prevalence populations, it may be preferable to dispense with a preliminary screen, and treat all women with the additional risk factors during labor.

As intrapartum prophylaxis of colonized pregnant women offers the possibility of reducing the incidence of infant sepsis, rapid methods for screening women in labor are desirable. A number of such methods of rapid diagnosis of colonization have been developed and evaluated, but thus far none are adequately sensitive.

13 Conclusions

Prenatal zidovudine treatment can help to reduce transmission of HIV infection from mother to baby. Treatment with more potent antiretroviral combinations, with or without planned delivery by cesarean section, may also have benefits but these are as yet unproven.

Congenital syphilis can be largely prevented by identification and treatment of the infected mother during pregnancy. Routine screening is justified by the simplicity of the test and the effectiveness of treatment with penicillin. The value of screening for other sexually transmitted diseases will depend on the prevalence in the community, and the effectiveness of the available treatments.

There is at present no evidence to warrant routine screening for bacterial vaginosis in pregnancy, but it may be helpful in women with a past history of preterm birth.

Screening pregnant women to detect asymptomatic bacteriuria and treating the condition with antibiotics is worthwhile. The practice will reduce the incidence of pyelonephritis and probably also the incidence of preterm labor and low-birthweight infants. The cost-effectiveness of this screening will depend on the prevalence of asymptomatic bacteriuria in the population.

Pyelonephritis in pregnancy requires intensive treatment with appropriate antibiotics, usually intravenously, but oral therapy may be appropriate for selected non-bacteremic women with acute pyelonephritis in pregnancy.

A high community level of rubella immunization should be obtained, and all rubella-susceptible women of childbearing age should be identified and vaccinated. Rubella vaccination in the early postpartum period is safe and effective. This opportunity for immunization should not be missed.

The optimal method of detecting colonization with group B streptococcus is by routine prenatal cultures. Antibiotics should be given to high-risk colonized women during labor.

Sources

Effective care in pregnancy and childbirth
Wang, E. and Smaill, F., Infection in pregnancy.

Cochrane Library
Brocklehurst, P., Interventions for treating gonorrhoea in pregnancy.
Interventions for reducing mother-to-child transmission of HIV infection.
Brocklehurst, P. and Rooney, G., Interventions for treating genital chlamydia trachomatis infection in pregnancy.

Brocklehurst, P., Hannah, M. and McDonald, H., Interventions for treating bacterial vaginosis in pregnancy.

Peyron, F., Wallon, M., Liou, C. and Garner, P., Treatments for toxoplasmosis during pregnancy.

Smaill, F., Antibiotics for asymptomatic bacteriuria in pregnancy.

Intrapartum antibiotics for group B streptococcal colonization.

Villar, J., Lydon-Rochelle, M.T. and Gulmezoglu, A.M., Duration of treatment for asymptomatic bacteriuria during pregnancy.

Walker, G., Antibiotics for syphilis diagnosed during pregnancy [protocol].

Diabetes in pregnancy

1 Introduction

Perinatal mortality in pregnancy associated with diabetes has dropped tenfold in the last four decades, compared with a fourfold to fivefold drop in perinatal mortality overall. Nowadays, some specialist centers report perinatal mortality rates close to those of non-diabetic populations but, in general, the risk of perinatal loss for the average diabetic woman remains higher than for non-diabetics, even after adjustment for fetal malformation. Population surveys suggest that the outcome of pregnancy overall is poorer than what would be inferred from the literature.

A number of factors have played a part in this remarkable improvement. These include, among others: increasing acceptance by physicians of the importance of tight control of diabetes; the introduction of programs to achieve this control; the development of home glucose-monitoring to facilitate such programs; gradual trends towards prolongation of pregnancy; and advances in neonatal care.

Although there is general consensus on the adverse impact of overt diabetes in pregnancy, the significance and appropriate management of lesser degrees of hyperglycemia are still widely debated. Diabetes is a disturbance of multiple metabolic pathways rather than of glucose metabolism alone, although the effects on carbohydrate metabolism are the most apparent. Generally accepted criteria for a diagnosis of diabetes in the presence of symptoms (polyuria, polydipsia, ketoacidosis) are random venous plasma glucose levels greater than 11 mmol/l (200 mg/dl) or fasting levels of greater than 8 mmol/l (140 mg/dl).

Normal values for plasma glucose values are defined as less than 8 mmol/l on a random sample, and less than 6 mmol/l fasting. Values between the normal and those of diabetes are considered to be 'equivocal', and evaluation with a glucose challenge is recommended (e.g. 75 g taken orally after an overnight fast). Values over 11 mmol/l 2 h post-challenge are taken to be diagnostic of diabetes, and those between 8 and 11 mmol/l are termed 'impaired glucose tolerance'.

2 Prepregnancy counseling and assessment

Increasingly, women with diabetes wish to discuss the implications of pregnancy before they conceive, and this should be actively encouraged by all health-care professionals before each pregnancy. While preconception clinics may fulfil an important role, the provision of adequate preconceptional care and advice does not necessarily depend on such specialized clinics. All who care for diabetic women should be aware of, and prepared to discuss, the importance of appropriate contraception and timing of pregnancy, the significance of pregnancy to the diabetic woman, the risks to the fetus and neonate as well as to herself, the importance of tight control of the diabetes just before and during pregnancy, and the need for accurate estimation of the date of conception.

Since diabetes is a chronic and progressive disease, the advice may need to include a discussion of the fact that postponement of pregnancy until a later age may worsen the prognosis.

The risks to the fetus are significant. Diabetes is associated with an increased incidence of congenital anomalies, up to three times as great as for the infants of non-diabetic mothers. Although no information is available from randomized trials, cohort studies suggest that tight control of the diabetes immediately before conception can reduce this risk significantly.

Macrosomia is still more common in the infants of diabetic mothers than in those of non-diabetic mothers, even with the best diabetic control currently available. Diabetes is not typically associated with intra-uterine growth restriction, unless the diabetes is complicated by microvascular disease. Women with vascular complications of diabetes will need particularly careful counseling.

Nephropathy without significant hypertension and a normal serum creatinine is not associated with a poor fetal outcome. The prognosis worsens in the presence of hypertension or impaired renal function. Renal disease that does not cause symptoms in non-pregnant individuals can jeopardize pregnancy outcome in some women. Although the majority of women with renal disease do not experience a deterioration of renal function during pregnancy, some women do suffer significant deterioration that does not improve after delivery.

There is also concern about the effect of pregnancy on women with proliferative retinopathy. Pregnancy appears to be associated with a deterioration in the condition. Cohort studies comparing pregnant and non-pregnant women with diabetic retinopathy show, however, that visual acuity can be maintained with intensive laser treatment throughout pregnancy, and the prognosis is no worse than for the non-pregnant woman.

The risk of spontaneous preterm birth is not increased. The apparent excess of preterm births relates either to delivery for complications, especially hypertensive disorders, or to policies advocating elective preterm delivery. Preterm births can be minimized by a reconsideration of such policies.

Diabetic women contemplating pregnancy will be reassured to learn that there is no good evidence of any long-term adverse effects of their diabetes on the development or intelligence of their offspring, and that the risk of their children developing juvenile diabetes is in the order of 2% or less.

Young diabetic women should have easy access to family planning services at all points of contact with the health-care system, both before and between pregnancies.

3 General care during pregnancy

Diabetic pregnant women should be cared for by both obstetricians and physicians with special interest in this field. Ideally this might be carried out at joint clinical sessions but other local arrangements can deliver quality integrated care. Such arrangements facilitate efficient deployment of other health-care professionals, such as dieticians and specialist liaison midwives or nurses.

The first few weeks of pregnancy are a period of readjustment, and many women require re-education about their diabetes and its control. Rotation of insulin injection sites, the interaction of diet and exercise, and the dietary requirements of pregnancy may be unfamiliar to many women. Specialist care in and for pregnancy should start as early as possible. Local organization should be such as to allow very rapid referral of diabetic women with suspected pregnancies. When the gestational age is in doubt, it should be estimated precisely by early ultrasound.

Hypoglycemia can be troublesome at this stage, and control of the diabetes may be difficult to achieve because of poor motivation, nausea and vomiting, or changes in the hormonal milieu. Considerable education is needed to resist over-treatment of impending hypoglycemic reactions. Glucose or sugar should be avoided; milk or a light snack, which can be repeated if necessary, are more appropriate. All diabetic women should be provided with glucagon for emergency situations.

In addition to routine prenatal assessment, obstetric care at this time should include assessment of renal function in diabetic women who have hypertension or proteinuria, and retinoscopy, particularly in women who have had diabetes for more than 10 years. This should be repeated once every trimester. Urine cultures should be repeated regularly in those with nephropathy. In view of the increased risk of malformation, detailed ultrasound is recommended. Additional expert fetal echocardiography is advisable given the high frequency of cardiac anomalies.

A diabetic woman without nephropathy or retinopathy, and with no other complications of pregnancy, usually experiences an uncomplicated second trimester. The educational and readjustment processes will hopefully be complete as far as possible and, unless there is a risk of compromised fetal growth or early pre-eclampsia, there is little need for intensive obstetric supervision at this time.

Women with associated hypertension may need to be followed closely and, if necessary, treated with hypotensive drugs. Serial assessment of renal function can be particularly useful in following these pregnancies.

4 Diabetic control

In the non-pregnant diabetic, intensive control using continuous subcutaneous insulin, or regimens with three or more injections daily, improves glycemic control. Randomized trials have demonstrated that such regimens significantly reduce the risk of progression to nephropathy and the long-term risk of retinopathy. In the short term, retinopathy may worsen and there is a trend towards more frequent severe hypoglycemic episodes. The incidence of diabetic ketoacidosis does not seem to be significantly higher using intermittent rather than continuous subcutaneous insulin regimens. These findings may be relevant to pregnancy where intensive regimens are commonly used. The aim of diabetic control is to establish normoglycemia, both fasting and before and after meals. Blood glucose levels can be monitored effectively and controlled by the woman at home, provided that she has readily available advice and support, predominantly through telephone contact. The use of home, instead of hospital, glucose monitoring can significantly reduce the time the woman spends in hospital, without affecting pregnancy outcomes.

The dose and type of insulin needed may require careful and frequent adjustment. Insulin may have to be given more frequently than before pregnancy, often requiring three and, occasionally, four injections a day. Pumps for continuous subcutaneous infusion of insulin are expensive and complex to use. Trials have shown no benefits for continuous infusion over conventional insulin administration in terms of metabolic control, use of cesarean section, or adverse pregnancy outcome. Temporary worsening of retinopathy may occur using such regimens. Despite the importance of the subject, to date the benefits and drawbacks of tight control of diabetes in pregnancy have been assessed in only one randomized trial. This trial compared the effects of very tight control (aiming to keep blood sugar levels below 5.6 mmol/l), tight control (blood sugar levels between 5.6 and 6.7 mmol/l) and moderate control (blood sugar levels between 6.7 and 8.9 mmol/l).

Best results were obtained with tight, rather than either very tight or moderate control. Very tight control was associated with episodes of hypoglycemia, and conferred no benefits in other pregnancy outcomes compared to tight control. On the other hand, a policy of only moderate control, in which blood sugar levels were allowed to rise up to 8.9 mmol/l, is associated with a higher incidence of macrosomia, urinary tract infection, and cesarean section, and a trend towards an increase in hypertension, preterm labor, respiratory distress syndrome, and perinatal mortality.

This evidence tends to confirm the conclusion from observational studies that keeping blood sugars within a well-controlled range, between 5.6 and 6.7 mmol/l, is better than either too strict or too lenient a regimen.

5 Obstetric care

As in any antenatal care program, much attention is focused on the early detection of gestational hypertension and in the identification of problems with fetal growth.

The incidence of pregnancy-induced hypertension is increased in pregnancies of diabetic women and it may occur earlier. Particularly at risk are those with pre-existing hypertension, those with nephropathy, and those with microvascular disease. There are currently no good predictors of pregnancy-induced hypertension and preventive therapy is untested in this population.

Problems with fetal growth divide into two groups – growth failure and macrosomia. Women with hypertension, nephropathy, or microvascular disease are at more risk of the complications of fetal growth failure. Women with moderate or poor diabetic control are at most risk of fetal macrosomia. Pregnancies in diabetic women should have additional ultrasound surveillance of growth in the late second and third trimester. Absolute size is not a good predictor of outcome and attention should be paid to growth velocity. As in the non-diabetic population, the precise value of screening for growth problems is not established.

Macrosomia can be assessed by ultrasound, but most formulae utilized to calculate fetal weight perform poorly in the larger fetus, and such estimates should be interpreted with caution.

Because of the increased perinatal mortality, most pregnancies are subjected to serial antepartum fetal assessment. Various regimens have been described, but to date there are no randomized trials addressing which is the most effective technique. Most studies are of a prospective interventional design and claims of improved outcome for any particular regimen of antepartum fetal surveillance must be interpreted within these limits.

6 Care in labor and delivery

Elective preterm delivery has long been one of the classical management strategies applied in diabetic pregnancy, based on an observation in one influential study that the stillbirth rate rose above the neonatal death rate after 36 weeks of gestation. Other cohort studies have shown, however, that this conclusion was flawed and that pre-emptive delivery does not result in an improvement in perinatal mortality. There is no valid reason to terminate an otherwise uncomplicated pregnancy in a diabetic woman before the expected date of delivery.

Assessment of pulmonary maturity has, until recently, been considered a prerequisite for planned delivery of the diabetic woman. There is increasing evidence to suggest that in well-controlled diabetics, the lecithin/sphingomyelin ratio reflects the same degree of pulmonary surfactant production and, therefore, the same risk of hyaline membrane disease, as in non-diabetics. The infants of poorly controlled diabetic mothers may have a disturbance in the development of pulmonary maturity. The problem becomes less important as delivery is delayed to a later gestational age, and as elective cesarean section is used less frequently.

Although cesarean section in diabetic women, as in all women, should only be performed for obstetrical indications, cesarean section rates tend to be much higher for diabetic women than for the general population. There seems to be little justification for this, except that the median birthweight for gestation is higher in diabetic pregnancies.

As blood glucose levels can be controlled confidently throughout labor with a glucose infusion with insulin added, the only increased hazard of vaginal delivery in diabetic women is that of birth trauma to the infant, particularly shoulder dystocia and brachial plexus injury secondary to macrosomia. In comparative studies, these risks appear unexpectedly higher in infants of diabetic mothers compared with similarly sized infants of non-diabetic mothers. The management of the second stage of labor in a diabetic pregnancy with suspected macrosomia should reflect this knowledge and appropriately skilled senior staff should be readily available.

7 Care after birth

After birth and delivery of the placenta, insulin requirements should be recalibrated according to blood glucose levels. All women will require significantly less insulin than during pregnancy.

Breastfeeding should be encouraged, although there must be an awareness of the increased caloric intake sometimes needed to support this.

Family planning is an important consideration. There is no contra-indication to the use of low-dose oral contraceptives, particularly in young, non-obese, non-hypertensive, non-smoking diabetics. The development of headaches or hypertension is an indication to change to alternative methods.

Intra-uterine contraceptive devices have, until recently, been a reasonable alternative, but concern over their effectiveness is making it less acceptable; barrier methods provide an acceptable second choice.

For all women, the risk of future pregnancy must be carefully weighed against the risk of the proposed method of contraception. Women with nephropathy or retinopathy should be counseled carefully about limiting family size.

Sterilization, if requested, is better not carried out at the time of cesarean section if this can be avoided, in view of the increased risk of still undiagnosed cardiac malformation in the newborn. The procedure can easily be performed by laparoscopy within the next few months.

8 Conclusions

Diabetic women embarking on pregnancy demonstrate a deep commitment to achieving a normal outcome. This involves much disruption of an already complex lifestyle. Their care must reflect this and should be individualized, so that disruption will be minimized and care tailored to meet the circumstances of each woman.

There is considerable evidence to suggest that pregnancy in diabetic women should be managed with fewer obstetric interventions than are currently practised. Specialized care and collaboration among various disciplines will achieve the best results, but good perinatal outcome is not confined to tertiary-care centers. Many diabetic women can be treated as normal pregnant women, with the one major addition of careful control of blood glucose levels. Tight, rather than either very tight or moderate control is required.

Allowing pregnancy to continue at least until the expected date of delivery, associated with a decreased need to assess pulmonary maturity and more judicious use of cesarean section, may allow pregnant women with diabetes to feel more like their non-diabetic counterparts.

Much has been achieved in improving the care for, and the outcome of, pregnancies in diabetic women without resort to randomized clinical trials. The lack of controlled studies, however, has resulted in a blurring of the contributions made by the various components of care, and in doubts about the utility of some. The need continues for well-designed trials to assess the value both of current treatments and of suggestions for their improvement. In addition, better survey data on the diabetic population are still needed, as data that refer only to women who attend specialist centers can be seriously misleading. Population based survey data may highlight deficiencies in the system of care and lead to improvements.

Sources

Effective care in pregnancy and childbirth

Hunter, D.S., Diabetes in pregnancy.

Cochrane Library

Boulvain, M., Stan, C. and Irion, O., Elective cesarean section or induction of labor at term for delivering women with diabetes [protocol].

Irion, O. and Boulvain, M., Induction of labour for suspected fetal macrosomia.

Walkinshaw, S.A., Dietary regulation for 'gestational diabetes'.

Very tight versus tight control for diabetes in pregnancy.

Pre-Cochrane reviews

Walkinshaw, S.A., Continuous subcutaneous infusion vs conventional insulin treatment in diabetic pregnancy. Review no. 04064.

Home vs intermittent clinic glucose monitoring of diabetes. Review no. 06647.

Home vs hospital inpatient glucose monitoring of diabetes. Review no. 06651.

CHAPTER 21

Bleeding in the latter half of pregnancy

1 Introduction

Bleeding in the second half of pregnancy is no longer a common cause of maternal death in the industrialized world, but it continues to be a major cause of perinatal mortality, and of both maternal and infant morbidity. Approximately half the women who present with bleeding in the second half of pregnancy are eventually found to have either placental abruption or placenta praevia. Often no firm diagnosis can be made for the other half.

2 Placental abruption

Placental abruption, or retroplacental hemorrhage, is a major contributor to perinatal mortality among normally formed fetuses. Although maternal mortality is fortunately rare now, maternal morbidity in the forms of hemorrhage, shock, disseminated intravascular coagulation, and renal failure is sufficiently frequent to justify intensive treatment.

The frequency with which placental abruption is diagnosed will vary with the criteria used for the diagnosis. The perinatal mortality rate with confirmed abruption is high, often over 300 per 1000. More than half the perinatal losses are due to fetal death before the mother arrives in hospital. Neonatal deaths are principally related to the complications of preterm delivery. Among surviving infants, rates of respiratory distress, patent ductus arteriosus, low Apgar scores, and anemia are more common than in unselected hospital series.

2.1 Clinical presentation

Abruption may occur at any stage of pregnancy. The diagnosis should be considered in any pregnant woman with abdominal pain, with or without bleeding. Mild cases may not be clinically obvious.

In severe abruption there may be heavy vaginal bleeding or evidence of increasing abdominal girth, if the blood is retained within the uterus. Uterine hypertonus is a common physical sign in the more severe grades of abruption, particularly when the fetus has died. In these cases the woman is usually in severe pain and may be shocked as a result of hypovolemia. Absence of clotting may be obvious in vaginal blood. Other signs of clotting defects may be bleeding from the gums or venepuncture sites, or hematuria.

The amount of blood loss may not be obvious – some may have been lost before admission, and large volumes of blood may be retained in the uterus. Clinical signs of hypovolemia may be masked by increased peripheral resistance. Cerebral and cardiac perfusion may be preserved, although renal blood flow is jeopardized. This will become manifest by diminished urine production.

Ultrasound examination of the uterus and contents has an important role in the differential diagnosis of antepartum hemorrhage. Most important is its ability to localize the placenta. A low-lying placenta brings placenta praevia into the differential diagnosis, while a posterior placenta might make the diagnosis of abruption more likely in a woman with back pain. The diagnosis of retroplacental hematoma by ultrasound is not always straightforward.

2.2 Treatment

In suspected mild abruption, the symptoms may resolve. If there has been bleeding, this may cease, with the fetal condition apparently satisfactory. It may be impossible to confirm the diagnosis. In this case, the woman may safely be allowed home after a period of observation, as is the case for bleeding of unknown origin.

In moderate and severe abruption, maternal resuscitation and analgesia are priorities. Restoration of the circulating volume and emptying the uterus are the cornerstones of treatment. The use of whole blood has become traditional in volume replacement in these women. It is likely, however, that a crystalloid infusion to precede the blood would be beneficial. It is probably best to use fresh frozen plasma, at the rate of 1 unit for every 4–6 units of red cells transfused, to replenish clotting factors. No systematic attempts have been made to study alternatives to blood transfusion in this condition. Plasma substitutes, such as plasma protein, dextran, gelatin, and starch, may produce adverse reactions, and dextran, in particular, can interfere with platelet function *in vivo* and cross-matching *in vitro*.

A clotting defect should be sought, although defects of clinical significance are rare when there is a live fetus. The process of disseminated intravascular coagulation usually starts to resolve after delivery.

When the fetus is alive, a decision should be made about the optimal time and mode of delivery to improve the chances of survival, based on the estimated fetal maturity. In former years, the usual policy was vaginal delivery at all reasonable costs, because the newborn's prognosis was so poor. More recently, policy has shifted to earlier resort to cesarean section in order to rescue the baby, and improved survival of the preterm newborn has often resulted. A recent series suggests, however, that an attempt to deliver vaginally, inducing or augmenting labor with oxytocin when necessary and using continuous electronic fetal heart rate monitoring, may result in a 50% reduction in the cesarean section rate without significant difference in the risk of perinatal mortality.

In severe abruption when the fetus is dead, vaginal delivery should be planned, except where there is an obvious obstetrical indication for cesarean section, such as transverse lie. Labor should be induced or augmented if needed, using oxytocin, or prostaglandins if there is no satisfactory response to oxytocin. Cesarean section is required in the rare cases in which uterine contractions can not be stimulated or when clinical shock associated with hemorrhage has been uncontrollable. Coagulation defects are common in this situation, and the maternal risks are considerable.

When cesarean section in a woman with disseminated intravascular coagulation is judged to be inevitable, it should be undertaken after close consultation with the anesthetist and a hematologist. Volume replacement and transfusions of whole blood, frozen plasma, and specific coagulation factors, should be given before and during the surgical procedure.

A well-equipped hospital should be able to provide adequate emergency treatment for the mother, and will often be able to achieve safe delivery of a fetus that is alive on admission. Survival of such live born infants depends to a large extent on the quality of neonatal care.

3 Placenta praevia

Placenta praevia is defined as a placenta that is situated wholly or partially over the lower pole of the uterus. The overall prevalence of the condition is slightly over 0.5%. The major cause of both mortality and morbidity is hemorrhage. Prevention and effective treatment of hemorrhage has reduced the gravity of the condition. With modern care, a perinatal mortality rate of 50–60 per 1000 is now attainable.

3.1 Clinical presentation

Although it is well recognized that a small proportion of women with placenta praevia do not bleed until the onset of labor, less than 2% of cases of placenta praevia present in this way. Painless vaginal bleeding in the absence of labor is the most common presentation. Some form of fetal malpresentation (transverse, oblique or unstable lie, and breech presentation) is found in approximately one-third of cases. In cephalic presentation, the presenting part is invariably high, and is often displaced slightly from the midline.

All placentae praeviae are asymptomatic before the first onset of bleeding. With routine ultrasound scanning in the early second trimester, approximately 5–6% of placentae are found to be low lying. Over 90% of asymptomatic placentae praeviae diagnosed by ultrasound in the early second trimester remain asymptomatic and become normally situated later as a result of anatomical changes in the lower-uterine segment in late pregnancy.

Women with low or cervical placental implantation found early in gestation should be rescanned between 30 and 32 weeks' gestation. Where an asymptomatic woman is found on ultrasound after 32 weeks still to have a placenta that appears to cross the cervix, she should be considered as having placenta praevia for purposes of subsequent care. Where there is a lesser degree of low placentation, the possibility remains that placenta praevia will not be present at the time of labor.

3.2 Treatment

A digital examination should never be performed when there is any possibility of placenta praevia, except in the operating room when termination of pregnancy is forced by bleeding or labor, or when the pregnancy has reached an adequate gestation for imminent childbirth to be safe. The really dangerous hemorrhage is often the one that has been provoked by ill-advised interference, such as digital examination of the cervical canal at, or very shortly after, the time of the warning hemorrhage. Rectal examination is even more dangerous than vaginal examination.

If bleeding is less severe or has stopped, confirmation of the diagnosis by ultrasound should be performed at the earliest opportunity. The early and accurate diagnosis of placenta praevia is imperative to spare women with a normally implanted placenta the economic, emotional, and social expense of long-term hospitalization.

The object of expectant care is to reduce the number of preterm births by allowing the pregnancy to continue until the baby has grown to a size and age that will give it a reasonable chance of survival. This form of care usually requires that the woman must remain in a fully equipped and staffed maternity hospital from the time of diagnosis until delivery, because of the risks to both mother and fetus from further major hemorrhage. Some clinicians have adopted a policy of permitting selected women to return home as part of expectant care, particularly when it can be assured that they will not be alone, and will have no difficulty in getting to hospital promptly if bleeding recurs. Many women sent home require re-admission to hospital for significant maternal bleeding, but no maternal deaths and no significant differences in perinatal outcome compared with those kept in hospital have been reported.

The two randomized trials that have compared policies of outpatient versus inpatient care for known placenta praevia, have not been large enough to permit definitive conclusions about safety.

Preterm birth continues to be a major problem, even when expectant management is used. Maternal and fetal well-being should be monitored. The mother should not be allowed to become anemic, and her hemoglobin should be maintained at a normal level by hematinics or, if necessary, by transfusion.

With every episode of bleeding, the Rh-negative woman should have a Kleihauer test performed for the presence of fetal blood cells, and be given prophylactic anti-D immunoglobulin.

The optimal timing for delivery remains controversial. Although expectant management until 37 weeks is most generally accepted, some clinicians have recommended elective preterm delivery after 34 weeks when amniocentesis has confirmed pulmonary maturity. No controlled trials to evaluate either approach have been reported.

3.3 Delivery

There is almost no indication for vaginal delivery for women with even marginal placenta praevia, whose babies have attained a viable age. The hazards of vaginal delivery include profuse maternal hemorrhage, malpresentation, cord accidents, placental separation, fetal hemorrhage, and dystocia, resulting from a posterior placental implantation. If the fetus is previable, malformed, or dead, vaginal delivery may occasionally be appropriate.

With improved ultrasound diagnosis, many authorities suggest elective cesarean section without prior digital confirmation. This approach has considerable merit, since digital examination may cause serious hemorrhage. Digital examination in the operating theatre does have a place, where ultrasound is not available, when the ultrasound appearances are equivocal, or the clinical signs of placenta praevia are not confirmed by ultrasound. If digital examination is indicated, it should be carried out only in the operating room, with the staff scrubbed and prepared for immediate cesarean section should catastrophic hemorrhage be provoked.

4 Bleeding of uncertain origin

Hemorrhage of undetermined or uncertain origin is the most common type of antepartum hemorrhage. Although in some cases the cause of bleeding later becomes clear, in the majority no cause can be demonstrated. The importance of this subgroup lies in its frequency, in the clinical problems it presents in diagnosis and management, and in the associated high fetal loss.

Hemorrhage of uncertain origin is a collective clinical category, and must include minor but unrecognized cases of all specific types of antepartum hemorrhage – localized abruption, marginal hemorrhage, cervical and vaginal lesions, and excessive show.

The clinical presentation of bleeding of unknown origin is painless antepartum hemorrhage, without evidence of placenta praevia. In the majority of cases the blood loss is not great enough to cause serious concern, and usually it settles spontaneously. The most serious threat to the fetus is preterm labor and birth, but this is relatively infrequent. The management of painless antepartum hemorrhage depends primarily on the gestational age of the fetus at the time of the initial bleed. An ultrasound examination for placental localization should be performed as soon as possible, and if placenta praevia is diagnosed or cannot be excluded, then care should follow the plan already discussed for placenta praevia. When the placenta is clearly defined in the upper segment, the woman should be allowed home after a period of rest and observation in hospital, provided that she has no recurrence of bleeding. The risk to the fetus in such cases is preterm birth and the great majority of perinatal deaths are due to preterm birth occurring within 7–10 days of the initial hemorrhage. After the bleeding has settled, and before discharge from hospital, both a speculum examination to exclude a local cause for the bleeding and a digital examination to exclude advanced cervical dilatation should be performed.

If a policy of expectant care is adopted, fetal well-being should be monitored. Although frequently recommended, routine induction of labor at 38 weeks should not be performed, and women should be allowed to go into spontaneous labor.

5 Conclusions

Bleeding in the second-half of pregnancy constitutes a possibly life-threatening condition. All professionals who care for women during pregnancy and childbirth must be aware of the causes and prognosis of such bleeding, and have a clear plan in mind for its differential diagnosis and management.

Sources

Effective care in pregnancy and childbirth

Fraser, R. and Watson. R., Bleeding during the latter half of pregnancy.

Cochrane Library

Neilson, J.P., Interventions for suspected placenta praevia during pregnancy.

CHAPTER 22

Suspected fetopelvic disproportion and abnormal lie

1 Fetopelvic disproportion

Fetopelvic disproportion exists when the capacity of the woman's pelvis is insufficient for the safe vaginal delivery of the baby. In the past, antenatal strategies to diagnose fetopelvic disproportion received considerable attention, with the objective of early induction of labor or delivery by planned cesarean section if disproportion was diagnosed. Attempts to predict the occurrence of fetopelvic disproportion have included measurement of maternal height and shoe size, and clinical and X-ray pelvimetry.

The correlations between maternal height or shoe size and cephalopelvic disproportion are of limited clinical use, because of the large overlap in obstetrical outcome between small and large women. There is a reasonable correlation between clinical and radiological assessment of pelvic dimensions, but neither are particularly accurate in predicting the outcome of labor. The effects of clinical pelvimetry have not been evaluated by randomized studies.

The meaning of non-engagement of the fetal head near term as an indicator of cephalopelvic disproportion is not well established. In black women having their first babies, in whom such non-engagement commonly occurs, it is associated with longer labors, but not with an increased rate of operative delivery or increased maternal or fetal morbidity. The most reliable predictor of pelvic adequacy remains the previous uncomplicated delivery of a baby of similar or greater birthweight than that estimated for the current pregnancy.

The formerly widespread use of X-ray pelvimetry to predict cephalopelvic disproportion has come under critical scrutiny since the reports of an association between prenatal irradiation and childhood leukaemia. As a general principle, irradiation that is not likely to benefit mother or baby should be avoided. The use of ultrasound for pelvimetry has been reported, but it has not been widely adopted. Computed tomographic pelvimetry, which greatly reduces the radiation exposure to the fetus, has been found in two small studies to be easier to perform, and in the measurement of a model pelvis, probably more accurate than conventional X-ray pelvimetry.

There is wide variation among individuals and institutions in the use of X-ray pelvimetry. Its utility has been questioned because of its poor predictive value as a screening test for cephalopelvic disproportion, and the infrequency with which the results influence management. Prospective randomized studies of X-ray pelvimetry, without and with previous cesarean section (two trials each), failed to detect any clear benefit of X-ray pelvimetry to either mother or baby. Their combined results show a substantial increase in the rate of cesarean section with the use of X-ray pelvimetry. The numbers studied were too small to evaluate perinatal outcome adequately.

Neither X-ray nor clinical pelvimetry have been shown to predict cephalopelvic disproportion with sufficient accuracy to justify elective cesarean section with cephalic presentations. Cephalopelvic disproportion is best diagnosed by a carefully monitored trial of labor, and X-ray pelvimetry should seldom, if ever, be necessary. Observational studies of labor induction for suspected macrosomia to reduce the likelihood of cesarean section and of difficult operative delivery cast doubts on the effectiveness of such a policy.

It is important to distinguish between the risk of disproportion related to the presenting fetal part and that related to a non-leading part of the fetus, because of the special hazards of obstructed labor to the partly born fetus, as in shoulder dystocia, or obstruction to the after-coming head in a breech presentation.

2 Shoulder dystocia

Shoulder dystocia (where the baby's head is delivered, but the shoulders remain stuck) is an obstetric emergency associated with considerable risk of fetal trauma and death. If a high likelihood of the condition could be predicted antenatally, it could be prevented by elective cesarean section. Cesarean section has been suggested for diabetic women with a fetal weight estimated to be above 4000 g and for non-diabetic women with an estimated fetal weight above 4500 g and slow progress of labor. Such a policy has not been subjected to randomized evaluation. Even if fetal weight estimation were accurate, this would prevent only a small proportion of potential cases of shoulder dystocia, while the majority of the cesarean sections would be unnecessary. Almost half of the cases of shoulder dystocia occur in infants weighing less than 4000 g.

Induction of labor in women thought to have large-for-gestational-age babies has not been shown to improve outcome, nor has detection of macrosomia by measurement of the distance from the symphysis to the fundus.

There is at present no reliable method for antenatal prediction of shoulder dystocia, and efforts to reduce the problem should be directed towards ensuring that birth attendants are skilled in the management of this condition when it occurs. The woman should be placed in the recumbent position with exaggerated flexion of her thighs and her knees pushed against her chest. A large episiotomy should be done. Attempts to then deliver the baby with maternal effort and downward traction, with or without suprapubic pressure or digital rotation of the shoulders, are often successful. Rarely, deliberate fracture of the baby's clavicles may be necessary.

Other methods of management of shoulder dystocia have been reported, including use of the squatting position. Symphysiotomy has been long practised in Africa. A maneuver in which the head is pushed back followed by cesarean section has been described.

3 Breech presentation

Breech presentation (where the baby's bottom, foot or feet present instead of the head), although sometimes associated with uterine, placental, or fetal abnormalities, is often simply an error of orientation that places a healthy mother and a healthy baby at risk. The prevalence of breech presentation decreases from about 15% at 29–32 weeks' gestation to between 3 and 4% at term. Spontaneous changes from breech to cephalic presentation occur with decreasing frequency as gestational age advances in the third trimester, and are more likely to occur at all gestational ages in women who have previously given birth. The risk of a breech presentation to the mother is an increased likelihood of cesarean section, and to the baby, the risk of cord prolapse and difficult vaginal or cesarean breech delivery. The perinatal outcome following breech birth is less favorable than for cephalic presentations, irrespective of the mode of delivery; childhood handicap is common following both vaginal and cesarean breech delivery. It is possible that breech presentation may be a marker for underlying impairment – a failure of the baby to achieve its first developmental milestone. The widespread use of cesarean section for term breech presentation has been based on the unproved assumption that the poorer outcome is at least in part the result of damage sustained during vaginal breech delivery.

Elective section for breech presentation makes a considerable contribution to cesarean section rates in many areas. It is important to determine whether cesarean section for term breech improves perinatal outcome sufficiently to justify the current and future risks to the mother. This is still unclear. The two small randomized trials that have been performed suggest that a policy of elective cesarean section for term breech presentation is associated with some decrease in short-term neonatal morbidity and an increase in maternal morbidity. The numbers studied are far too small to address the important issues of perinatal mortality or morbidity, nor has the question of long-term neonatal morbidity been addressed. The use of cesarean section for breech delivery in the belief that it is safer may become a self-fulfilling prophecy, as attendants become less skilled at breech delivery. A large international trial of planned vaginal delivery versus elective cesarean section for term breech is currently under way.

Cephalopelvic disproportion, if present, is perilous in a breech presentation because of the risk that the after-coming head may be trapped. There is no reason to expect that X-ray pelvimetry should be more accurately predictive of cephalopelvic disproportion for breech than it is for cephalic presentations. In breech presentations, however, it is usual to avoid vaginal delivery when pelvic dimensions are even slightly reduced, in an attempt to exclude all potential cases of cephalopelvic disproportion. If vaginal birth of an infant presenting as a breech is planned, fetopelvic relationships should be carefully monitored as labor progresses. If the frank or complete breech passes easily through the pelvis, the head can be expected to follow without difficulty. For women admitted in advanced labor, tocolysis may be used to allow time for careful assessment before proceeding to vaginal or cesarean delivery. The rare condition of deflexion of the head with a breech presentation may add additional risk to vaginal delivery. Ultrasound examination in early labor can diagnose or exclude the condition.

During vaginal breech delivery, expulsion by maternal effort is encouraged as traction on the breech may cause extension of arms and head. One quasi-random trial of routine expedited breech delivery (aimed at completion of delivery with a single uterine contraction), was methodologically inadequate to support firm conclusions. The fact that traction is usually used for cesarean breech delivery may account for cases of trauma due to delivery of the after-coming head.

4 External cephalic version for breech presentation

Over the years, many postural techniques have been used by midwives, doctors, and traditional birth attendants to turn the baby so that the head presents (cephalic version). Little, however, has appeared in the medical literature on this subject. A midwifery technique claimed to be effective is to ask the mother to lie on her back, with her hips slightly elevated, and hips and knees flexed. She then rolls gently through 180 degrees from side to side for 10 min, and repeats this three times a day. Another example of traditional practice is to attempt to correct abnormal presentations during labor by manually shaking the uterus, while the mother is in the knee–elbow position on the floor.

Uncontrolled studies have suggested that use of the knee–chest position is associated with a high rate of spontaneous version and normal vaginal birth. The woman is instructed to kneel with her hips flexed slightly more than 90 degrees, but with her thighs not pressing against the abdomen, while her head, shoulders, and upper chest lie flat on the mattress. This is done for 15 min every 2 waking hours for 5 days. The small reduction in non-cephalic births found in controlled studies, and the marginally lower overall cesarean section rate and rate of low Apgar score at 1 min, could all be the result of chance. They are consistent with anything between a large positive and a large negative effect. Larger studies are needed to establish whether or not postural management is effective.

There are fundamental differences between external cephalic version (where the attendant attempts to turn the baby by rotating its body through the mother's abdominal wall) attempted before term and at term, and these two approaches must be considered separately. While external cephalic version before term can be readily accomplished, it serves little purpose. A high proportion of fetuses revert to breech presentation. Three controlled trials (one randomized and two quasi-randomized) failed to demonstrate any effect of external cephalic version before term on the incidence of breech birth, cesarean section, or perinatal outcome. Although there was no overall difference in perinatal mortality rate for treatment and control groups, the close to 1% fetal mortality rate, thought to be associated with the procedure, led to a decline in its use.

Interest in external cephalic version for breech presentation was revived by a 1975 report that cephalic version could be achieved after 37 weeks' gestation, provided that the uterus was relaxed with betamimetic agents, when necessary. In contrast to external cephalic version before term, version at term shows better results. The procedure, with or without tocolysis, results in a 58% reduction in the relative risk of a non-cephalic presentation at birth, and a 48% reduction in the risk of cesarean section. Delay of external cephalic version attempts until term allows time for a maximal number of spontaneous versions to take place, and for obstetrical complications that may require delivery by cesarean section to become apparent. Thus, by waiting until term, fewer unnecessary attempts at external cephalic version are required. At term complications of the version can be readily managed by prompt abdominal delivery of the mature infant. Following successful external cephalic version, fewer reversions to breech presentation occur. The disadvantage of delaying external cephalic version until term is that the opportunity to attempt external cephalic version may be missed when the breech descends in the pelvis, when the membranes rupture, or when labor commences before term.

Routine use of tocolysis for external cephalic version at term reduces the rate of failed and difficult procedures and fetal heart rate slowing. These advantages must be weighed against the risk of maternal cardiovascular side-effects. Tocolysis should be used at least in women with high uterine tone or failed initial attempt, if not routinely.

Fetal vibro-acoustic stimulation, to stimulate movement of the fetus from the dorso-anterior to the dorso-lateral position, has been used in one small trial to facilitate external cephalic version, as have epidural analgesia and transabdominal amnio-infusion. Theoretically, oral hydration might achieve similar amniotic fluid expansion. None of these procedures has been investigated sufficiently to be recommended for general use.

Several authors have investigated which factors are associated with an increased chance of successful external cephalic version. Successful version at term rates are low in some populations, particularly in North America and Europe, and amongst nulliparous women. For this reason, there may be a role for external version to be commenced before term for selected breech pregnancies. This procedure should not be undertaken except as part of a randomized controlled trial.

External cephalic version at term in women with previous cesarean section has not been studied in controlled trials, but observational data are encouraging.

External cephalic version in early labor is worthy of consideration as an extension of the trend towards version later in pregnancy. Earlier reports have included occasional references to attempted external cephalic versions during labor, and success rates up to almost 75% have been reported. In theory, this approach has several advantages. Maximum time would be allowed for spontaneous version to take place and for possible contra-indications to external cephalic version to appear, thus limiting the number of versions that would be necessary. The risks of external cephalic version may be reduced further by performing the procedure in the labor ward, with continuous monitoring of the fetal condition until delivery. In cases assessed as unsuitable for vaginal breech birth, the external cephalic version may be attempted in the operating theatre, and in the event of failure followed immediately by cesarean section.

Because waiting for the onset of labor would involve the inconvenience of performing version as an emergency rather than as an elective procedure, and because the breech may be well engaged in some cases, it is unlikely that external cephalic version during labor will become a first-line approach for breech presentation. When breech presentation is encountered during labor while the membranes are still intact, however, the limited data available suggest that external cephalic version with tocolysis is a reasonable procedure to consider.

The randomized trials reported have not been of sufficient size to address issues of maternal or fetal safety. The risk of attempted external cephalic version to the mother is exceedingly small. It consists of the possibility of adverse effects from any of the drugs used to facilitate version and the hazards of placental abruption, a rare but recognized complication.

Attempted external cephalic version must be recognized as an invasive procedure that involves some risk to the fetus. Fetal risks are related to gestational age and to the methods employed. Findings from observational data suggest that the complication rate is greater when external cephalic version is attempted before 37 weeks' gestation, when general anesthesia is employed, and when the placenta is situated anteriorly. Provided that fetal well-being is confirmed and monitored, and provided that appropriate precautions are observed (including administration of anti-D immunoglobulin to Rh-negative women), the risk to the mature fetus appears to be small.

Moxibustion (burning herbs to stimulate acupuncture points), a traditional Chinese method to promote version of fetuses in a breech presentation, has recently been evaluated in a randomized controlled trial. Despite the fact that more subjects in the control group received subsequent external cephalic version, significantly more fetuses in the intervention group had a cephalic presentation at birth.

5 Oblique and transverse lie

Oblique and transverse lies differ fundamentally from breech presentation in that factors maintaining a longitudinal lie are not present. They are associated with multiparity, abdominal laxity, uterine and fetal anomalies, shortening of the longitudinal axis of the uterus by fundal or low-lying placenta, and conditions that prevent the engagement of the presenting part, such as pelvic tumours and a small pelvic inlet. Abnormal lie, particularly oblique lie, may be transitory and related to maternal position.

When non-longitudinal lie is encountered after 32 weeks' gestation, underlying abnormalities should be sought. Further care options include antenatal attempts at external version, version at term followed by induction of labor, or expectant care with or without intrapartum attempts at version, if the abnormal lie persists.

The role of external version in the management of oblique and transverse lie has not been assessed in a randomized trial. A number of descriptive case series have been reported. With expectant care, most cases of abnormal lie will revert to the longitudinal lie by the time of delivery. Less than 20% of transverse lies observed after 37 weeks' gestation persist to delivery. Given the high spontaneous version rate and the unstable nature of the non-longitudinal lie, with a high probability of reversion following external version, there is no firm case for external version prior to labor or planned delivery. Care of the woman with a transverse or oblique lie encountered during labor is more straightforward, as the choice lies between cesarean section and external version. A prospective but uncontrolled study of external version for transverse lie in labor showed a modest rate of success. There were no fetal or maternal complications associated with the procedure, though larger studies would be needed to evaluate potential risks.

In the absence of controlled trials, the timing of intervention in pregnancies complicated by non-longitudinal lie must remain a matter of clinical judgement. The advantage of gaining fetal maturity, allowing time for spontaneous version to take place and allowing labor to begin spontaneously, must be weighed against the risk of membrane rupture or cord prolapse before the version can be attempted. Once labor has begun or the decision has been made to deliver the baby, attempted version with immediate recourse to cesarean section if necessary, is a reasonable option.

6 Conclusions

No reliable methods are available for accurate prediction of fetopelvic disproportion before labor. Labor is the best test of pelvic adequacy in cephalic presentations. The place of pelvimetry in breech presentations has not been established, and a trial to determine its benefits, if any, is warranted if this common practice is to be continued.

There is at present inadequate evidence either to substantiate or refute the effectiveness of routine cesarean section for term breech presentation in improving perinatal outcome.

The controlled trials reported to date are too small to support or refute the alleged benefits of postural management for breech presentation. External cephalic version for breech presentation before term is not warranted. External cephalic version at term, on the other hand, substantially reduces the incidence of breech presentation at birth and of cesarean section.

Sources

Effective care in pregnancy and childbirth

Hofmeyr, G.J., Suspected fetopelvic disproportion.

Hofmeyr, G.J., Breech presentation and abnormal lie in late pregnancy.

Cochrane Library

Hofmeyr, G.J., Maternal hydration for increasing amniotic fluid volume in oligohydramnios and normal amniotic fluid volume.

Hofmeyr, G.J. and Hannah, M.E., Planned caesarean section for term breech delivery.

Hofmeyr, G.J. and Kulier, R., Cephalic version by postural management for breech presentation.

Expedited versus conservative approaches for vaginal delivery in breech presentation.

External cephalic version for breech presentation before term.

External cephalic version for breech presentation at term.

External cephalic version facilitation for breech presentation at term.

Hands/knees posture in late pregnancy or labor for fetal malposition (lateral or posterior).

Irion, O. and Boulvain, M., Induction of labor for suspected fetal macrosomia.

Neilson, J.P., Symphysis-fundal height measurement in pregnancy.

Pattinson, R.C., Pelvimetry for fetal cephalic presentations at term.

Walkinshaw, S A., Very tight versus tight control for diabetes in pregnancy.

Other sources

Cardini, F. and Weixin, H. (1998). Moxibustion for correction of breech presentation: a randomized controlled trial. *JAMA*, **280**, 1580–4.

Cheng, M. and Hannah, M.E. (1993). Breech delivery at term: a critical review of the literature. *Obstet. Gynecol.*, **82**, 605–18.

Danielian, P.J., Wang, J. and Hall, M.H. (1996). Long term outcome by method of delivery of fetuses in breech presentation at term: population based follow up. *BMJ*, **312**, 1451–3.

Gifford, D.S., Morton, S.C. and Kahn, K. (1995). A meta-analysis of infant outcomes after breech delivery. *Obstet. Gynecol.*, **85**, 1047–54.

CHAPTER 23

Prelabor rupture of the membranes

1 Introduction

Prelabor rupture of the membranes is defined as spontaneous rupture of the membranes before the onset of regular uterine contractions. It is often referred to as 'premature rupture of the membranes', but that name may be misleading, because the word 'premature' has also been associated with low birthweight and preterm birth. The expression 'prelabor rupture' is more appropriate and precise.

When prelabor rupture of the membranes occurs before 37 weeks gestation, we refer to it as 'preterm prelabor rupture of the membranes'; at or after 37 weeks, it is referred to as 'term prelabor rupture of the membranes'. The distinction, while arbitrary, is important both for prognosis and for care.

2 Diagnosis

2.1 Ruptured membranes

It is important to be certain whether or not the membranes are ruptured. Sometimes the diagnosis is obvious from the sudden gush of clear amniotic fluid from the vagina and its continued leaking thereafter. Sometimes it can be difficult to differentiate rupture of the membranes from other leaks of body fluid, such as vaginal discharge or urine. If the rupture has occurred recently, it may be possible to confirm the diagnosis by collecting some fluid, either by asking the woman to sit on a suitable receptacle or obtaining a sample from a pool of amniotic fluid in the posterior fornix on speculum examination.

The nitrazine test is probably the most widely used test for differentiating amniotic fluid from other body fluids, but it has a false-positive rate of about 15%. For this reason an additional test, usually microscopic observation of ferning, is worthwhile. The fern test is less likely to produce false-positive results, although it has a higher rate of false-negatives.

If the suspected rupture has occurred some hours previously and most of the fluid has escaped from the vagina, it may be not be possible to establish or confirm the diagnosis with any degree of confidence. In these circumstances, much depends on taking a careful history from the woman. Information can be obtained as to when and how the gush of fluid occurred; whether anything like it has ever happened before; approximately how much fluid was lost; what the colour was like; whether it smelled of anything; and whether there was anything else remarkable. The latter question may elicit a comment on the presence of white or greasy particles. The ultrasound finding of oligohydramnios is strong confirmatory evidence of prelabor rupture of membranes, when there is a history of sudden release of fluid.

It is not clear whether or not high (hindwater) rupture of the membranes should be considered as clinically distinct from low rupture. There is little information about how these two types of rupture can be differentiated, or whether or not they warrant different forms of care. In the absence of such data, the only practical approach is to consider them as equivalent.

2.2 Vaginal examination

It is likely that vaginal examinations can introduce or increase the risk of intra-uterine infection, although no controlled comparisons have been conducted to substantiate or refute this belief. A vaginal examination should only be performed to obtain information that would be useful in determining further care, and that cannot be obtained in a less invasive way. There is probably little benefit to be derived from performing both digital and speculum examinations. The information that can be obtained by speculum examination is likely to be superior to that obtained by digital examination. It may include visualization of amniotic fluid 'pooling' in the posterior fornix, and collection of some of that fluid for nitrazine test, and microscopic examination for ferning to confirm that the membranes are ruptured. There may be sufficient fluid for phosphatidylglycerol determination as a measure of fetal lung maturity. Material may be collected for culture or screening for pathogens, including group B streptococci. On the other hand, speculum examination is likely to be more unpleasant for the mother than digital examination. No controlled comparisons have been conducted to establish the benefit, if any, of either digital or speculum examination.

2.3 Assessing the risk of infection

Any woman with prelabor rupture of the membranes, at any period of gestation, should be assessed for signs of intra-uterine infection. These include fever and maternal or fetal tachycardia. If any one of these is accompanied by a tender uterus and foul-smelling liquid, there will be no doubt about the diagnosis. Uterine tenderness and fetid discharge are, however, late signs of intra-uterine infection.

The earliest clinical signs of intra-amniotic infection are fetal tachycardia and a slight elevation of maternal temperature, but both these signs are rather nonspecific. The estimation of C-reactive protein in the maternal circulation, which is used in some settings, may be a reasonably reliable early sign of intra-uterine infection, but the value of this test has never been assessed in a controlled comparison.

Although intra-uterine infection may on occasion precede rupture of the membranes, the main risk is infection ascending from the vagina into the uterine cavity. Information on the presence of pathogens in the vagina may, therefore, be useful, particularly about those organisms that are responsible for the majority of fetal infections, such as the group B streptococci, *Escherichia coli*, and *Bacteroides*. Intrapartum antibiotic treatment of mothers carrying group B streptococci in the vagina reduces the incidence of neonatal sepsis and neonatal death from infection due to group B streptococci. In populations with a high prevalence of group B streptococci carriers, either screening for the organism or routine intrapartum antibiotic treatment after prolonged rupture of membranes should be adopted as standard care. In other populations, an initial culture should be part of the care provided after preterm prelabor rupture of the membranes.

Amniocentesis has been advocated to assess the risk of infection particularly in the preterm period. Problems with amniocentesis include the invasiveness and risks associated with the procedure, failure to obtain amniotic fluid in a proportion of cases, and, most importantly, the poor correlation between the results of diagnostic tests applied to the fluid and the development of fetal infection. Bacteria are not found in all women with clinical signs of intra-amniotic infection, nor are they always absent in women without signs of infection. Some observational studies have suggested that white cells in the amniotic fluid are more predictive of infectious morbidity than bacteria, but this has not been confirmed by others.

There has been only one controlled trial to assess the value of amniocentesis for detection of intra-uterine infection by Gram stain and culture after preterm prelabor rupture of the membranes. The use of amniocentesis did not reduce the proportion of women delivered because of clinical amnionitis or the number of perinatal deaths. It did result in a reduced frequency of abnormal fetal heart patterns in labor and a reduction in the average number of days that the infants remained in hospital after the mother had been discharged. On the whole, there is inadequate evidence to judge whether the use of amniocentesis in women with prelabor rupture of the membranes preterm confers more benefit than harm to mother and baby.

A number of observational studies suggest that fetal breathing movements and gross body movements cease when intra-amniotic infection develops. These changes in fetal behavior require further assessment, but may prove to be as reliable for the detection of intra-uterine infection as the more invasive technique of amniocentesis.

2.4 Assessing the risk of fetal immaturity

Assessing the risk of fetal immaturity largely depends on a careful determination of gestational age, including ascertainment of any ultrasound assessments made in early pregnancy. There will usually be little difficulty in identifying fetuses who are either profoundly immature or who are clearly close to term. In between these two categories, and most typically between 26 and 34 weeks of gestation, weighing the risk of relative immaturity is considerably more difficult.

Pulmonary maturity, as determined by analysis of amniotic fluid, is associated with a decreased risk of mortality and morbidity from respiratory disorders, but does not necessarily imply that other hazards associated with preterm birth, most notably periventricular hemorrhage, will be avoided.

3 Preterm prelabor rupture of the membranes

3.1 Risks

The most serious, and most common, consequence of preterm prelabor rupture of the membranes is preterm birth. The risk associated with this is directly related to the gestational age and maturity of the fetus. At the extreme lower end of the gestational age range, improvement in perinatal outcome will depend entirely on continuing the pregnancy. At the other end of the preterm gestational age range, care policies should differ little, if at all, from those that apply after rupture of the membranes at term. Prelabor rupture of the membranes at gestational ages between these two extremes (roughly between 24 and 34 weeks) presents the difficult dilemma of balancing the risks of immaturity against those of infection.

Infectious morbidity, mostly due to ascending intra-uterine infection, is the second most important hazard for the baby. This risk is greater at lower gestational ages, possibly because of the relative immaturity of antibacterial defense mechanisms, and the underdeveloped bacteriostatic properties of amniotic fluid at early gestational age.

In addition to these two main risks, other hazards of preterm prelabor rupture of the membranes include: prolapse of the umbilical cord; cord compression due to the loss of the protective amniotic fluid; pulmonary hypoplasia and various deformities associated with persistent oligohydramnios; placental abruption; and the mechanical difficulties (if cesarean section becomes necessary) of delivering a baby from a uterus that contains little, if any amniotic fluid and has a poorly developed lower segment.

Prolapse of the umbilical cord may occur either at the time of membrane rupture or later with the onset of labor. Any change in an apparently stable situation, such as a recurring loss of amniotic fluid or the onset of uterine contractions, should alert the caregiver to this possibility. Frequent assessments of the fetal heart rate, either by auscultation or cardiotocography and a careful ultrasound examination may be useful in these circumstances.

Compression of the umbilical cord may occur due to the loss of the protective effect of amniotic fluid. The risk of local increase in pressure escalates with the onset of uterine contractions, and the incidence of severe fetal heart rate decelerations is directly related to the degree of oligohydramnios.

Prolonged rupture of the membranes with oligohydramnios for several weeks may lead to a spectrum of fetal postural and compression abnormalities. Adequate amounts of amniotic fluid are necessary for normal lung development. Early onset and prolonged rupture of the membranes may lead to pulmonary lung hypoplasia and when severe, to neonatal death. It is not clear whether the presence of fetal breathing movements or ultrasonographic chest measurements are useful to indicate that lung growth is preserved; the reported observational studies have yielded conflicting results.

Placental abruption should be considered whenever blood loss or abdominal pain occur in a woman with preterm ruptured membranes.

3.2 Care before the onset of labor

Preterm birth is *the* main consequence of preterm prelabor rupture of the membranes. Where adequate facilities for intensive perinatal and neonatal care are lacking, the most effective form of care is referral of the woman to a perinatal center, where such facilities are readily available.

Most women will go into labor within hours or a few days after rupture of the membranes in the preterm period. In some women, however, labor will be delayed much longer. Among these women will be some in whom the diagnosis of ruptured membranes may have been made in error; in others a high leak may have sealed over, so that amniotic fluid returns to normal. This, however, is the exception rather than the rule. Renewed accumulation of amniotic fluid may imply that the woman can return home with a reasonable degree of safety, although this has never been assessed in a controlled comparison.

Provided that mother and fetus are well at the initial assessments, the main concerns in the first few days after rupture of the membranes relate to detecting the onset of infection or uterine contractions. Care should center on detecting these by regular assessments of maternal temperature and pulse, fetal heart rate, and uterine contractility. It is not clear whether serial leukocyte counts or C-reactive protein levels provide additional accuracy to this surveillance. Variation in leukocyte counts and C-reactive protein levels can be quite large, particularly when the influences of labor or corticosteroid administration are added.

Other elements of surveillance are guided by the need to detect other complications that may occur after preterm prelabor rupture of the membranes.

3.2.1 Prophylactic antibiotics

Treatment with prophylactic antibiotics reduces the risk of preterm birth occurring within one week, of infections in the mother before delivery, and of infection in the baby. No effect has been shown on the overall incidence of preterm birth (less than 37 weeks), on maternal postpartum infectious morbidity, or on the risk of neonatal pneumonia.

One would expect that the reduction in neonatal infection, coupled with the improved fetal maturity achieved by prolonging the time until birth, would increase neonatal survival. Although controlled trials so far have failed to demonstrate this, the cumulative evidence would be in favor of antibiotic treatment. It is not clear which antibiotics would provide the best results, nor what duration of treatment is necessary. Treatment probably should be guided by bacterial culture, and continued until delivery.

3.2.2 Prophylactic tocolytics

Two small studies on the use of oral ritodrine have addressed the question of whether the administration of tocolytic drugs might improve outcome in women not in labor after preterm prelabor rupture of the membranes. There was no difference in the proportion of women who delivered within 10 days. The number of women involved was too small to assess the influence, if any, on neonatal infection, respiratory distress syndrome, or perinatal mortality.

These data, and data from placebo-controlled trials on the prophylactic use of betamimetic drugs in women without ruptured membranes, offer no support for suggestions that prophylactic tocolysis before the onset of uterine contractions is worthwhile.

3.2.3 Corticosteroid administration

The theoretical concerns that corticosteroids might be both superfluous and hazardous in women with prelabor rupture of the membranes have not been confirmed by the results of controlled trials. These concerns were based on the observation that rupture of the membranes *per se* may enhance fetal pulmonary maturity, and thus make the use of other agents to promote maturity unnecessary. In addition, there were fears that the immunosuppressive effects of corticosteroids might both increase susceptibility to intra-uterine infection and mask early signs of infection in women with prelabor rupture of the membranes.

These concerns are not supported by the evidence. A systematic review of the randomized trials of corticosteroid administration to women with preterm prelabor rupture of the membranes clearly shows that the incidence of respiratory distress syndrome is further reduced by corticosteroid administration, irrespective of any effects that prelabor rupture of the membranes itself may have on fetal pulmonary maturity. Overall, the frequency of maternal infection is not increased after corticosteroids, although maternal infection may be increased in women whose membranes have been ruptured for longer than 24 h.

The risk of neonatal infection was not statistically significantly increased in the corticosteroid-treated group, compared with the control group. Nevertheless, neonatal infection following maternal corticosteroid treatment remains a possible risk. The concomitant use of antibiotics may be appropriate (see Chapter 25).

3.2.4 Induction of labor

Controlled comparisons between an 'active' policy of elective delivery after preterm prelabor rupture of the membranes and a control policy without elective induction show no protective effect of the active policy against any adverse outcome. Indeed, there is a tendency for outcomes to be less favorable in the 'active' policy group. These adverse outcomes include maternal sepsis and several forms of infant morbidity (neonatal infection, respiratory distress syndrome, intracranial hemorrhage, and perinatal death from causes other than congenital malformations).

Even when corticosteroids, to improve pulmonary maturity, are used along with induction of labor, the active policy confers no benefit on the infant. In this case, the beneficial effects of prenatal corticosteroids in preterm prelabor rupture of the membranes appear to be offset by shortening the duration of pregnancy with elective delivery.

3.3 Care after the onset of labor

The onset of uterine contractions may be the result of intra-uterine infection. Whether or not the fetus is mature, preterm labor starting after the membranes have been ruptured for some time should probably be allowed to proceed to preterm birth, because of the risk of infection. When the fetus is so immature as to have no chance of extra-uterine survival, attempts to prolong pregnancy should depend not only on what little might be gained in terms of infant outcome, but even more on the maternal risks and the opinions of the parents. Decisions about the method of delivery and whether cesarean section will be necessary, should differ little from those for other preterm births (see Chapter 37).

3.3.1 Antibiotics

Whether or not antibiotics should be administered at once in these circumstances has not been addressed adequately by controlled studies. Both clinical common sense and data from studies that have compared intrapartum with immediate postpartum antibiotic treatment for intra-amniotic infection tend to support the use of antibiotic treatment as soon as a diagnosis of intra-uterine infection is suspected.

3.3.2 Tocolysis

The small controlled trials that have compared tocolysis with no tocolysis in preterm labor following prelabor rupture of the membranes show no differences in any of the outcomes examined. These include delay of birth, recurrence of preterm labor, preterm birth, birthweight, mortality, and respiratory morbidity.

There is no evidence that tocolytic agents *per se* improve perinatal outcome and they are not innocuous. They should be used only when the benefits of prolonging the pregnancy by a few days clearly outweigh the risks. Examples of this would be when the inhibition of labor permits implementation of other measures that are effective in improving outcome for the preterm infant, such as administration of maternal corticosteroids or transfer of the mother to a perinatal centre with adequate facilities for care around preterm birth and the preterm infant.

3.3.3 Amnio-infusion

Decelerations of the fetal heart rate during preterm labor occur more frequently if the membranes have ruptured before the onset of labor. Many of the abnormal fetal heart-rate patterns are suggestive of umbilical cord compression, and may well be due to the loss of the protective effect of amniotic fluid. The relative merits and hazards of using amnio-infusion during labor in women with preterm prelabor rupture of the membranes have not yet been thoroughly assessed. Available data, thus far, suggest a significant reduction in the number of severe fetal heart rate decelerations per hour during the first stage of labor, and increased umbilical artery pH, with amnio-infusion. The merits and hazards of this approach warrant further evaluation.

4 Term prelabor rupture of the membranes

Prelabor rupture of the membranes occurs in 6–19% of all term births. Most women with term prelabor rupture of membranes will go into labor soon after the membranes rupture. Almost 70% of these women will give birth within 24 h and almost 90% will do so within 48 h. A remarkably constant 2–5% will be undelivered after 72 h, and almost the same proportion will remain undelivered after 7 days. It is possible that these women may have a deficiency in prostaglandin production or in their prostanoid biosynthesis pathway, and that this is responsible, not only for their failure to go into spontaneous labor, but also for the frequently observed poor progress in cervical dilatation when labor is induced with oxytocin.

Infection, both maternal and neonatal, has been the main concern. This concern relates back to reports in the 1950s, when prelabor rupture of the membranes at term was associated with a high risk of maternal and perinatal mortality. Not surprisingly, immediate induction of labor was advocated to reduce this risk.

The prognosis of prelabor rupture of the membranes at term has changed considerably in the later decades of this century. Data collected over long periods, some of which include women who gave birth more than 25 years ago, are of questionable relevance to current obstetric practice. The maternal deaths noted in former years mostly occurred in women with prolonged, severe intra-uterine infection, who often had inadequate antibiotic therapy judged by today's standards. Maternal mortality is almost never found in more recently conducted studies of prelabor rupture of the membranes at term, and perinatal death from infection has also become a rarity. With the changed prognosis for women and their infants, and concern about the perceived increased risk of operative delivery after induction of labor, a more expectant approach has recently become popular.

The key question about the care of women with ruptured membranes, at or near term, is whether it is better to induce labor promptly after the membranes rupture or to delay induction in the expectation that labor will start spontaneously. The next question, in the event that prompt induction is chosen, is the method of induction: oxytocin or prostaglandins. Women need to be informed about the effects of the care options available to them, and encouraged to choose the treatment option they would prefer.

4.1 Induction of labor with oxytocin

Induction of labor with oxytocin, at or near term (when the main dangers of pulmonary immaturity have been overcome), decreases the risk of maternal infection (chorioamnionitis and endometritis) and shows a trend towards lowering the risk of neonatal infection compared to expectant care. Most of the controlled trials that have assessed neonatal infection, however, were of poor methodological quality, and the beneficial effect of induction of labor with oxytocin on neonatal infection may have been overstated. Induction of labor with oxytocin decreases the rate of admission to neonatal intensive care.

Induction with oxytocin carries a slightly, but not statistically significant, increased risk of operative delivery or cesarean section. It is associated with more frequent use of epidural analgesia and of internal fetal heart-rate monitoring.

4.2 Induction of labor with prostaglandins

The effects of induction of labor with prostaglandins, with or without concomitant oxytocin, for term prelabor rupture of the membranes, are similar to those for induction with oxytocin alone. Compared with expectant care, prostaglandin induction results in a lower risk of maternal infection and a trend towards less infection in the newborn, along with a decreased use of admission to the neonatal intensive care unit. There are no significant differences in the rates of operative vaginal delivery or cesarean section. The use of analgesia/anesthesia and of maternal side-effects (diarrhea) is more frequent in women induced with prostaglandins than in women managed expectantly.

4.3 Comparison of prostaglandins and oxytocin

Direct comparisons between oxytocin alone and prostaglandins (with or without oxytocin) for induction of labor for term prelabor rupture of membranes show little difference between the two methods with respect to the rates of operative delivery or cesarean section. Fewer epidurals are used in association with prostaglandins but no effect is seen on the overall use of analgesia/anesthesia.

The use of prostaglandins results in more frequent maternal infections, possibly related to an increased number of vaginal examinations. It also appears to increase the risk of neonatal infection, particularly if women are known to be colonized with group B streptococcus (although, as the assessment of neonatal infection was made blind to treatment allocation and duration of membrane rupture in only one of the 18 controlled trials, the harmful effect on this outcome may be less than that suggested by the data). Overall admissions to neonatal intensive care are more frequent with prostaglandin induction.

The evidence thus suggests that if early induction of labor after term prelabor rupture of the membranes is chosen, induction with oxytocin rather than with prostaglandins would offer the greatest benefit with the least harm.

4.4 Prophylactic antibiotics

That appropriate therapeutic antibiotics are required when there are signs of infection with prelabor rupture of membranes goes without saying. The place of antibiotics in the care of women with no evidence of infection is much less clear. The two controlled trials of prophylactic antibiotics conducted in the 1960s, utilized antibiotic treatments that are no longer in use. Although they failed to show any effect on the incidence of fetal and neonatal infection, a statistically significant reduction in the incidence of postpartum infectious maternal morbidity was observed after antibiotic prophylaxis. In some centers, this has led to the adoption of policies involving routine administration of antibiotics *after* delivery to women with prolonged rupture of the membranes at term. Although the utility of this approach has not been addressed in randomized comparisons, it would be worth assessing which women, without overt signs of infection, might benefit from postpartum administration of antibiotics.

One small randomized trial has addressed the question of whether prophylactic antibiotics should be given to the baby after birth in women with prolonged prelabor rupture of membranes. There was some support for the idea that prophylactic antibiotics reduced the risk of infection, but the trial requires replication on a larger sample, with blind assessment of infant outcomes.

5 Conclusions

Any woman with a history suggestive of prelabor rupture of the membranes should be assessed as soon as possible. Attention should be directed to whether the membranes are indeed ruptured; to a careful review of the menstrual history and assessment of gestational age; to possible signs of incipient or established infection; to signs of fetal distress due to cord compression or prolapse; and to signs of uterine contractions.

For the woman with preterm prelabor rupture of the membranes who is not in labor, is not infected, and shows no evidence of fetal distress or other fetal or maternal pathology, continuation of the pregnancy is more likely to be beneficial than harmful. Administration of antibiotics prophylactically to women with preterm prelabor rupture of the membranes delays the birth and reduces the risk of both maternal and neonatal infection. No effect has yet been demonstrated on perinatal mortality. In women known to be carrying group B streptococci, intrapartum antibiotics should be adopted as standard care (see Chapter 19).

There is no evidence that the prophylactic use of betamimetic agents before uterine contractions begin is of value in preventing the onset of preterm labor.

Because preterm birth frequently follows preterm prelabor rupture of the membranes, corticosteroids should be administered if there is no evidence of sufficient pulmonary maturity, to reduce the risk of respiratory distress syndrome. Although there is no evidence from controlled trials, combining antibiotics with corticosteroids may do more good than harm.

The routine use of measures to effect early delivery after preterm prelabor rupture of the membranes does not reduce the risk of infection, and is more harmful than beneficial. If there are signs of intrauterine infection, however, antibiotic treatment should be started and delivery effected as soon as possible. A skilled neonatologist should be present at birth.

For women with term (or near term) prelabor rupture of the membranes, the effects of induction over expectant care must be carefully weighed. The risks of infection (both maternal and neonatal) are somewhat higher with expectant management. If early induction of labor is chosen, oxytocin rather than prostaglandins offers the greatest benefit with the least harm.

Sources

Effective care in pregnancy and childbirth

Grant, J. and Keirse, M.J.N.C., Prelabour rupture of the membranes at term.

Keirse, M.J.N.C., Ohlsson, A., Treffers, P. and Kanhai, H., Prelabour rupture of the membranes preterm.

Cochrane Library

Crowley, P., Prophylactic corticosteroids for preterm delivery.

Hofmeyr, G.J., Amnio-infusion for preterm rupture of membranes.

Kenyon, S. and Boulvain, M., Antibiotics for preterm premature rupture of membranes.

Tan, B.P. and Hannah, M.E., Oxytocin for prelabour rupture of membranes at or near term.

Prostaglandins versus oxytocin for prelabour rupture of membranes at term.

Prostaglandins versus oxytocin for prelabour rupture of membranes at or near term.

Prostaglandins for prelabour rupture of membranes at or near term.

Pre-Cochrane reviews

Crowley, P., Corticosteroids and induction of labour after PROM preterm. Review no. 06871.

Elective delivery after preterm prelabour rupture of membranes. Review no. 04473.

Keirse, M.J.N.C., Betamimetics after preterm prelabour rupture of membranes. Review no. 04396.

Other sources

Hannah, M.E., Ohlsson, A., Wang, E.E., Matlow, A., Foster, G.A., Willan, A.R. *et al.* (1997). Maternal colonization with group B streptococcus and prelabor rupture of membranes at term: the role of induction of labor. Term PROM Study Group. *Am. J. Obstet. Gynecol.*, 177, 780–5.

Preterm labor

1 Introduction

Preterm birth remains the major cause of mortality and of both short- and long-term morbidity in normally formed babies. Prevention and treatment of preterm labor is important, not as an end in itself, but as a means of preventing preterm birth and its consequences (see Chapter 37). Preterm labor, by definition labor beginning before 37 completed weeks of gestation, is a continuum, with the more serious consequences of preterm birth occurring before 34 weeks of gestation.

Prevention of preterm birth is not always wise; many preterm births occur as a result of conditions such as prelabor rupture of the membranes with its inherent risk of amnionitis, or as a planned intervention to end a pregnancy because of serious maternal illness or problems with fetal well-being or growth. These situations are discussed in other chapters.

Physiologically, preterm labor differs little from labor at term, except that it occurs too early. It will, however, be accompanied by increased anxiety for the women and her partner. It is not always easy to tell whether preterm labor really has or has not commenced. In many instances, apparently progressive preterm labor stops, irrespective of whether any treatment is instituted. An overly expectant attitude while watching for signs of progress can be dangerous, as more advanced preterm labor is more difficult to stop.

Successful suppression of uterine contractions does not necessarily improve the outcome for the infant. Birth may not be postponed to a clinically useful extent, while any treatment that is powerful enough to suppress uterine contractions may have other effects on the women or the baby, some of which may be undesirable or dangerous.

2 Prevention of preterm labor

2.1 Social interventions
There is a strong association between a woman's social and economic circumstances, and her risk of preterm birth. This association has prompted a number of social programs with the aim of reducing that risk. However well-intentioned these interventions are, controlled evaluation (discussed in Chapter 3) has not detected any effects on the rate of preterm birth.

2.2 Physical measures

2.2.1 Home uterine-activity monitoring
Several trials have addressed the question of whether electronic monitoring of uterine activity at home, with daily transmission to a

monitoring center by telephone, can reduce the frequency of preterm birth by early identification of women at risk for preterm labor. Unfortunately, there was enormous potential for bias in the initial reports. More recent, better-quality trials in pregnancies at higher risk of preterm labor, failed to show that home uterine-activity monitoring resulted in earlier diagnosis of preterm labor or in reduced rates of preterm birth or neonatal morbidity.

2.2.2 Bed-rest

Bed-rest, in the hope of reducing the incidence of preterm birth, has been used predominantly in multiple pregnancies. The intervention has not been demonstrated to be effective for this purpose (see also Chapter 17.)

2.2.3 Cervical cerclage

Cervical cerclage may be useful for preventing preterm birth in a small proportion of women but, unfortunately, there are no satisfactory methods of identifying the women who are likely to benefit from this intervention. Benefits are more likely to occur in women who have had two or more past pregnancies that ended preterm.

The intervention should be avoided in women who are unlikely to benefit, because of potential hazards associated with the surgery and the additional risk of stimulating uterine contractions.

2.2.4 Cervical assessment

A few small trials, and one large multicenter trial, have addressed the question of whether vaginal examination or ultrasound assessment of cervical length may help to recognize women who are likely to give birth too early, in time to institute useful preventive measures. No benefits have been demonstrated. While some of these approaches may be promising, there are also distinct disadvantages both to the procedures themselves and to the interventions that may be precipitated by their results.

2.3 Prophylactic pharmacological approaches

2.3.1 Betamimetic drugs

Many clinicians prescribe betamimetic drugs to prevent uterine contractions in women who, for one reason or another, are considered to be at increased risk of preterm labor. Trials of prophylactic betamimetics, both in multiple pregnancy and in singleton pregnancies believed to be at high risk of preterm birth, have failed to detect any reduction in the risk of preterm birth, low birthweight, or perinatal mortality.

2.3.2 Magnesium

The effects of routine magnesium supplementation on a number of adverse pregnancy outcomes, including preterm labor, have been addressed in a few trials. Overall they are of too poor quality to provide a reliable assessment of magnesium supplementation.

2.3.3 Calcium

Calcium supplementation of at least 1 g daily during pregnancy reduces the risk of women developing hypertension and pre-eclampsia. The effect is greatest for women at high risk of hypertension and women with a low baseline dietary calcium intake. Whether lower doses of calcium may have similar benefits needs assessment. Overall, no reduction in the risk of preterm birth is evident.

2.3.4 Progestogens

Regular intramuscular injections of 17α-hydroxyprogesterone caproate may reduce the incidence of preterm labor and preterm birth in women considered to be at high risk of preterm labor, but they have not been shown to decrease perinatal mortality or morbidity. The findings may warrant further evaluation, preferably with less invasive forms of administration.

2.3.5 Other agents

Prophylactic dietary supplementation with fish oils, and with zinc compounds, have both been evaluated in randomized trials. The use of fish oils shows a promising increase in the length of gestation and birthweight (see Chapter 6).

3 Tocolytic treatment for active preterm labor

3.1 Betamimetic drugs

Betamimetics to suppress uterine contractions preterm are used more extensively than any of the other labor-inhibiting agents that are employed. A variety of betamimetics have been introduced in the hope of developing agents that would have a maximal effect on uterine relaxation, with minimal effect on the heart or other body organs.

Only three of the many betamimetic agents available have ever been compared with a placebo or a no-treatment control group for inhibition of preterm labor. Some of the drugs that are widely used, such as salbutamol or fenoterol, have never been so tested. The majority of the controlled trials relate to ritodrine. Data from these trials show that betamimetics reduce the proportion of births that occur within the first 24 hours and within 48 hours after beginning treatment. Betamimetics also reduce the incidence of preterm birth. No decrease in perinatal mortality or serious morbidity, such as respiratory distress syndrome, has been detected.

At least three factors may contribute to this lack of effect on important adverse outcomes. First, the trials may have included too many women who were already sufficiently advanced in gestation, so that postponement of birth and prolongation of pregnancy were unlikely to confer any substantial benefit to the baby. Second, the time gained by betamimetic drug treatment may not have been used to implement measures with direct beneficial effects, such as promoting fetal lung maturity or transfer to a center with adequate perinatal care facilities (see Chapter 37). Third, there may be direct or indirect adverse effects of the drug treatment (including prolongation of pregnancy when this is contrary to the best interests of the baby), which counteract their potential gain.

The placebo-controlled trials do not suggest that betamimetic drug treatment frequently poses great hazards to either the woman or her baby, but other data in the literature show that these drugs are not harmless. The most frequently observed symptoms associated with betamimetic use are palpitations, tremor, nausea, and vomiting. Headache, vague uneasiness, thirst, nervousness, and restlessness may occur.

The most common, and dose-related, side-effect observed in all betamimetic treated women is an increase in heart rate. Only rarely will effective labor inhibition be achieved with maternal heart rates below 100 beats per minute. Heart rates of 130–140 beats per minute, on the other hand, should preclude further increases in the dose of betamimetics administered. Chest discomfort and shortness of breath should alert those providing care to the possibility of pulmonary congestion.

Pulmonary edema is a well-recognized complication of beta-mimetics. Most cases are associated with aggressive intravenous hydration and neglecting signs of fluid accumulation. It is safer to administer betamimetic drugs in a small volume of fluid with the use of an infusion pump than to rely on intravenous infusion of dilute solutions of the drug. Pulmonary edema is more likely in women with twin pregnancies. Plasma volume expansion is larger in women with multiple pregnancies, and these women are at greater risk of developing pulmonary edema during treatment with betamimetics than women with singleton pregnancies.

Myocardial ischemia has been described as the other serious, albeit rare, complication of betamimetic drug treatment. Betamimetic drug administration in pregnancy results in a marked increase in cardiac output, of the same order as that observed in moderate exercise. The additional work imposed on the myocardium may be too much for women with pre-existing cardiac disease. These women should not be given betamimetic drug treatment, as the hazards for them are likely to be greater than any possible benefits that might be derived.

All betamimetic agents show a clear tendency to lower diastolic blood pressure. This is usually accompanied by an increase in systolic blood pressure, with the effect of a net increase in pulse pressure. Clinically significant hypotension is less frequently encountered with currently used betamimetic drugs, such as ritodrine and terbutaline, than with earlier agents, such as isoxsuprine, but the problem has not been eliminated.

Other drugs, including calcium antagonists (verapamil) and beta-1 blockers (atenolol, metoprolol), have been tried as adjuncts to betamimetics in attempts to reduce the cardiovascular side-effects. The use of these agents has not been shown to achieve the desired effects, and the available data do not justify their use.

All betamimetic agents influence carbohydrate metabolism: blood sugar levels increase by about 40% and there is an increase in insulin secretion. In women with diabetes the rise in glucose levels is even more pronounced. Thus a woman with well-controlled diabetes is likely to become deregulated when betamimetics are administered. This applies even more forcibly when betamimetics are combined with corticosteroids, which also have diabetogenic effects.

There is no doubt that betamimetic agents cross the placenta. Stimulation of beta receptors in the fetus evokes roughly the same effects as it does in the mother. The cardiovascular effects result in fetal tachycardia, although this is usually less pronounced than in the mother. Since the metabolic effects in mother and fetus may result in hypoglycemia and hyperinsulinism after birth, assessment of blood sugar levels is advisable in infants born during or shortly after use of betamimetics to inhibit labor.

A few studies have compared long-term outcomes between infants whose mothers had received betamimetic drugs and infants whose mothers had not received such treatment. All of these studies have been small, and the control groups have been variously constructed. No long-term ill effects have as yet been observed.

None of the studies comparing one betamimetic drug with another has been large enough to have had a chance of detecting or excluding important differences in the outcomes that really matter. Nor have any of the trials shown any clear differences in serious maternal outcomes, such as pulmonary edema. Taken together, the trials comparing different betamimetic agents show no reason to prefer one agent over another.

3.2 Inhibitors of prostaglandin synthesis

As prostaglandins are of crucial importance in the initiation and maintenance of human labor, suppression of prostaglandin synthesis is a logical approach to the inhibition of preterm labor. Several agents with widely different chemical structures inhibit prostaglandin synthesis. Those that have been used to treat preterm labor include naproxen, flufenamic acid, aspirin, and sulindac, but the most widely used has been indomethacin.

These drugs all act by inhibiting the activity of the cyclooxygenase enzyme necessary for the synthesis of prostaglandins, prostacyclin and thromboxane, but the mechanisms of inhibition may be different. Aspirin, for example, causes an irreversible inhibition of the enzyme, whereas indomethacin results in a competitive and reversible inhibition.

Prostaglandin synthesis inhibitors are effective inhibitors of myometrial contractility, both during and outside pregnancy. They are more effective in this respect than any of the betamimetic drugs. No case has been reported in which a betamimetic drug resulted in suppression of uterine contractility after inhibition of prostaglandin synthesis had failed; the reverse has been observed repeatedly. Trials of indomethacin, although of a heterogeneous nature, show that this drug reduces the frequency of delivery within 48 hours, and within 7–10 days, of beginning treatment. The incidence of preterm birth and low birthweight are reduced. There is a trend, towards a reduction in the incidence of perinatal death and respiratory distress syndrome.

Only a few reports on the use of naproxen, flufenamic acid, and aspirin have appeared in the literature. These drugs have not been as widely used as indomethacin, and there have been no controlled trials of their use.

Inhibitors of prostaglandin synthesis are not innocuous. The most serious potential maternal side-effects are peptic ulceration, gastro-intestinal and other bleeding, thrombocytopenia and allergic reactions. Nausea, vomiting, dyspepsia, diarrhea, and allergic rashes have all been observed in women treated, even briefly, with prostaglandin synthesis inhibitors in preterm labor. Headache and dizziness may occur at the very start of treatment.

Gastro-intestinal irritation is common with the use of prostaglandin synthesis inhibitors, and it can occur irrespective of the route of administration. With indomethacin, it is less frequent with rectal than with oral administration; as the drug is equally well absorbed with both routes of administration, the rectal route offers some advantage.

Signs of infection may be masked by administration of prostaglandin synthesis inhibitors and this could hamper or postpone the diagnosis of incipient intra-uterine infection. The prolongation of bleeding time seen with prostaglandin synthesis inhibitors may be important, especially when epidural anesthesia is considered.

Prostaglandin synthesis inhibitors, including indomethacin and sulindac, cross from the mother to the fetus, and influence several fetal functions. The areas of major concern relate to the cardiopulmonary circulation, renal function, gastro-intestinal function, and coagulation. Constriction of the ductus arteriosus has been identified as a serious concern. This probably has little effect on fetal oxygenation in the short term, but with prolonged treatment, may result in changes similar to those seen in persistent pulmonary hypertension in the newborn. Several reports have linked persistent pulmonary hypertension in the neonate to the prenatal use of prostaglandin synthesis inhibitors.

Indomethacin treatment may reduce both fetal and neonatal renal function. The effect is dose-related and appears to be transient. Several reports have noted impaired renal function in fetuses and in the neonates at birth following administration of prostaglandin synthesis inhibitors to the mother. Long-term maternal treatment may influence fetal urine output enough to alter amniotic fluid volume, although other mechanisms may be involved in the reduction of amniotic fluid volume that can be seen during indomethacin treatment. There is no evidence, however, that the use of this drug in preterm labor leads to permanent impairment of renal function in the infant.

Several reports have linked the prenatal use of prostaglandin-synthesis inhibitors to the development of necrotizing enterocolitis.

Inhibitors of prostaglandin synthesis all inhibit platelet aggregation and prolong bleeding time. They do so in the mother, in the fetus, and in the neonate at birth. Since neonates, and particularly preterm neonates, eliminate these drugs far less efficiently than their mothers, these effects will last longer in the baby than in the mother. Indomethacin, like betamimetics, may prove to be a useful drug for obtaining sufficient delay of delivery to improve infant outcome. More and better controlled data will be needed before an adequate assessment of its usefulness in care for preterm labor can be made.

The lasting effect of salicylates on platelet function and the large doses required to arrest uterine contractions preclude the use of these drugs for preterm labor.

3.3 Ethanol
Ethanol, for a long time one of the main labor-inhibiting drugs, is now only of historical interest. It is less efficacious than other drug treatments and has serious side-effects in both mothers and babies.

3.4 Progestogens
The small amount of controlled research on the use of progesterone in established preterm labor has not demonstrated any useful labor-inhibiting effects.

3.5 Magnesium sulphate
Magnesium sulphate has been used for inhibition of preterm labor, although the placebo-controlled trials have not shown it to be effective in reducing the frequency of any adverse outcomes. It can have serious side-effects. Pulmonary edema has been reported in association with magnesium sulphate and corticosteroid administration in preterm labor. As magnesium is primarily excreted by the kidney, hypermagnesemia can occur if renal function is impaired. This may lead to impaired reflexes, respiratory depression, alteration in myocardial conduction, cardiac arrest, and death. Regular examination of the tendon reflexes is said to offer protection against such complications, since these reflexes disappear at less elevated magnesium levels than those that cause respiratory depression and cardiac conduction defects.

Magnesium levels in the fetus closely parallel those in the mother. Infants born during or shortly after treatment are reported to be drowsy; they have reduced muscle tone, low calcium levels and may take 3 or 4 days to eliminate the excess magnesium.

3.6 Calcium antagonists

'Calcium channel blockers' or 'calcium antagonists' include a wide range of different and apparently unrelated compounds, some of which, such as verapamil and nifedipine, have been used in the treatment of ischemic heart disease and arterial hypertension, and have also been used for the treatment of hypertension in pregnancy.

In the few small trials to evaluate these agents in preterm labor, fewer maternal side-effects, longer postponement of delivery, and fewer admissions to the neonatal intensive care unit, have been reported. Further well-designed, randomized trials are needed to establish whether these effects lead to improved neonatal and infant outcome.

3.7 Oxytocin antagonists

Several oxytocin analog antagonists are currently under investigation. Results to date suggest that maternal side-effects may be fewer compared with betamimetics, while effects on uterine activity are similar.

3.8 Diazoxide

Diazoxide is a powerful antihypertensive agent, which also inhibits uterine contractions. It shares many of the properties of the betamimetic drugs, both on the cardiovascular system and on carbohydrate metabolism. No controlled trials of this drug in preterm labor have been reported, although it is said to be the principal tocolytic agent in at least a few centers in North America. The available evidence does not justify its use in pregnancy and certainly not for the inhibition of preterm labor.

4 Other treatments for active preterm labor

4.1 Hydration

Hydration with intravenous fluid, with or without sedation, is frequently used as a primary approach to stop preterm labor, particularly in North America. This approach has not been well evaluated and the available data show that hydration is not more useful than no treatment at all. There is an increased risk of pulmonary edema if labor inhibiting-drugs are subsequently used. This practice should be abandoned unless evidence is brought forward to substantiate it.

4.2 Antimicrobial agents

Subclinical infection and bacterial colonization may cause preterm labor with or without prior rupture of the membranes. A wealth of data in support of these suggestions has, for many years, been described in various epidemiological, microbiological, and histological associations between preterm birth and infections of the reproductive tract. The hypothesis that antibiotic therapy might be of benefit in the care of women in preterm labor is thus attractive.

The evidence from the few trials that have been conducted is conflicting. When membranes are intact, the data demonstrate no significant benefit from antibiotic treatment on the rate of preterm birth, prolongation of pregnancy, respiratory distress syndrome, or neonatal sepsis, although maternal infection (chorioamnionitis/endometritis) and neonatal necrotizing enterocolitis were reduced. Overall there appears to be a slight increase in perinatal related mortality associated with the use of antibiotics. A large pragmatic multicenter trial is underway and should help to clarify some of these uncertainties.

Antibiotic treatment following preterm prelabor rupture of the membranes is associated with prolonging pregnancy, reduced chorioamnionitis, and reduced neonatal infectious morbidity. No difference on other measures of neonatal morbidity or mortality in the short or long term could be detected from the trials that have been reported.

4.3 Magnesium sulphate

Infants born very, or extremely, preterm are at increased risk of cerebral palsy; the earlier the gestational age at birth the greater the risk. From case-controlled studies there is a strong association between prenatal exposure to magnesium sulphate before very preterm birth and a reduced risk of cerebral palsy, but there are also concerns about a potential increase in perinatal mortality with the use of magnesium sulphate. Several multicenter international controlled trials are currently in progress to assess whether prenatal administration of magnesium sulphate to women immediately prior to very preterm birth reduces the risk of cerebral palsy for the infant.

5 Maintenance of preterm labor inhibition

Successful arrest of preterm labor does not imply that the problem may not reoccur before adequate fetal maturity has been achieved. Thus, attention has been devoted to detecting recurrences and to maintaining labor inhibition for as long as necessary.

Home uterine-activity monitoring has been used for early detection of recurrences in women in whom contractions were said to have been effectively stopped by treatment of preterm labor.

Betamimetics given orally to maintain labor inhibition after uterine contractions had been arrested by intravenous therapy will reduce the risk of recurrent preterm labor, but they have not been shown to reduce the incidence of preterm birth. The few reported trials of oral maintenance of labor inhibition failed to detect any effect on the incidence of respiratory distress syndrome or perinatal death.

Oral magnesium maintenance treatment has not been shown to reduce the risk of preterm birth or perinatal mortality, although the few trials have been of poor quality.

6 Conclusions

Social and physical interventions have proved to be disappointing in their lack of effect in preventing preterm labor. Enhanced social support, despite its promise, has not been shown to be effective in reducing the risk of preterm labor and birth. Home uterine-activity monitoring is an expensive and invasive intervention, which has not been demonstrated to result in any substantive benefit. Bed-rest, which has been evaluated mainly in multiple pregnancy, does not reduce the risk of preterm birth. No benefits (or hazards) have been shown for repeated vaginal examinations or ultrasound assessment of cervical length.

There is no evidence that the prophylactic use of oral betamimetic agents does more good than harm. Because long term-treatment with these agents cannot be assumed to be free from adverse effects on the baby, they should not be used outside the context of controlled trials. There is reasonable evidence, however, that oral maintenance treatment after inhibition of active preterm labor with intravenous betamimetics, reduces the frequency of recurrent preterm labor and the need for repeated hospitalization, and intravenous treatment with betamimetic agents, although no reduction in the risk of preterm birth or in substantive neonatal outcomes have been demonstrated.

At present, only two categories of drugs merit consideration for the inhibition of preterm labor: betamimetic agents and inhibitors of prostaglandin synthesis. All the others are either obsolete, excessively hazardous, or still in an experimental stage. There is no longer a place for ethanol or progesterone in the treatment of preterm labor. Oxytocin analogs and calcium antagonists have been insufficiently studied to assess whether they are beneficial. Magnesium sulphate, although widely used in some centers, has never been adequately evaluated. Other drugs, such as diazoxide, should not be used in attempts to inhibit preterm labor because of their potential for serious side effects.

The rejection of other agents does not imply strong endorsement of either betamimetic agents or the inhibitors of prostaglandin synthesis. Although both are effective in temporarily postponing delivery, there is no evidence that the use of these drugs *per se* reduces infant morbidity. They can be useful when the time that is gained before delivery is used to implement effective measures, such as transfer of the mother to a center with adequate facilities for intensive perinatal and neonatal care, the administration of prenatal corticosteroids to reduce neonatal morbidity, or judicious use of 'expectant management' in the period of gestation in which the infants chances of intact survival are very poor. Treatment with these powerful drugs may be dangerous for the women and can occasionally result in maternal death.

The potential benefits of betamimetics, weighed against the risk of adverse effects, does not justify their use in women with heart disease, hyperthyroidism, or diabetes. If labor needs to be inhibited in these women, prostaglandin synthesis inhibitors are the logical choice. For other women who require labor inhibition, betamimetic drugs are currently the drugs of choice.

Oral maintenance therapy with betamimetics or magnesium after inhibition of active preterm labor does not reduce the risk of preterm birth.

The roles of antimicrobial agents in active preterm labor, and magnesium sulphate administered immediately before preterm birth for the prevention of cerebral palsy, are under evaluation.

Sources

Effective care in pregnancy and childbirth

Keirse, M.J.N.C., Grant, A. and King, J., Preterm labour.

Crowther, C. and Chalmers, I., Bed-rest and hospitalization during pregnancy.

Grant, A., Cervical cerclage to prolong pregnancy.

Cochrane Library

Atallah, A.N., Hofmeyr, G.J. and Duley, L., Calcium supplementation during pregnancy for preventing hypertensive disorders and related problems.

Crowther, C.A. and Moore, V., Magnesium for preventing preterm birth after threatened preterm labour.

Crowther, C.A., Hiller, J.E. and Doyle, L., Magnesium sulphate for preventing preterm birth in threatened preterm labour [protocol].

Hodnett, E.D., Support during pregnancy for women at increased risk.

Kenyon, S. and Boulvain, M., Antibiotics for preterm premature rupture of membranes.

King, J. and Flenady, V., Antibiotics for preterm labour with intact membranes.

Makrides, M. and Crowther, C.A., Magnesium supplementation during pregnancy.

Pre-Cochrane reviews

Grant, A.M., Cervical cerclage (all trials). Review no. 04135.

Stutz pessary vs cervical cerclage. Review no. 03282.

Kaufman, K., Weekly vaginal examinations. Review no. 06818.

Keirse, M.J.N.C., Ultrasound vs pelvic examination for prevention of preterm delivery. Review no. 06817.

Betamimetic tocolytics in preterm labour. Review no. 03237.

Prophylactic oral betamimetics in pregnancy. Review no. 04401.

Oral betamimetics for maintenance after preterm labour. Review no. 04380.

Tocolytic treatment during preterm labour after PROM. Review no. 04397.

Prophylactic oral betamimetics in twin pregnancies. Review no. 03462.

Ethanol tocolysis in preterm labour. Review no. 04377.

Progesterone in active preterm labour. Review no. 04381.

Indomethacin tocolysis in preterm labour. Review no. 04383.

Prendiville, W.J., 17alpha-hydroxyprogesterone caproate in pregnancy. Review no. 04399.

Other sources

Buekens, P., Alexander, S., Boutsen, M., Blondel, B., Kaminski, M. and Reid, M. (1994). Randomised controlled trial of routine cervical examinations in pregnancy. European Community Collaborative Study Group on Prenatal Screening. *Lancet,* **344,** 841–4.

CHUMS (The Collaborative Home Uterine-Monitoring Study) Group (1995). A multicenter randomized controlled trial of home uterine monitoring: active versus sham device. *Am. J. Obstet. Gynecol.,* **173,** 1120–7.

Dyson, D.C., Danbe, K.H., Bamber, J.A., Crites, Y.M., Field, D.R., Maier, J.A. *et al.* (1998). Monitoring women at risk for preterm labor. *N. Eng. J. Med.,* **338,** 15–9.

Promoting pulmonary maturity

1 Introduction

Respiratory distress syndrome is the most common complication of preterm birth, affecting over 50% of babies born before 32 weeks' gestation. It remains a significant cause of death and severe morbidity in preterm infants.

A number of agents can promote fetal lung maturation and thereby reduce the risk of respiratory distress syndrome in the newborn. Only three of these have been evaluated in controlled trials: corticosteroids, ambroxol, and thyrotropin-releasing hormone (TRH) administered in combination with corticosteroids. Of these, corticosteroids and TRH in combination with corticosteroids have been evaluated thoroughly, and only prenatal corticosteroids are of benefit.

2 Benefits of prenatal corticosteroid administration

2.1 Respiratory distress syndrome

Prenatal administration of corticosteroids that pass through the placenta to the fetus results in a clinically important and statistically significant decrease in the risk of respiratory distress syndrome. Betamethasone (24 mg) and dexamethasone (24 mg) are both associated with an important and statistically significant reduction of respiratory distress syndrome. The risk reduction is approximately 40–60%. Hydrocortisone has been evaluated in only a few small trials, without sufficient power to demonstrate a statistically significant effect.

Maximum benefit is achieved for babies delivered more than 24 hours and less than 7 days after commencement of the medication. The reductions in the incidence of respiratory distress seen for babies born outside of this optimum period do not achieve statistical significance in the trials conducted, although the trend suggests a benefit.

No beneficial treatment effect has been demonstrated from the trials for babies born more than 7 days after the first course of prenatal steroids. Because of this, it has become widespread practice to administer prenatal corticosteroids at weekly intervals to women who remain undelivered and at risk of preterm birth. Whether or not prenatal steroids should be repeated if the woman remains undelivered and at risk of preterm birth 7 days or more after an initial course, is still unknown and is currently being evaluated by randomized trials (see also Section 3.2).

Corticosteroid administration to infants born at less than 28 weeks' gestation, produced similar reductions in the risk of respiratory distress to that observed for preterm babies as a whole, although the numbers available for analysis were not sufficient to demonstrate statistical significance. Respiratory distress is uncommon among babies born after 34 weeks' gestation, so the beneficial effects will be less in absolute terms, but the relative reduction of risk is similar to that found at earlier gestational ages. Gender of the baby does not modify the effects of prenatal corticosteroid administration.

2.2 Other neonatal morbidity and mortality

An important secondary benefit of corticosteroids has been a reduction in the duration and cost of neonatal hospital stay. The need for use of surfactant is reduced. Corticosteroids reduce the risk, not only of respiratory morbidity, but also of other serious forms of neonatal morbidity. The risk of periventricular hemorrhage is less than half that seen without the use of corticosteroids. This effect is probably related to the reduced risk of respiratory distress, although it might also reflect an effect of corticosteroids on the periventricular vasculature. No statistically significant effects have been observed on the risk of necrotizing enterocolitis or of chronic lung disease.

The marked reductions in risk of respiratory distress syndrome and periventricular hemorrhage are reflected in a substantial reduction in the risk of early neonatal mortality. As there is no concomitant increase in the risk of fetal death with corticosteroid use, this represents a decrease in overall perinatal mortality.

3 Potential risks of prenatal corticosteroid administration

3.1 Risks to the mother

Instances of pulmonary edema have been reported in pregnant women receiving a combination of corticosteroids and labor-inhibiting drugs. It is difficult to estimate the magnitude of this risk, or to differentiate the separate effects of corticosteroids and the labor-inhibiting drugs.

Infection is another potential risk of prenatal corticosteroid administration. Maternal infection is not increased overall, although infection is increased in women with rupture of the membranes for more than 24 hours prior to birth.

Other pharmacological effects of corticosteroid administration in adults relate to long-term treatment, and they provide few grounds for concern when a single course of prenatal corticosteroids is used for a period of 24–48 hours to promote fetal maturation.

3.2 Risks to the baby

The immunosuppressive effects of corticosteroid therapy could, in theory, result in an increased susceptibility to infection or to a delay in its recognition. This concern has received a great deal of attention, especially in pregnancies complicated by prelabor rupture of the membranes. Data from the trials show no evidence that corticosteroid therapy increases the risk of fetal or neonatal infection overall or in cases of preterm prelabor rupture of the membranes.

A fetus may be exposed to corticosteroids throughout pregnancy if the mother is receiving long-term steroid therapy for ulcerative colitis, asthma, rheumatoid arthritis, or other conditions. A review of the literature shows no striking excess over expectation for any adverse outcomes.

The most reliable evidence about the long-term effects of a single course of prenatal corticosteroid therapy comes from follow-up of children whose mothers had been treated in the randomized trials. None of the studies indicate that prenatal corticosteroid therapy affects physical growth, lung growth, or development. Because of the reduced neonatal mortality rate in corticosteroid-treated babies, survivors from the corticosteroid groups had a lower mean gestational age at birth than survivors from the control group. Despite this, the available evidence suggests that prenatal corticosteroids may protect against the long-term neurological sequelae of hemiparesis, diplegia, and quadriplegia. This is plausible in the light of the complications that sometimes accompany both respiratory distress and its treatment.

No controlled data are available on the risk of a repeat course of prenatal corticosteroids on the baby, although poorly controlled data suggest a reduction in birthweight. Animal studies have suggested other concerns, such as an effect on the fetal adrenals, and prompt caution against repeated use of prenatal corticosteroids until the results of trials are available.

4 Prenatal corticosteroid administration in special situations

Elective preterm delivery differs from spontaneous preterm birth in at least four main ways. First, the timing of elective preterm delivery can be controlled, thus securing the delay required to gain maximum benefit from corticosteroid administration. Second, cesarean section, which predisposes to respiratory distress, is a common route of delivery in this group of babies. Third, elective preterm birth usually takes place somewhat later in gestation than spontaneous preterm birth, so that the absolute risk of respiratory distress is usually lower. Finally, elective preterm birth is often undertaken for conditions such as diabetes, in which corticosteroid administration may have unwanted effects.

4.1 Hypertensive disease
Hypertensive disorders in pregnancy constitute one of the major indications for elective preterm birth. The initial concern about the use of steroids in women with pre-eclampsia was based on the statistically

significantly increased risk of fetal death associated with corticosteroid use in the 90 women with pre-eclampsia studied in the first reported trial. This early finding was not based on a plausible hypothesis, and came from a subgroup analysis. All 12 deaths occurred in women with proteinuria of more than 2 g per day for more than 14 days, a severity of disease that was not found in any of the placebo-treated women. There were no fetal deaths of babies of a similar number of hypertensive women in the three other trials from which data are available to address this issue. A consistent adverse effect of corticosteroids would have resulted in an increased incidence of stillbirth overall, but this did not occur. Thus, there is no good reason to deny women with pre-eclampsia the benefits of steroid therapy.

Even in the absence of any adverse effect of corticosteroids in women with pre-eclampsia, the clinician may be faced with the possible risks of postponing delivery for the few hours required to achieve a useful effect of corticosteroid administration. In some cases this delay may constitute an unacceptably high risk of complications, such as eclampsia or cerebral hemorrhage in the mother. Delivery should not be delayed at the expense of maternal health, but even an incomplete course of steroids may help the baby.

4.2 Intra-uterine growth restriction

Intra-uterine growth restriction, like hypertensive disease in pregnancy, is a common indication for elective preterm birth. Moreover, the two conditions often co-exist. The lungs of fetuses with growth restriction in the absence of maternal hypertension may have accelerated maturation, but there might still be benefit from corticosteroid administration.

A potential disadvantage of prenatal corticosteroid therapy with intra-uterine growth restriction is the risk of neonatal hypoglycemia, which is an important complication in growth restricted infants. Although one trial reported more cases of neonatal hypoglycemia among corticosteroid-treated babies compared with controls, without information from other trials it is difficult to know whether this is anything more than a chance difference.

4.3 Diabetes mellitus

Maternal diabetes mellitus may predispose to the development of respiratory distress syndrome. The results of the randomized trials do not clarify whether or not the use of corticosteroids is of benefit for diabetic women who deliver preterm, as only 35 such women were included in the trials. Insufficient data are available to allow an evidence based recommendation.

While the efficacy of prenatal corticosteroids to women with pregnancies complicated by diabetes mellitus is unknown, the potential side-effects should be a source of concern. Fetal hyperinsulinism may or may not cause cortisol resistance in the fetal lung. Administration of corticosteroids causes insulin resistance in the diabetic. Loss of diabetic control is to be expected with the doses of corticosteroids administered to promote fetal pulmonary maturation. Therefore, prenatal corticosteroid therapy in the diabetic woman would require exceptionally close supervision, possibly with continuous intravenous insulin and frequent blood glucose estimation. Failure to maintain control of the mother's diabetes may result either in ketoacidosis, which carries a high perinatal mortality rate, or in a state of fetal hyperinsulinism, which may increase the likelihood of failure to respond to corticosteroid therapy. Corticosteroid administration, if used at all in diabetic women, should be used with great caution, as it is not certain that it will do more good than harm.

4.4 Rhesus iso-immunization

Elective preterm delivery plays an important role in the management of rhesus iso-immunization. Unlike other conditions associated with chronic intra-uterine stress, rhesus disease is not thought to provoke an acceleration of pulmonary maturation. While there is a trend towards a reduction in perinatal mortality and in the incidence of respiratory distress syndrome in steroid-treated infants compared with controls, the numbers reported in the trials are too small to provide any secure estimates of the likely effects. However, there are no specific contra-indications to the administration of corticosteroids in women with rhesus iso-immunization.

5 Other agents to promote pulmonary maturity

5.1 Ambroxol

Treatment with prenatal ambroxol compared with placebo shows a tendency towards reducing the risk of respiratory distress syndrome, but the results are not statistically significant. Direct comparisons of ambroxol with corticosteroids show no clear differential effect, although there were methodological weaknesses in the trials that examined this. The main disadvantage with ambroxol is the 5-day period required to complete therapy. Because the evidence in favor of prenatal corticosteroids in anticipated preterm birth is so strong, they remain the prophylactic strategy of choice.

5.2 Thyrotropin-releasing hormone

Prenatal administration of thyrotropin-releasing hormone (TRH) in addition to corticosteroids, prior to very preterm birth, does not reduce the risks of respiratory distress syndrome or of chronic lung disease, and is associated with an increased risk of maternal side-effects of nausea, vomiting, light headedness, and elevation of pulse and blood pressure.

Systematic review of the randomized trials available shows not only no benefit but an increase in the risk of respiratory distress syndrome, need for ventilation, and death or need for oxygen by day 28 after birth, in babies exposed to prenatal TRH who deliver 10 or more days later. In view of this, prenatal TRH cannot be recommended.

6 Conclusions

Prenatal treatment with 24 mg betamethasone, or 24 mg dexamethasone, for lung maturation, is associated with a significant reduction in the risk of respiratory distress syndrome in preterm infants. This reduction is independent of gender, and applies to babies born at all gestational ages at which respiratory distress syndrome may occur. It is accompanied by reductions in the risk of periventricular hemorrhage, lower neonatal mortality rate, and in a reduced cost and duration of neonatal care.

These benefits are achieved without any detectable increase in the risk of maternal, fetal, or neonatal infection. Although maternal infection is increased in women with rupture of membranes for more than 24 hours prior to birth, prenatal corticosteroid administration does not increase the risk of stillbirth.

Every effort should be made to treat women with corticosteroids prior to preterm birth, either as a result of preterm labor or planned elective preterm birth. The only possible exception is for women with diabetes. Treatment should commence at presentation in women with any symptoms or signs that suggest the onset of preterm labor or indicate a potential need for elective preterm birth in the near future. Treatment should not be withheld because birth appears imminent. There are no controlled data to recommend or refute the widespread use of repeat doses of prenatal corticosteroids for women who remain at risk of preterm birth but undelivered after an initial course. Until the results from the trials currently in progress are available, multiple doses of prenatal corticosteroids should be avoided. TRH should not be used for the promotion of pulmonary maturation.

Sources

Effective care in pregnancy and childbirth

Crowley, P., Promoting pulmonary maturity.

Cochrane Library

Crowley, P., Prophylactic corticosteroids for preterm delivery.

Crowther, C.A., Alfirevic, Z. and Haslam, R. Prenatal thyrotropin-releasing hormone (TRH) for preterm birth.

Pre-Cochrane reviews

Crowley, P. Ambroxol vs placebo prior to preterm delivery. Review no. 03276.

Ambroxol vs betamethasone prior to preterm delivery. Review no. 03852.

Ambroxol vs intralipid prior to preterm delivery. Review no. 03853.

Corticosteroids + induction of labour after PROM preterm. Review no. 06871.

Corticosteroids prior to preterm delivery. Review no. 02955.

Post-term pregnancy

1 Introduction

The reported frequency of post-term pregnancy (defined as pregnancy lasting 42 completed weeks or more), varies from 4 to 14%, depending on the nature of the population surveyed, the criteria used for assessment of gestational age, and the proportion of women who undergo elective delivery. The more accurate determination of gestational age made possible by routine early pregnancy ultrasound reduces the number of women who receive induction of labor for apparently post-term pregnancy.

Contradictory findings and conclusions about the risks associated with post-term pregnancy have led to opposing views on the most effective form of care. A variety of policies for care of a woman with a post-term pregnancy have evolved, ranging from routine induction of labor at or around 40 weeks, 41 weeks, or 42 weeks gestation, through selective induction of labor based on abnormalities detected by antenatal fetal surveillance, to an intention to await spontaneous labor.

Semantic problems have also contributed to the confusion in understanding of post-term pregnancy. The words 'post-term', 'prolonged', 'post-dates', and 'post-mature' are all used as synonyms but are laden with different evaluative overtones. The name 'post-maturity' has also been given to a clinical syndrome in the infant with a hierarchy of features ranging from loss of subcutaneous fat and dry cracked skin, through meconium staining and birth asphyxia, to respiratory distress, convulsions, and fetal death. Confusion is bound to arise when a clearly pathological syndrome is described by a word that is used as well to make a simple statement about the chronological duration of a pregnancy.

2 Risks in post-term pregnancy

Post-term pregnancy is associated with an increase in perinatal mortality. Part of this increase is due to congenital malformations, which are more frequent among post-term births than among births at term. The other main cause of death is asphyxia.

The risk of perinatal death with post-term pregnancy increases with the onset of labor. It occurs mainly during the intrapartum and neonatal period, rather than during the pregnancy. Meconium-stained amniotic fluid is a common feature among the intrapartum and asphyxial neonatal deaths.

The incidence of early neonatal seizures, a marker of perinatal asphyxia, is between two and five times higher in infants born after 41 weeks.

3 Prevention of post-term pregnancy

Stripping or sweeping of membranes (digital separation of the fetal membranes from the lower pole of the uterus) in pregnancies at or beyond term reduces both the incidence of formal induction of labor and the frequency of the pregnancy continuing beyond 42 weeks. It does not appear to have any effect on the mode of delivery or on the risk of infection. Women have reported increased discomfort during vaginal examination with 'sweeping', as well as other side effects of bleeding and irregular contractions (see Chapter 40).

Advice advocating breast stimulation for women from 39 weeks until the onset of labor has been compared with avoiding breast stimulation in two small trials. One of these suggested a decrease in the number of women who remained undelivered at 42 weeks, the other showed no difference. Neither trial showed a difference in any other outcome. For the present, breast and nipple stimulation cannot be recommended to prevent post-term pregnancy. It should not be implemented without further trials to assess the efficacy and acceptability to women.

4 Routine induction of labor

Obstetricians have, for many years, expressed irreconcilably different opinions on the role of induction of labor for post-term pregnancy. The results of even large observational studies shed little light on the question, because of inherent selection biases and the influence of both duration of pregnancy and other aspects of care on outcome. The best evidence supporting a policy of routine induction at 41 weeks or beyond, versus a selective induction of labor, comes from randomized trials. Fortunately, the results of a number of trials are now available. Some trials have examined the effects of induction at or about 40 weeks, other trials have dealt with induction during or after the 41st week.

4.1 Perinatal death

A policy of routine induction of labor reduces the risk of perinatal death in normally formed babies. This is due to a reduction in perinatal mortality in pregnancies with induced labor after 41 weeks. Although none of the trials individually was large enough to show a statistically significant difference, the combined results of the 19 randomized trials that have assessed this outcome show a clear picture. There was one such death among more than 4000 women allocated to elective delivery, compared to nine among the similar number of women in the surveillance arm of the trials; that is, one perinatal death was prevented for each 500 inductions performed. This difference is both clinically important and statistically significant. There is no evidence of a beneficial effect of induction at less than 41 completed weeks gestation.

4.2 Perinatal morbidity

Routine induction of labor reduces the risk of meconium-stained fluid but the risk of meconium-aspiration syndrome and neonatal seizures is not affected. No consistent effect of elective induction on the incidence of neonatal jaundice has been demonstrated in the available trials. There is no evidence that routine induction of labor influences the rate of fetal heart-rate abnormalities during labor.

During the 1970s, there were several reports of an association between elective induction of labor and unintended preterm birth, followed by respiratory distress and other neonatal morbidity. By the 1980s, this had become less of a problem, because of greater awareness of the dangers of elective induction of labor without firm grounds for being certain about the duration of gestation. No cases of iatrogenic respiratory distress syndrome are reported in the randomized trials of routine induction of labor, but it must be realized that well-documented fetal maturity was an entry criteria for most of them.

4.3 Effects on the mother

In the one trial that assessed maternal satisfaction, this was not found to be affected by induction of labor. Policies of active induction of labor do not show any effect on the use of opiate or epidural analgesia.

Routine induction of labor is not associated with an increased use of cesarean birth; indeed, the trials of induction after 41 weeks show a small, but statistically significant decrease in the frequency of cesarean section for women in whom labor is induced. Subgroup analysis shows this to be true regardless of parity, state of the cervix, method of induction or overall cesarean section rates in the trials. Subgroup analyses also show a significant decrease in the use of cesarean section for primigravid women in whom labor is induced, when prosta-glandins are used for induction, and when the overall cesarean section rates in the trial was 10% or more. This challenges a widely held belief that there is an inherent association between induction post-term and an increased risk of cesarean section.

5 Surveillance

In all randomized trials of routine induction of labor at 41+ weeks, some form of fetal surveillance was used in the conservatively managed arm of the trial. This surveillance usually involved consultations at 2–3-day intervals after 41+ weeks, and varied from the mildly intrusive use of ultrasound or cardiotocography, to the highly invasive procedures of amnioscopy or amniocentesis. There is some evidence that these tests can detect pregnancies in which there is 'something wrong', but less evidence that their use improves outcome, or can elim-inate the additional risk of post-term pregnancy. The only controlled trial shows no advantages of complex fetal monitoring with comput-erized cardiotocography, amniotic fluid index, assessment of fetal breathing tone, and gross body movements over simple monitoring with standard cardiotocography and ultrasound measurement using maximum amniotic fluid pool depth.

6 Conclusions

Post-term pregnancy, in most cases, probably represents a variant of normal, and is associated with a good outcome, regardless of the form of care given. In a minority of cases there is an increased risk of perinatal death and early neonatal convulsions.

Where reliable early pregnancy ultrasound is available at an acceptable cost this should be offered routinely to confirm expected date of delivery and avoid unnecessary induction of labor for a mistaken diagnosis of post-term pregnancy.

A policy of induction of labor after 41+ weeks gestation slightly reduces the risk of perinatal death, in the range of one death saved for each 500 inductions. It also reduces the rate of meconium staining of the amniotic fluid, and is not associated with any major disadvantage. Provided that appropriate induction methods are used, there is a small reduction in the risk of cesarean section for women with a post-term pregnancy.

Induction of labor before 41 weeks gestation is not associated with any advantage apart from a small reduction in meconium staining of the amniotic fluid. The reduction in perinatal death associated with induction of labor appears to be confined to pregnancies of 41+ weeks' duration. A policy of routine induction at 40–41 weeks in normal pregnancies cannot be justified in the light of this evidence from controlled trials, and is unacceptable to many mothers.

Obstetricians, midwives, and women should be aware of the poor quality of the evidence available to support the use of all methods of fetal surveillance commonly offered to women with prolonged pregnancies. The best policy is to provide women with the most accurate information available, including the small reduction in risk in perinatal mortality with induction. Once the duration of pregnancy has with certainty attained 41 completed weeks, women who choose to be induced should be offered induction of labor by the best available method.

Sources

Effective care in pregnancy and childbirth

Bakketeig, L.S. and Bergsjo, P., Post-term pregnancy: magnitude of the problem.

Crowley, P. Post-term pregnancy: induction or surveillance?

Cochrane Library

Alfirevic, Z. and Neilson, J.P., Biophysical profile for fetal assessment in high risk pregnancies.

Boulvain, M. and Irion, O., Stripping/sweeping the membranes for inducing labour or preventing post-term pregnancy.

Chambers, H.M. and Chan, F.Y., Support for women/families after perinatal death.

Crowley, P., Interventions for prevention or improving the outcome of delivery at or beyond term.

Neilson, J.P., Ultrasound for fetal assessment in early pregnancy.

Fetal death

1 Introduction

The interval between a diagnosis of antepartum fetal death and birth is a time of great distress. When the diagnosis of fetal death has been made and confirmed by ultrasound examination, women require the time and opportunity to adjust. Rushed decisions are unnecessary, except for complications such as placental abruption or severe hypertension. Women should be made aware of the options available to them, given time to consider these options and to decide what they want. They must be allowed the time to start to grieve, and to make decisions in an environment in which they feel secure. Many women will want to return home, even if only for a brief period. It is important to remember to ask the woman how she came to the hospital or clinic. It may be preferable for her not to drive at such a time, or go home unaccompanied.

2 Choosing between active and expectant care

From the physical standpoint, given appropriate means to induce labor after fetal death, there are no overwhelming benefits or hazards for induction of labor over expectant care. The advantages and the disadvantages of both these approaches relate almost exclusively to their emotional and psychological effects. The woman herself is the best judge of these, and she is the one who should make the choice. Her caregivers should assist her by providing her with the information needed to make an informed choice. They should ensure that whatever option she chooses is provided in an empathetic environment with as little psychological and physical discomfort as possible (see Chapter 49).

It is wrong to assume that all women desire the most rapid method of delivery when their babies have died *in utero*. For some women, the uncertainty and the learning of the death are the worst moments; carrying the dead fetus still permits them a feeling of closeness to the baby, that will be lost once it is born.

Many women, on the other hand, are anxious to give birth as quickly as possible. Some may even suggest that this should be done by cesarean section. Discussing the facts and alternatives with the woman and her partner conveys compassion and understanding. Often it will help to defuse initial feelings of anger, suspicion, inadequacy, and guilt, which are typically felt by all, caregivers and women alike, after the sad diagnosis is made.

The main advantage of the expectant option is the absence of any need for intervention. The woman can stay at home, and she will avoid procedures that might turn out to be less effective and more risky than anticipated.

The disadvantages of expectant care are mainly psychological, and relate to the unpredictable and usually long time during which the woman may have to carry the dead baby. Sometimes, she or her relatives may be under the impression that the baby will rot inside her and exude toxins that can poison her. It is important to dispel such fears, although this may not always be successful.

The only physical hazard of the expectant policy relates to a possible increase in the risk of disturbances in blood coagulation. These are most likely to occur when fetal death has been caused by placental abruption. Disorders of coagulation in association with other causes of fetal death are rare. The hypofibrinogenemia that is held responsible for these disorders occurs very slowly and is rarely clinically significant in the first 4–5 weeks after fetal death. By the time that clinically significant alterations in coagulation mechanisms could arise, the chances are that birth will have occurred.

The main advantages of an active policy to effect delivery in the care of women with a dead fetus are that it offers the option of ending a pregnancy that has lost its purpose and that a post-mortem diagnosis may be easier to achieve in the absence of maceration. The disadvantages of an active policy relate to the means through which it is effected. If labor is induced, the efficacy and safety of the method used will be the most influential factor in considering the relative merits of the policy.

3 Choice of methods for inducing labor

A variety of agents and methods have been used for inducing labor after antepartum fetal death. Agents used include saline, oxytocin, the natural prostaglandins, prostaglandin analogs such as 15-methyl-prostaglandin $F_{2\alpha}$, sulprostone, and misoprostol, and the progesterone antagonist mifepristone. Consideration must be given to the route of administration, the choice of prostaglandin, and the choice of other agents where prostaglandins are not readily available.

When intra-uterine fetal death occurs in late pregnancy it is usually possible to induce labor with any of the prostaglandin regimens that are employed for other inductions (see Chapter 40). Methods with which one is thoroughly familiar tend to perform better than those that are only rarely needed and require careful study before being applied. These methods may be less effective, however, at the earlier gestational ages when the sensitivity of the uterus to prostaglandins is lower than it is at term.

Intravenous administration of natural prostaglandins has been superseded because of a high incidence of side-effects compared with local routes. The intra-amniotic route of administration has also been largely superseded by local preparations.

Vaginal administration of prostaglandins or prostaglandin analogs in the form of suppositories, gels, or pessaries, is widely used at present because of its convenience and ease of administration. Prostaglandin E_1 (gemeprost, Cervagem) and PGE_2 analogs, such as sulprostone, are often used.

When prostaglandins are not available, extra-amniotic infusion of saline, or simply placement of an extra-amniotic balloon without any infusion may be used.

The prostaglandin E_1 analog misoprostol has been shown to be effective for the induction of labor at all stages of pregnancy, administered orally or vaginally. As it is not registered for use in obstetrics and gynecology, no manufacturer's guidelines for route of administration or dosage are available. The main problem is uterine hyperstimulation, which may even result in uterine rupture. Its use at present should be restricted to research protocols to determine optimum and safe regimens

Mifepristone, a steroid compound that antagonizes progesterone action, has shown promise for induction of labor after fetal death, possibly in combination with prostaglandins to further enhance the success rate. With improvements in techniques with prostaglandins and prostaglandin analogs alone, the place of mifepristone appears to be limited.

4 Conclusions

In the case of fetal death, the decision whether or not to induce labor should be made on psychological or social grounds, and the woman herself is the best judge of these. Should induction be chosen, the most effective method in the later weeks of pregnancy is likely to be one with which the caregiver has adequate experience from inducing labor in other pregnancies. Earlier in gestation, vaginal administration of prostaglandin analogs appears to be the treatment of choice. Methods employing an extra-amniotic catheter bulb may be considered when prostaglandin analogs are unavailable, unaffordable, or ineffective. In the future, misoprostol may become a useful alternative.

Sources

Effective care in pregnancy and childbirth

Keirse, M.J.N.C. and Kanhai, H.H.H., Induction of labour after fetal death.

Cochrane Library

Chambers, H.M. and Chan, F.Y., Support for women/families after perinatal death.

Pre-Cochrane reviews

Keirse, M.J.N.C., 15-methyl-prostaglandin F2alpha after fetal death. Review no. 06188.

Low vs high dose sulprostone for induction after fetal death. Review no. 04474.

Mifepristone for induction of labour after fetal death. Review no. 05533.

Other sources

Bulgalho, A., Bique, C., Machungo, F. and Bergstrom, S. (1995). Vaginal misoprostol as an alternative to oxytocin for induction of labor in women with late fetal death. *Acta. Obstet. Gynecol. Scand.*, 74, 194–198.

Cabrol, D., Dubois, C., Cronje, H., Gonnet, J.M., Guillot, M., Maria, B., Moodley, J., Oury, J.F., Thoulon, J.M., Treisser, A., Ulmann, D., Correl, S., Ulmann, A. (1990). Induction of labor with mifepristone (RU 486) in intrauterine fetal death. *Am. J. Obstet. Gynecol.*, 163, 540–542.

Ghorab, M.N. and El-Helw, B.A. (1998). Second-trimester termination of pregnancy by extra-amniotic prostaglandin F2alpha or endocervical misoprostol. A comparative study. *Acta. Obstet. Gynecol. Scand.*, 77, 429–32.

Kanhai, H. and Keirse, M.J.N.C. (1989). Induction of labour after fetal death: a randomized controlled trial of two prostaglandin regimens. *Br. J. Obstet. Gynaecol.*, 96, 1400–1404.

Mahomed, K. and Jayaguru, A.S. (1997). Extra-amniotic saline infusion for induction of labour in antepartum fetal death: a cost effective method worthy of wider use. *Br. J. Obstet. Gynaecol.*, 104, 1058–1061.

Toppozada, M.K., Shaala, S.A., Anwar, M.Y., Haiba, N.A., Addrabbo, S., el Abey, H.M. (1994). Termination of pregnancy with fetal death in the second and third trimesters – the double balloon versus extra-amniotic prostaglandin. *Int. J. Gynaecol. Obstet.*, 45, 269–273.

Childbirth

CHAPTER 28

Social and professional support in childbirth

1 Introduction

Support during childbirth can be provided by the professionals responsible for the clinical care of the woman in labor, by other individuals specifically designated to provide support other than clinical care, or by the woman's partner, family, or friends. Controlled studies thus far have examined the contribution of the first two groups: persons specifically designated to provide support in labor. Insights into the nature and value of support by partners, family members, and friends have been gleaned from data from observational studies.

2 The nature of support in childbirth

A central feature of support in childbirth is the promise that the laboring woman will not, at any time, be left without available support. The mere physical presence of a support person is not enough. That person must also provide supportive activities, which encompass both physical comfort measures and emotional support.

Physical comfort measures should be provided in response to the woman's own needs and wishes. These will vary from culture to culture, and from individual to individual. Her supportive companion may, for example, walk with her, massage her back, offer food and fluids, help her to find a comfortable position, or assist her with a bath or shower. He or she can provide analgesic measures, such as counterpressure, cold with an ice pack or heat with a hot water bottle to painful areas of her body. The companion can help the woman to use breathing patterns that may help her relax, or other rituals that she may have practised during the pregnancy.

Emotional support may include maintaining eye contact, and providing information, praise, and encouragement. The supporting companion can help ensure that the woman understands the purpose of every procedure and the result of every examination, that she is kept informed of the progress of her labor, and that she is praised for her efforts and encouraged to continue.

The extent to which support may be seen as an integral component of care during childbirth depends on the orientation of the caregivers. Some professionals may give priority to the technical tasks of caring for a woman in labor. Others may feel that technical tasks and emotional/physical support are intimately related in helping the woman to progress successfully throughout labor, and cannot be separated. Modern technology may make support difficult for caregivers who hold the latter view, as their time and attention may be distracted away from the woman towards the monitor or the intravenous drip.

Every woman should be able to choose her source of social support in labor. This may be her partner, another family member, or a friend. Midwives, doctors, and nurses should respect her choice and provide, in addition to clinical care, appropriate physical and emotional support where it is needed.

3 The birth environment: implications for support

For much of this century, in much of the world, the subjective experiences of labor and birth were submerged by narcotic analgesia and general anesthesia, in a vain attempt to render labor painless. While women were unconscious, questions of physical and psychological support were irrelevant. When the natural childbirth movement redefined the experience of giving birth as potentially positive, these aspects of the birth environment took on a new significance.

Many aspects of the birth environment in hospitals can induce stress. The setting and the people in it may be strange to the laboring woman. Common procedures, such as restriction of fluids and foods, vaginal examinations, electronic fetal monitoring, and confinement to bed, can further add to the stress. Fear, pain, and anxiety may be increased by a mechanized, clinical environment and by unknown attendants, and this can have potentially adverse effects on the progress of labor. Women appreciate a constantly available, supportive companion in labor, together with appropriate care from a small number of professionals. This form of continuous support is not always provided. A woman's feeling of isolation can be compounded by the intermittent appearance and disappearance of unknown people, including obstetricians, midwives, nurses, and medical, nursing, or midwifery students. One study reported that a low-risk mother having her first child in a teaching hospital was attended by 16 people during 6 hours of labor, but was still left alone most of the time. A Canadian study found that women giving birth in hospital encountered an average of over six unfamiliar professionals during labor, with some women reporting up to 14 attendants. Several work-sampling studies have shown that on average less than 10% of the labor nurse's time was spent in supportive activities.

Five controlled trials have compared the effects of labor and birth in a home-like institutional settings, i.e. birth rooms or hospital birth centers, to that in a conventional hospital labor ward. Over 8000 women have participated in these trials. The women allocated to labor and to give birth in a home-like birth setting used, on average, less pain medication during labor, were slightly less likely to have their labors augmented with oxytocin, and had a slightly greater chance of being very satisfied with their birth experience.

In the years since these trials were published, many hospitals have allocated scarce resources towards renovating their labor wards, to provide more attractive, home-like settings for birth. Such settings are undoubtedly attractive, and also provide more pleasant work environments for caregivers. It is quite possible that happier caregivers may provide better care. Nevertheless, hospitals that are considering renovations of their labor wards should be aware that there is much stronger evidence to support the need for changes in caregivers' behavior than there is to support the need for cosmetic or structural changes to labor wards. If renovations are desired, they should be targeted towards factors that would encourage changes in behavior, such as removing lithotomy poles and replacing uncomfortable delivery beds with comfortable furniture and cushions.

Efforts to change caregivers' behavior, to help them to provide appropriate support to laboring women, should also be introduced. Such changes do not come easily. A multicenterd trial of a marketing strategy using opinion leaders to encourage nurses to provide labor support did not have the hoped-for outcome. A follow-up study in those hospitals where the hypothesized improvements did occur showed that a highly involved nurse manager was critical to its success.

4 Place of birth

Most doctors and many other health professionals strongly believe that hospital births are safer than home births. This opinion, which is shared by many childbearing women, may in part stem from the poor perinatal outcomes of unplanned, precipitate home births, which include a high proportion of preterm and low-birthweight babies. These unfortunate statistics do not, however, apply to planned home-birth for eligible women attended by caregivers experienced in home birth, backed up by a modern hospital system.

Several methodologically sound observational studies have compared the outcomes of planned home-births (irrespective of the eventual place of birth) with planned hospital-births for women with similar characteristics. A meta-analysis of these studies showed no maternal mortality, and no statistically significant differences in perinatal mortality between the groups. The number of births included in the studies was sufficiently large to rule out any major difference in perinatal mortality risk in either direction. Significantly fewer medical interventions occurred in the home-birth groups (including women transferred to hospital), and there were significantly fewer low Apgar scores, neonatal respiratory problems, and instances of birth trauma among the babies.

Only one small randomized trial, involving 11 women, has been mounted to compare home with hospital birth. This was done more to demonstrate the feasibility of randomizing women to home or hospital than concern about outcomes. The majority of the women in the hospital group were disappointed by the allocation. This finding was not surprising. Choosing a home (or hospital) birth is a very individual and personal choice for a woman based on her own priorities and values.

Maternal and perinatal mortality are so low in low-risk pregnancies that these cannot be the primary outcome measures for a trial. Yet they are the outcomes of real interest and the source of the polarized concerns. A study looking at issues of less importance would not provide data that are relevant to those who wish to make a choice based on considerations of safety. Women who have no factors that contra-indicate a home birth, and who prefer a planned, attended home-birth with facilities for prompt transfer to hospital if necessary, should not be advised against this.

5 Men during labor and at birth

The acceptance of men, as husbands and partners, into labor and birth is a recent phenomenon in industrialized countries. As women in these countries have begun to reclaim birth as a positive experience, the exclusion of a woman's sexual partner and the baby's father has come to be seen as incongruous.

Partners are now expected to reinforce what has been taught in childbirth education classes and, if necessary, to act as advocates for the childbearing woman. They are also expected to fill the gaps in care. More and more women planning a hospital birth feel that nurses are too busy or view the nurse's role as purely technical in nature. They tend to rely on their partners for support, assistance with breathing techniques, and comfort measures.

Realizing that midwives and nurses often have little time to give adequate psychological support, hospitals have increasingly permitted and encouraged husbands or partners to assume active roles in women's care during labor. In many countries in the industrialized world, the presence of women's partners during labor has, within 20 years, gone from being occasionally permitted to being normative and virtually universal.

There has been almost no research on the support actually provided by husbands and partners. Also unresearched are the expectations that women bring to labor about the support that they will have and that they will need. In a Canadian trial, the group of women who received continuous labor support from a lay midwife reported higher levels of support from their husbands, than did women who had the usual nursing support during labor. The husbands in the 'additional support' group provided more physical comfort measures and emotional support to their wives (apparently as a result of the encouragement and advice they received from the trained support person), and their satisfaction with their experience was higher than that of the husbands in the control group. Studies of the impact of the father's presence on labor and birth have been limited by small sample sizes and self-selection.

Some doubts have been expressed about handing over the supportive role to fathers. One concern relates to whether they are equipped for tasks that were formerly the responsibility of an experienced and professionally trained person. Another is the issue that the father should not be expected to provide the majority of the support when he, too, is emotionally involved. He is sharing the experience and may need support himself. Other questions relate to the possibility that the father's presence might negatively influence the laboring woman and interfere with the normal progress of labor. When there are tensions in the couple's relationship, practical and emotional support in labor may be both difficult for the partner to provide, and for the woman to accept.

6 Other support people

Apart from institutionally employed support persons, midwives, and partners, two other categories of people are currently providing support in labor: other family members and friends, and paid or volunteer companions currently referred to as labor coaches or 'doulas'. Hospitals vary greatly in the extent to which they permit these other support people in labor wards.

At home, and in alternative birth settings such as birthing centers, it is customary for several people to be present for at least some of the time. The freedom to choose who will be present, and when, is often a factor in a woman's choice to give birth outside hospital. It would be unwise to assume, though, that the presence of several people will necessarily provide additional support. Family and friends, like husbands and partners, may be there to share in the experience rather than to provide support.

Just as the role of support persons arose from the splitting of care into management and support, so the role of the doula comes from the splitting of support from assessment of maternal and fetal well-being during labor. Once support becomes a separate activity, those responsible for care and management in labor may not know what women or couples have been taught during antenatal classes, and may be unwilling or unable to support laboring women in the use of the skills that they have learned. They may belittle the usefulness of the education program, at the same time complaining about the unreal expectations that it has created.

The potential for territorial rivalries over the provision of support is great indeed. When a labor coach or doula is recruited as an advocate for the laboring woman, rivalries with hospital staff are almost inevitable and the intended support may end up as a casualty of the conflict.

One can legitimately ask if, given the constraints posed by institutional norms and policies, an employee of the hospital can provide the same quality of support and advocacy that a professional 'outsider' can. On the other hand, the presence of an outsider can pose a threat to the institution, which may have a negative influence on the quality of care received by the laboring woman.

The role of a special support person in labor has now been assessed by 14 controlled trials in several countries, in a variety of settings. There was remarkable consistency in the descriptions of the experimental intervention in the various trials. 'Support' included continuous presence, if not for all of labor, then at least during active labor, and in 13 trials, specific mention was made that support included comforting touch and words of praise and encouragement.

The results of the trials were also remarkably consistent, despite the disparities in obstetrical routines, hospital conditions, the obstetrical risk status of the women, the differences in policies about the presence of significant others, and the differences in the professional qualifications of the persons who provided the support. The continuous presence of an experienced support person who had no prior social bond with the laboring woman reduced the likelihood of: medication for pain relief, cesarean delivery, operative vaginal delivery, and a 5-min Apgar score <7. Another beneficial effect found in six trials was the decreased likelihood of negative evaluations of the childbirth experience, of feeling very tense during labor, and of finding labor worse than expected. Individual trials have found many other benefits of intrapartum support, including less perineal trauma, a reduced likelihood of difficulty in mothering, and of early cessation of breastfeeding.

7 Conclusions

Given the clear benefits and the absence of known risks associated with intrapartum support, every effort should be made to ensure that all laboring women receive support, not only from those close to them but also from experienced caregivers. The support that should be routinely offered to women should include continuous presence (when wished by the mother), the provision of hands-on comfort, and verbal encouragement. Depending upon the circumstances, ensuring the provision of appropriate support may necessitate alterations in the current work activities of midwives and nurses, so that they are able to spend less time on ineffective activities and more time providing support for women.

Sources

Effective care in pregnancy and childbirth

Keirse, M.J.N.C., Enkin, M.W. and Lumley, J., Social and professional support in childbirth.

Cochrane Library

Hodnett, E.D., Caregiver support during childbirth.
Home-like versus conventional institutional settings for birth.
Olsen, O. and Jewell, M.D., Home versus hospital for birth.

Other sources

Gagnon, A. and Waghorn, K. (1996). Supportive care by maternity nurses: a work sampling study in an intrapartum unit. *Birth*, 23, 1–6.

Hodnett, E.D. (1989). Personal control and the birth environment: comparisons between home and hospital settings. *J. Envir. Psychol.*, 9, 207–16.

Hodnett, E.D. (1996). Nursing support of the laboring woman. *J. Obstet. Gynec. Neon. Nursing*, 25, 257–64.

Hodnett, E.D. (1997). Commentary: are nurses effective providers of labor support? Should they be? Can they be? *Birth*, 24, 78–80

Olsen, O. (1997). Meta-analysis of the safety of home births. *Birth*, 24 4–13.

Simkin, P. (1989). *The Birth Partner*. The Harvard Common Press, Boston, Massachusetts.

Hospital practices

1 Introduction

Most births now take place in hospitals. Like other large institutions, hospitals (and the professionals working in them) depend on rules and routines for efficient functioning; it is probably essential that they continue to do so. Professionals need a structure within which to do their work. This structure necessarily involves working rules and at least some routines intended to serve the interests of other people working in and using the institution. Change can be slow because familiar rules and routines are comforting, and because it takes time to develop and agree on new policies – time that may be seen as better spent providing clinical care.

The marked variations in the type of care women receive, therefore, tend to depend more on which maternity unit a woman happens to attend, and which professional she consults, than on her individual needs or preferences. These differences in practice, which may occur in remarkably similar settings, are often so dramatic that they cannot possibly be explained by differences in medical indications or by the characteristics of women attending different hospitals.

2 First impression

A woman entering a hospital in labor may have experienced months or even years of anticipation, fear, and uncertainty about childbirth. Much of that anticipation, fear, and uncertainty is focused on the moment when she enters the labor ward. This is the time when she feels, and is, most vulnerable. She needs to be welcomed into the strange environment, and given comfort and care. It may be especially difficult to meet these needs if the woman has not met any of her caregivers before.

The midwife or labor-room nurse may have an entirely different set of priorities. Her main concerns are probably to discover what stage of labor the woman is in, and to reassure herself that the mother and baby are well. She will also have record-keeping tasks and, sometimes, may be responsible for other women in labor. Providing appropriate care for each individual woman, with her own distinct needs, is a daunting task.

Various recommendations for changes in admission practices have been made to help alleviate the anxiety and fear felt by women entering the hospital labor ward. Caregivers should welcome and support mothers and their companions from the moment of arrival. They should introduce themselves and give information about others whom the mother might see during labor. It would be helpful if midwives or nurses also asked women how they wish to be addressed. This is common courtesy and should be universal.

Admission in labor provides an opportunity to discuss a woman's requests and plans for (and worries and concerns about) labor and birth. Sometimes these discussions are formalized by completing a written 'birth plan'. The birth plan may help to facilitate communication of the woman's wishes to all members of the health care team.

The support of a partner or other companion may be particularly important to a woman when she first arrives and during the initial examination. Unfortunately, some hospitals have policies that exclude companions at this time. Surveys show that only a small proportion of women prefer not to have anyone with them at this point. Most women interviewed expressed pleasure and relief when their partner or companion could stay, and disappointment when they were unable to do so, whether because of work or childcare responsibilities, or because they were excluded as the result of a hospital regulation. A woman is usually asked to undress when she first arrives in labor. If this is done insensitively, it can be a humiliating experience for her. Many women prefer the option of bringing a comfortable nightdress from home, rather than having to wear a hospital gown; this gives them a little more dignity and individuality.

3 Clinical assessment

The main clinical tasks when a woman comes into hospital are to assess her progress in labor, her condition and that of her baby, and to make decisions about care. To do so, caregivers may use a variety of measures, including a discussion with the woman about her history, symptoms, and obstetric records; observation of her temperature, blood pressure, and general condition; abdominal and vaginal examination; and some form of monitoring of the fetal heart. Most women want to be involved in decisions about their care, and almost all will appreciate an explanation of what is being done and why.

The 'diagnosis' of labor has received relatively little research attention. The advice given to a woman antenatally about the onset of labor, what she is told over the telephone when she calls in, and whether or not a caregiver can assess her at home first, will influence her decision on when to come to hospital. What she experiences when she arrives will depend on hospital policies and the decisions made by her caregivers. If she is judged not to be in labor, she may be sent home or to another hospital ward. A small trial in the USA showed that a specific education program can reduce the number of admissions of women who are not in active labor.

In North American hospitals 'early labor assessment' or 'triage' areas have become popular. Rather than being directly admitted to the hospital labor ward, women who believe they are in labor are assessed in a homelike area that is usually near to the labor ward. The goal is to ensure that only women in active labor are admitted to the labor ward, on the assumption that women who do not 'need' to be in a labor ward should not be there (either because they may be exposed to unnecessary procedures, become more anxious, or because they add to the workload of the labor ward staff). Depending on the results of the initial assessment, women are either admitted and sent to the labor ward, observed for several hours in the assessment area, or sent home. A Canadian trial of 209 women found that women in the early-labor assessment group were less likely to use analgesia or anesthesia during labor and birth, less likely to have oxytocics during first stage labor, and rated their birth experiences more positively, than those who were admitted directly to the labor ward. The trial was not large enough, however, to determine whether pre-admission labor assessment reduces the cesarean section rate, or is associated with important adverse events such as unplanned out-of-hospital birth. Hospital administrators tend to believe that pre-admission labor assessment reduces costs (in that labor ward nurses are not giving care to those who are not in active labor), but no formal economic evaluations have been reported. Furthermore the assumption that women who are not in active labor do not require ongoing professional support and advice is open to question. Highly anxious women may have great need for, and benefit from, extra support during the latent or early phase of labor. Further research on this practice is required.

4 Preparation procedures

At one time, admission to hospital in labor included the routine use of bowel preparation with enemas or suppositories, and the shaving of the pubic and perineal area. Although these practices are only of historical interest in many countries, in others they still continue.

4.1 Enemas

The supposed benefits of bowel preparation were to allow the fetal head to descend, to stimulate contractions and thereby shorten labor, and to reduce contamination at delivery thereby minimizing the risks of infection in mother and baby. The practice is uncomfortable, and not without risk. Cases of rectal irritation, colitis, gangrene, and anaphylactic shock have all been reported.

Two randomized, controlled trials have evaluated the effects of routinely giving enemas on admission to hospital in labor. Without an enema, the fecal soiling was mainly slight and it was easier to remove than the soiling after an enema. No effects on the duration of labor or on neonatal infection or perineal wound infection were detected. Of the women who had enemas or suppositories, a small number were pleased or had requested this, half of the remainder either did not mind or were prepared to have whatever was necessary, while the other half expressed negative feelings such as embarrassment, discomfort, or reluctance. The majority of women who did not have an enema were pleased or relieved.

As routinely administering enemas to women in labor confers no benefit, the results of trials of different types of enema are largely irrelevant. Nevertheless, for situations in which an enema is deemed necessary, or is requested by the mother, it is worth noting that no advantages have been shown for a medicated over a tap-water enema, and that soapsuds enemas should not be used because they frequently cause cramps and griping.

4.2 Pubic shaving

Predelivery shaving was formerly believed to lessen the risk of infection and to make suturing of perineal trauma easier and safer. As early as 1922, these assumptions were challenged by a controlled trial. That trial and the only other controlled trial that examined this practice, were unable to detect any effect of perineal shaving on lowering puerperal morbidity; rather there was a tendency towards increased morbidity in the shaved groups.

The results of these trials are supported by those of non-randomized cohort studies, and of randomized trials of pre-operative shaving in surgical patients. Other writers have drawn attention to the disadvantages in terms of women's embarrassment during the procedure, their discomfort during the weeks in which the hair grows back, as well as to the minor abrasions caused by shaving.

5 Nutrition

The belief that food and drink should be withheld or severely restricted once labor has commenced is widely accepted in current hospital care. A small minority hold equally strong views that, except for women at high risk of needing general anesthesia, the benefits of nourishment in accordance with women's wishes far outweigh the possible benefits of more restrictive policies.

Surveys of labor ward policies in England and the United States showed that in the late 1980s most units prohibited all solid foods. Almost 50% allowed no oral intake except ice chips; most of the remainder allowed only sips of clear fluids; and only about one in ten units allowed women to drink as much fluid as they desired. None of the hospitals surveyed in the United States permitted women to eat and drink as they wished. Policies about oral intake have come under scrutiny in recent years, and have been liberalized in many units, with no detrimental effects on mother or baby reported. Nevertheless, restrictive policies remain in force in many centers.

For many women, these restrictions do not present a problem. Most women do not want to eat during the active phase of labor. For those who are in the early phase of labor and do want to eat, enforced hunger can be a highly unpleasant experience. Enforced fasting may also lead to poor progress in labor, the diagnosis of dystocia, and a cascade of interventions culminating in a cesarean delivery. The work of labor has been likened to the work of continuous moderate exercise. In longer labors in which oral intake is prohibited, there is a progressive rise in urinary ketones. In an American study of women who had had elevated ketones in labor, women reported that hunger was one of their most unpleasant sensations during labor. Why then are such restrictive policies employed when some women so obviously find them distressing? The explanation lies in the widespread concern that eating and drinking during labor will put women at risk of aspirating stomach contents during regurgitation.

5.1 Risks of aspiration

This concern is real and serious, but perhaps misguided. The risk of aspiration is almost entirely associated with the use of general anesthesia. The degree of risk, therefore, relates directly to the frequency with which general anesthesia accompanies childbirth, and to the care and skill with which the anesthetic is administered. The level of risk has always been low and is now very low. Aspiration plays a very small role in maternal mortality, although it remains a largely unquantified factor in maternal morbidity.

Policies that restrict oral intake during labor have the laudable aim of reducing the risk of regurgitation and inhalation of gastric contents. Aspiration of food particles of sufficient size to obstruct a main stem or segmental bronchus may result in a collapse of lung tissue beyond the obstruction. Even in the absence of food particles, if the stomach contents are sufficiently acidic they can cause chemical burns in the airways. It is this syndrome of acid aspiration in particular, described by Mendelson over 50 years ago, that constitutes the greatest risk in pregnant women who undergo general anesthesia.

Over the years, a number of specific measures have been introduced to avoid aspiration. It has been pointed out repeatedly that failure to apply proper anesthetic technique is the major reason that deaths from aspiration of gastric contents still occur. Most cases of aspiration could be prevented by a combination of decreasing the frequency of procedures that require anesthesia (particularly cesarean section), the use of regional anesthesia whenever feasible, and meticulous attention to safe anesthetic technique.

5.2 Measures to reduce volume and acidity of stomach contents
Measures to reduce the volume and acidity of gastric contents cannot compensate for inadequate anesthetic technique. Such measures are, however, widely used.

5.2.1 Restriction of oral intake
Fasting is the most commonly used measure to reduce the stomach contents. Fasting during labor does not have the desired effect of ensuring an empty stomach. To quote the conclusions of one study 'the myth of considering the time interval between the last meal and either delivery or the onset of labor as a guide to gastric content volume should now be laid firmly to rest'. Withholding food and drink during labor will not ensure an empty stomach, should general anesthesia become necessary. No time interval between the last meal and the onset of labor guarantees a stomach volume of less than 100 ml.

The use of a low residue, low-fat diet with the aim of providing palatable, attractive, small meals at frequent intervals is a reasonable alternative to fasting. Such a diet could consist of tea, fruit juice, lightly cooked eggs, crisp toast and butter, plain biscuits, clear broth, and cooked fruits. Some women prefer high-calorie snacks and drinks.

Nor can fasting during labor be relied on to lower the acidity of the gastric contents. One author commented provocatively: 'Is it not intriguing that, in England and Wales, the number of maternal deaths from acid-aspiration apparently rose only after the institution of severe dietary restriction in labor, amounting in most units almost to starvation?'

Restricting food and drink during labor may result in dehydration and ketosis. Whether the degree of ketosis that occurs in some women during labor is a harmless physiological state or a pathological condition that interferes with uterine action is uncertain. There are no published data about the nutritional needs of laboring women. For some women, these are likely to be similar to those of an individual engaged in strenuous athletic activity.

The most common response to the problems of dehydration and ketosis in maternity units where eating during labor is prohibited is the use of intravenous glucose and fluid. The effects of this practice should be carefully weighed against those of the alternative option of allowing women to eat and drink as they desire. The first controlled trial to compare a policy of encouraging women to eat and drink during labor involved 328 women in a Canadian hospital. Women enjoyed being able to control their own oral intake; no other benefits or harmful effects were found.

5.2.2 Routine intravenous infusions

The biochemical effects of intravenous glucose solutions during labor have been evaluated in a number of controlled trials. The rise in the mother's blood sugar level is accompanied by a rise in the production of insulin. The available data show no consistent effect on either maternal pH or lactate levels.

Infusions of glucose solutions to the mother result in increased blood sugar levels in the baby, and also in a decrease in umbilical arterial blood pH. Excessive insulin production in the fetus occurs when women receive more than 25 g glucose intravenously during labor, and this can result in low blood sugar and raised levels of blood lactate in the baby. A further danger is that the excessive use of salt-free intravenous solutions can result in serious hyponatremia, in both the mother and the fetus. Thus, the use of intravenous glucose and fluids to prevent or combat ketosis and dehydration in the mother may have serious unwanted effects on the baby.

Currently, intrapartum intravenous protocols typically involve the use of Ringers Lactate, a non-glucose based solution that does not provide a source of energy. The potential hazards of intravenous infusions might be obviated by the more natural approach of allowing women to eat and drink during labor.

5.2.3 Pharmacological approaches

The frequency of unpredictably large volumes and equally unpredictable acidity of the stomach contents, whether women fast or do not fast during labor, has led to the use of a number of agents in attempts to decrease both the content and the acidity of the stomach in laboring women.

The stomach contents can be emptied mechanically with a stomach tube, or vomiting can be induced with pre-operative apomorphine. A comparison of these two methods for women in labor who required a general anesthetic, showed no statistically significant difference in the mean gastric aspirate during the operation. Most women having the stomach tube passed found it 'very unpleasant', whereas the majority of those receiving apomorphine found the procedure only 'slightly unpleasant'. Neither method guarantees that the stomach will be empty. Hydrogen ion inhibitors, such as cimetidine and ranitidine, can increase the rate of gastric emptying and thus result in quite striking decreases in stomach contents.

The stomach contents can be made less acid by the use of antacids such as aluminium hydroxide, magnesium trisilicate, or sodium citrate, and by acid suppressing agents such as cimetidine, ranitidine, or omeprazole. Randomized comparisons between different agents have provided no evidence that any particular agent or class of agents influences gastric pH more effectively than others.

The effectiveness of these agents in reducing acidity, however, does not necessarily mean that they will have an effect on the incidence or severity of Mendelson's syndrome. Although from 1966 onward there has been a movement towards the routine administration of antacids to all women before cesarean section, cases of Mendelson's syndrome still occur in women who had a full regimen of antacid treatment.

6 Maternal position during the first stage of labor

Interest in maternal position during the first stage of labor has existed throughout the twentieth century, but until recently there has been little well-controlled research to assess the validity of the various strongly held opinions. Lying down in labor continues to be routine practice in many maternity units. The available data cast doubt on the wisdom of this policy.

6.1 Effects on blood flow and uterine contractility

The supine position (lying flat on the back) causes a reduction in cardiac output. It is associated with a greater decline in femoral than in brachial arterial pressure, which does not occur in the lateral position or when the uterus is tilted to the left. This observation suggests that the supine position can compromise uterine blood flow during labor.

Contraction intensity is consistently reduced, and contraction frequency is often increased, when the laboring woman sits or lies supine after being upright. Standing and lying on the side are associated with greater contraction intensity. The efficiency of the contractions (their ability to accomplish cervical dilatation) is also increased by standing and by the lateral position.

The results of several studies suggest that the supine position can adversely affect both the condition of the fetus and the progression of labor, by interference with the uterine blood supply and by compromising the efficiency of uterine contractions. Frequent changes of maternal position may be a way of avoiding the adverse effects of supine recumbency. No evidence from controlled studies suggests that the supine position should be encouraged.

6.2 Effects on the mother and the baby

The results of controlled trials show that women who were asked to stand, walk, or sit upright during labor had, on the average, shorter labors than women asked to remain lying flat. Trials in which an upright position was compared with lying on the side showed no striking differences in the length of labor.

In the only trial in which labor was found to be longer in the ambulant than in the non-ambulant group, women in the recumbent group were permitted to get up if they desired and women in the ambulant group were allowed to rest in bed 'whenever they wanted'. Women in the upright group preferred to recline in bed as labor progressed, often at about 5–6 cm dilatation. This suggests that free choice of position may be the most important consideration.

Women allocated to an upright posture used less narcotic analgesics or epidural anesthesia, and received fewer oxytocics to augment labor. In part this may be because it was easier to administer such drugs to women who were lying in bed. The available data provide no evidence of a consistent effect of position during the first stage of labor on the likelihood of instrumental delivery.

Similarly, there is no consistency in the findings with respect to the condition of the baby. Only one trial reported significantly lower incidences of fetal heart-rate abnormalities and depressed Apgar scores associated with an upright position. Other investigators, some of whom used telemetry (a means of electronically monitoring the fetal heart while the woman is mobile) in conjunction with ambulation, did not detect differences in fetal heart-rate patterns or Apgar scores. No information is available about the effect of position during the first stage of labor on more substantive indicators of the babies' well-being.

7 Conclusions

Hospital routines are necessary for efficient functioning. The challenge faced by professionals working in maternity units is firstly to introduce or maintain only those routines and rules that have been shown, on balance, to do more good than harm, and secondly, to apply those routines flexibly in a way that takes the needs of each individual child-bearing woman into account.

The presence of a companion when women first come into hospital and during the initial examination is important to many women. The presence of companions whom women choose should be encouraged and facilitated.

Caregivers should pay attention to ways of maintaining the woman's dignity, of providing privacy, and of treating women as adults, for example, in styles of address and introductions. Abandoning the traditional hospital gown is a step towards this goal.

Women appreciate the efforts of caregivers to inform and consult them about their progress in labor and the care they are to receive. When choices about care are offered, they should be presented in a manner that allows women to ask for what they want, and discuss their uncertainties.

There is no evidence to support outmoded practices, such as administering enemas routinely or perineal shaving, which cause discomfort and embarrassment for women.

No presently known measures can ensure that a laboring woman's stomach is empty, or that her gastric juices will have a pH greater than 2.5. Enforced fasting in labor, the use of antacids, or pre-anesthetic mechanical or chemical emptying of the stomach are only partially effective. All of these have unpleasant consequences and are potentially hazardous to the mother, and possibly her baby.

The syndrome of aspiration of stomach contents under general anesthesia is rare but serious. It is wise to avoid general anesthesia for delivery whenever possible, and to use a proper anesthetic technique with meticulous attention to the known safeguards when general anesthesia must be used.

Professional requirements that women lie flat during the first stage of labor are less widespread than they used to be, but they still exist. The available evidence suggests that this policy compromises effective uterine activity, prolongs labor, and leads to an increased use of oxytocics to augment contractions.

Controlled trials are required, not only to evaluate the effects of routine hospital policies and practices, but also to evaluate methods of implementing changes when these practices are ineffective, inefficient, or counter-productive.

Sources

Effective care in pregnancy and childbirth

Chalmers, I., Garcia, J. and Post, S., Hosptial policies for labour and delivery.

Johnson, C., Keirse, M.J.N.C., Enkin, M.W. and Chalmers, I., Nutrition and hydration in labour.

Roberts, J., Maternal position during the first stage of labour.

Cochrane Library

Basevi, V. and Lavender, T., Routine perineal shaving for labour [protocol].

Cuervo, L.G., Rodriguez, M.N. and Delgado, M.B., Routine enema for labour.

Lauzon, L. and Hodnett, E., Antenatal education for self-diagnosis of the onset of active labour at term.

Caregivers' use of strict criteria for diagnosing active labour in term pregnancy.

Olsen, O. and Jewell, M.D., Home versus hospital for birth.

Other sources

Broach, J. and Newton, N. (1988). Food and beverages in labor. Part I: Cross-cultural and historical practices. *Birth*, 15, 81–5.

Broach, J. and Newton, N. (1988). Food and beverages in labor. Part II: The effects of cessation of oral intake during labor. *Birth*, 15, 88–92.

Flamm, B., Berwick, D. and Kabcenell, A. (1998). Reducing cesarean section rates safely: lessons from a 'breathrough series' collaborative. *Birth*, 25, 117–24.

Heston, T.F. and Simkin, P. (1991). Carbohydrate loading in preparation for childbirth. *Med Hypotheses*, 34, 97–8.

Ludka, L.M. and Roberts, C.C. (1993). Eating and drinking in labor. A literature review. *J. Nurse Midwifery*, 38, 199–207.

Tranmer, J.E. (1999). Nutritional support during labour: a randomized controlled trial of patient controlled oral intake during labour. Unpublished PhD thesis, University of Toronto.

Care of the fetus during labor

1 Introduction

The principal aim of monitoring the fetus during labor is to identify fetal hypoxia, which, if uncorrected, might cause death or short-term or long-term morbidity. In theory at least, it should then be possible to avert the adverse outcomes by appropriate and timely measures.

Several methods of monitoring fetal well-being have been evaluated in randomized trials. Although these trials have generated consistent evidence about the effects of alternative methods of monitoring on fetal and maternal outcome, controversy still remains about how monitoring should be performed and about the appropriate response to an 'abnormal' result.

2 Clinical methods of fetal monitoring during labor

2.1 Intermittent auscultation of the fetal heart

Intermittent auscultation (listening with a fetal stethoscope or hand-held Doppler ultrasound monitor) of the fetal heart has been the predominant method of monitoring the fetus during labor during most of this century. It is still widely used, despite a trend that began during the 1970s to replace it with continuous electronic monitoring.

As evaluated in the randomized trials, auscultation is performed every 15 min during the first stage of labor, and more often during the second stage. The criteria for 'fetal distress' are a fetal heart rate above 160 or below 100–120, or an irregular heart beat. Although some authorities feel that changes in fetal heart rate during contractions might give an earlier warning sign, auscultation is usually performed after contractions.

2.2 Assessment of the amniotic fluid

Passage of meconium is associated with an increased risk of intrapartum death, neonatal death, and various measures of neonatal morbidity, such as low Apgar score or lowered acid-base status. Part, but by no means all, of this association is explained by respiratory problems due to meconium aspiration.

Thick meconium recognized at the onset of labor carries the worst prognosis, and is associated with a five to sevenfold increased risk of perinatal death. Thick, undiluted meconium also reflects reduced amniotic fluid volume at the onset of labor, which in itself is a significant risk factor. Slight staining of the liquor at the onset of labor probably reflects a small increase in risk, but this has been disputed.

Meconium-staining of the fluid at the onset of labor reflects events that occurred prior to the onset of labor. It may be a sign of impaired placental function that exposes the fetus to the risk of hypoxia during labor. Passage of meconium for the first time after the onset of labor is less common, and it seems to carry an associated risk intermediate between heavy and light early passage of meconium. Whatever the degree or time of passage of meconium, the risks associated are increased if fetal heart-rate abnormalities are also present.

Because of these associations between liquor status and adverse outcomes, routine assessment of the amniotic fluid in early labor, if necessary by amnioscopy or artificial rupture of the membranes, has been recommended as a screening test for identifying fetuses at increased risk. Unfortunately, no controlled evaluation of such a policy has been reported.

3 Continuous assessment of the fetal heart

The development in 1960 of an electrode that could be attached to the fetal scalp led to a great deal of research into the relationship between fetal heart-rate changes and events during labor. Various fetal heart-rate changes were deemed to indicate 'fetal distress'. These changes were of three types: changes in baseline rate, periodic changes related to uterine contractions, and changes in the variability of the baseline rate. Although tachycardia (abnormally rapid fetal heart rate) and bradycardia (abnormally slow fetal heart rate) were classical signs of 'fetal distress', a distinction could be made between constant or 'baseline' bradycardias, which were almost invariably associated with good fetal outcome, and bradycardias that represented a change in rate from a previously higher heart rate. Periodic changes included late fetal heart-rate decelerations that followed, repetitively, the peaks of contractions and which were thought to be due to uteroplacental insufficiency; and variable decelerations, which had a varying shape and relationship to contractions that were ascribed to umbilical cord compression. A reduction in the normal 'beat to beat' variation of the fetal heart rate was attributed to fetal 'depression', reflecting a reduced influence of the central nervous system on control of the heart.

Continuous electronic fetal heart monitoring during labor is now most commonly achieved either 'externally' by Doppler ultrasound or 'internally' by electrocardiography. Doppler ultrasound provides the most reliable method for monitoring the fetal heart rate during late pregnancy, and for external monitoring of the fetal heart rate during labor. Ultrasound fetal heart-rate monitors are satisfactory for determining the fetal heart rate, but may be less satisfactory for determining fetal heart-rate variability than the internal monitor. Problems that may arise are that a maternal heart rate may occasionally be counted in error (which may lead to an inappropriate diagnosis of fetal distress) and that, when the fetus or mother moves, the signal may be lost or artefactual, necessitating frequent repositioning of the transducer.

External monitoring is usually employed during early labor, particularly before the membranes have ruptured. In many centers internal monitoring by scalp electrode application is preferred later in labor because it provides a more reliable trace and allows the mother greater freedom of movement.

4 Fetal scalp blood acid-base assessment

The technique of sampling blood from the fetal scalp for assessment of the acid-base status during labor was first described in the early 1960s. A scalpel or stylette is passed through the cervical os to make a small incision in the fetal scalp. A sample of blood is then collected in a heparinized capillary tube and analyzed to determine its acid-base status. The technique has changed little since it was first described, requires readily available blood gas machine availability, and remains somewhat cumbersome, time-consuming, and difficult and uncomfortable for the woman.

5 Comparison of auscultation and electronic fetal monitoring

The two broad approaches to fetal monitoring during labor currently practised are first, the use of electronic monitoring in as high a proportion of women as possible, and second, its use only in women whose pregnancies are deemed to be at high risk.

Continuous electronic fetal heart-rate monitoring provides more information than intermittent auscultation with a fetal stethoscope. Listening for 1 min every 15 min between contractions, as is commonly employed with intermittent auscultation during the first stage of labor, samples the fetal heart rate for only about 7% of the time, and provides relatively little information about the relationship between changes in the fetal heart rate and uterine contractions, or about fetal heart-rate variability. The important question is whether or not the increased information provided by continuous electronic monitoring during labor leads to any improvement in outcome for the baby.

Although continuous electronic fetal heart monitoring gives substantially more information about the fetal heart rate, the interpretation of fetal heart-rate traces is open to great variation. Tracings are often interpreted differently by different obstetricians, or even by the same obstetrician at different times. The problem with electronic fetal heart monitoring is not with its ability to measure, but in its interpretation.

5.1 Effects on labor and delivery

Twelve randomized, controlled trials comparing electronic fetal monitoring with intermittent auscultation of the fetal heart rate, involving over 58 000 women in 10 centers, have been reported. Cesarean section and operative vaginal delivery rates were both higher in all the electronically monitored groups. The increase in cesarean section rate is much greater when scalp pH estimations are not available.

One concern about the use of continuous electronic monitoring (without telemetry, which allows the woman to be mobile), has been the possibility that it prolongs labor by restricting women's movement, but data from the trials, when considered together, do not support this. There is no clear effect of the monitoring method on either the use or the method of analgesia.

5.2 Effects on the fetus and neonate

There is little evidence that the extra cesarean sections associated with continuous electronic fetal monitoring lead to any substantive benefits for the baby. The number of perinatal deaths that occurred among the births in the trials of electronic fetal heart monitoring with fetal pH estimation were evenly distributed between the electronically monitored and control groups. There is no evidence that intensive fetal heart-rate monitoring, with or without fetal pH estimation, reduces the risk of Apgar score less than 7, or the rates of admission to special care nurseries.

The one measure of neonatal outcome that does seem to be improved by more intensive intrapartum monitoring is neonatal seizures. This effect seems to be restricted to electronic fetal monitoring backed by fetal pH estimation. For babies monitored in this way, the odds of neonatal seizures appears to be reduced by about one-half. No effect was seen in preterm babies, and so the estimated protective effect may be even greater in term babies. A secondary analysis of the largest trial suggested that the reduced risk of neonatal seizures was limited to labors that were induced or augmented with oxytocin, or that were prolonged.

The finding of a 50% reduction in the risk of neonatal seizures, associated with continuous monitoring of the fetal heart and fetal acid-base estimation, is potentially very important. Indeed, between a quarter and a third of babies who suffer neonatal seizures die, and a further quarter to a third are seriously impaired in childhood. Nevertheless, the follow-up data available suggest that the neonatal seizures prevented by intensive monitoring are not those associated with long-term impairment.

Neonatal infection was uncommon in all the trials, but there is no evidence to suggest that intensive monitoring increased this risk. The data are insufficient to explore differences between types of electrode in this respect.

5.3 Mother's views

Most studies of women's opinions of intrapartum fetal monitoring have been uncontrolled surveys of their views. These surveys suggest that continuous monitoring is acceptable to most women, but that it can also have important adverse consequences for some.

Many women reported that continuous monitoring and recording of the fetal heart rate was reassuring because it demonstrated that the baby was alive, and provided the information that caregivers need during labor. These feelings are enhanced if women are given a clear view of the monitor during labor. Women at relatively high risk of problems during labor, and those most knowledgeable about continuous monitoring, seem most likely to be reassured. Detailed information given just before the start of labor, however, appears to have little positive effect on women's perceptions of intrapartum monitoring.

Continuous electronic monitoring of the fetal heart rate can generate anxiety in a number of ways that cannot be predicted in advance for individual women. Some women interviewed in the surveys reported discomfort and restriction of movement, or worries that an electrode would damage the baby's scalp. Others found the monitor a distraction that interfered with their relationships with caregivers and their companion in labor. The trace may become worrying, and this may be particularly disquieting if there is uncertainty about the significance of the 'abnormality' among caregivers. It may be of poor quality or even artefactual, or the monitor itself may malfunction, sometimes repeatedly. An external abdominal transducer may become displaced or a scalp electrode detached. These problems are not uncommon.

How much weight should be given to the various maternal views of electronic fetal heart-rate monitoring revealed in these uncontrolled surveys? Three of the randomized, controlled trials included an assessment of women's views of the alternative approaches. There were no clear differences between the groups but there was a tendency for women allocated auscultation to have a more positive experience of labor. Women in the electronically monitored group tended to be left alone more often but nearly all women interviewed reported that they were able to get in touch with a nurse or doctor at any time. No difference was detected in the proportions of women who reported 'worries or anxieties' during labor, or that labor had been 'unpleasant'. In line with the observational studies, more women in the continuously monitored group felt 'too restricted' during labor. Overall, the method of monitoring was less important to women than was the support that they received from staff and companions during labor.

5.4 Technique of electronic fetal monitoring

Direct comparisons of electronic fetal monitoring, with and without fetal blood sampling as an adjunct, show that access to scalp sampling reduces the number of cesareans for fetal distress, with no clear differences in neonatal outcome. Data from indirect comparisons point both to better maternal and better neonatal outcome if fetal blood sampling is used.

Electronic fetal heart-rate monitoring is now often performed intermittently (e.g. for 15 min each hour). A randomized trial showed no evidence that intermittent cardiotocography was less safe than continuous monitoring.

One trial compared cardiotocography plus simultaneous analysis of the fetal electrocardiogram (ECG) waveform, with cardiotocography alone. Operative delivery for 'fetal distress' was markedly reduced in the cardiotocography plus ECG waveform group, but this effect was to some extent attenuated by operative deliveries for other reasons; there was a lesser need for scalp sampling. Overall there is, as yet, little reason to recommend this approach and further evaluations are necessary.

Fetal pulse oximetry is, at present, being assessed in a randomized trial.

5.5 Comment

Although a number of trials of electronic monitoring have now been completed, these collectively have not been sufficiently large to remove uncertainty about the impact, if any, of this technique on the rare, but important, problems of intrapartum fetal death and cerebral palsy.

Evidence from the randomized comparisons of alternative methods of fetal heart-rate monitoring suggests that intrapartum death is prevented equally effectively by intermittent auscultation as by continuous electronic fetal heart-rate monitoring, provided that importance is attached to the prompt recognition of intrapartum fetal heart-rate abnormalities, whatever the monitoring policy is. (During the 2 years of the Dublin trial, for example, the intrapartum death rate was lower than in the preceding and following years.)

The reliability of intermittent auscultation may be increased by the use of a hand-held ultrasound monitor rather than conventional fetal stethoscopes. There are arguments for always using these devices, partly because they cause less maternal discomfort than a fetal stethoscope. Compliance with intermittent auscultation should be straightforward, if a caregiver has responsibility for only one woman during labor. Such individualized attention is likely to have other benefits for a woman. It is to be deplored that staffing and other policies for intrapartum care in many delivery wards make this ideal impossible to meet. The implication is that auscultation may not be performed as frequently or regularly as it should be to provide safe fetal surveillance in labor.

The complexity of continuous electronic monitoring makes it susceptible to technical and mechanical failures. Machine maintenance and replacement, and in-service training of personnel, are therefore important. Electronic fetal monitoring may also provide suboptimal surveillance, if it reduces the frequency with which the caregiver formally checks the fetal heart rate. A fetal heart monitor should be an adjunct to, not a substitute for, personal care.

The wide variation in the interpretation of continuous fetal heart-rate records demonstrates that this is a major problem with current methods of continuous monitoring.

Implications for policy depend on the importance attached to a reduction in the risk of neonatal seizures. Limited follow-up of the children in the Dublin trial who suffered neonatal seizures suggests that the neonatal seizures that are potentially preventable by more intensive monitoring are not associated with long-term problems. Nevertheless, some people will consider that neonatal seizures are sufficiently important in their own right for their prevention to form the basis for current policy. On this basis, there is a good case for using more intensive monitoring when labor ceases to be 'physiological', for example, during induction or augmentation of labor, if labor is prolonged, if there is meconium-staining of the liquor, or with multiple pregnancy.

For the majority of labors for which no such indications apply, the current evidence suggests that more intensive monitoring increases obstetric intervention with no clear benefit for the fetus. Regular auscultation by a personal attendant, as used in the randomized trials, therefore seems to be the policy of choice in these labors. Such a policy will be difficult to re-implement in the many hospitals whose current policy is universal electronic monitoring. First, individualized care during labor is often perceived as not possible; and second, midwives and others may have lost the ability and confidence to monitor labor by intermittent auscultation.

The choice of technique for fetal heart monitoring has much wider implications than the direct effects on surveillance and physical health of the fetus. Depending on the prevailing system of care for women during childbirth, it may influence the roles and relationships of those involved. With intermittent auscultation, the midwife is the center of care giving, with the obstetrician playing a consultative role if the midwife is worried that there may be problems. In contrast, use of continuous electronic monitoring changes the delivery room into an intensive-care unit. The midwife takes on a more technical role with obstetricians becoming more centrally involved in routine care. The presence of a monitor may also change the relationships between the woman and her partner on the one hand, and the woman, midwife, and doctor, on the other. These wider implications must be recognized.

6 Other methods of fetal monitoring and diagnosis in labor

6.1 Admission test

Intrapartum 'fetal distress' commonly reflects problems that predate the onset of labor. For this reason, there is a strong case for careful risk assessment at the beginning of labor. A short (15–20 min) period of external electronic fetal-heart monitoring upon admission in labor has been recommended as a screening test for women who are deemed to be at low risk. The rationale for this practice is that it would identify a subgroup of fetuses who would benefit from more intensive monitoring, and might identify major fetal problems that would be missed by intermittent auscultation.

In principle, a screening test on admission in labor as a basis for deciding on selective intensive monitoring is attractive, because it should identify fetuses that embark on labor in an already compromised state. There are, however, two other components of monitoring that must be fulfilled if the policy is to be effective: first, whether the test is interpreted accurately; and second, whether the test results are acted on appropriately when used in clinical practice. These questions can only be addressed satisfactorily in trials to compare the outcomes for women randomly allocated to a policy of screening test plus appropriate response or to a control group wherein the test is not used.

6.2 Intrapartum fetal stimulation tests

Fetal heart-rate acceleration is commonly accepted as an indicator of fetal well-being in antepartum non-stress testing. These accelerations in a non-stress test are commonly associated with fetal movements or uterine contractions, but may be evoked by other stimuli, such as sound. The observations that fetal heart-rate accelerations sometimes coincided with fetal scalp blood sampling, and that scalp blood pH tended to be normal if an acceleration occurred, has prompted consideration of intrapartum stimulation tests by applying a clamp to the scalp, or by using a sound stimulus. These tests could reduce the need for scalp blood sampling, or be used as an alternative when scalp sampling is either not available or technically impossible. They have not, however, been evaluated rigorously. On the basis of currently available evidence, a non-reactive stimulation test should be followed by fetal scalp blood acid-base estimation.

7 Conservative management of 'fetal distress'

The most common treatment for intrapartum 'fetal distress', diagnosed by persistent fetal heart-rate abnormalities or depressed fetal scalp blood pH, is prompt delivery. Many fetal heart-rate abnormalities, however, will resolve with simple conservative measures, such as a change in maternal position (to relieve aortocaval compression and pressure on the umbilical cord), interruption of oxytocin administration to increase uteroplacental blood flow and short-term maternal oxygen administration (to improve oxygen transport to the placenta).

Maternal hypotension often follows the induction of epidural anesthesia, with consequent fetal heart-rate abnormalities. Preloading with intravenous fluids has been shown to counteract the relative hypovolemia that follows epidural block, and to reduce substantially the frequency of fetal heart-rate abnormalities.

Intravenous betamimetics are a useful treatment for 'buying time' when persistent fetal heart-rate abnormalities indicate a need for elective delivery. In a randomized, controlled trial involving 20 labors characterized by both ominous fetal heart-rate changes and a low fetal scalp blood pH, 10 of the 11 treated with intravenous terbutaline showed improvement in the heart-rate pattern, compared with none in the control group. At birth, the babies were less likely to be acidotic and to have low Apgar scores. The results of this trial are supported by other less well-controlled studies. This short-term improvement could be very useful in situations where facilities for emergency cesarean section are not immediately available. The improvement in the trace pattern is sometimes sustained. In these circumstances, labor may be allowed to continue without urgent delivery.

Another temporizing maneuver, amnio-infusion to correct oligohydramnios, may be useful as a method of preventing or relieving umbilical cord compression during labor. Saline or Ringers lactate is infused through a catheter into the uterine cavity. The technique has been used prophylactically in various conditions that are commonly associated with oligohydramnios, and therapeutically for repetitive variable fetal heart-rate decelerations during labor, which are attributed to umbilical cord compression. The use of amnio-infusion for intrapartum umbilical cord compression, potential or diagnosed by cardiotocography, or for meconium-stained liquor in labor, has been evaluated in several controlled trials. This procedure significantly decreases the rate of persistent variable decelerations of the fetal heart. It also improves more substantive outcomes, such as the rate of cesarean section (both overall and for 'fetal distress') and postpartum endometritis for the mother, and results in fewer babies with birth asphyxia, low Apgar score, or low umbilical cord pH. In the presence of meconium stained liquor, amnio-infusion also reduces the incidence of meconium aspiration syndrome. No clear adverse effects of the procedure have been noted but the trials have not been sufficiently large to exclude the possibility of uncommon but serious maternal complications.

The prophylactic use of amnio-infusion for women with intrapartum oligohydramnios but no cardiotocographic abnormalities has not shown any advantages over its therapeutic use triggered by the appearance of variable decelerations.

A third approach to the conservative treatment of persistent 'fetal distress' has been to 'treat' the fetus to prevent any adverse effects. Piracetam, a derivative of gamma-aminobenzoic acid given intravenously, is thought to promote the metabolism of the brain cells when they are hypoxic. It has been evaluated in a single placebo-controlled trial. The results suggest that piracetam treatment reduces the need for cesarean section, and improves neonatal outcome as judged by the Apgar score and neonatal 'respiratory problems and signs of hypoxia', but these results must be confirmed by other studies before the approach can be applied clinically. Pyridoxine administration during labor appears to decrease oxygen affinity in cord blood. This may have therapeutic implications, but no information is available as to is clinical importance.

Maternal oxygen administration is widely used for suspected 'fetal distress' in labor but has not been subjected to randomized evaluation.

An interesting trial, reported in 1959, which compared operative with conservative policies of management for 'fetal distress', may still be of more than historical interest. In this study, operative delivery rates for 'fetal distress' were 61% in the operative group and 20% with the conservative policy. The rate of perinatal mortality was similar in the two groups. The changes in obstetric practice and methods of fetal evaluation since this trial was carried out make it difficult to relate the results to contemporary obstetric practice. For those working in situations without modern obstetric facilities, however, it is useful to note that the ready use of operative delivery in the event of meconium-stained liquor or slowing of the fetal heart causes a considerable increase in operative deliveries, and has not been shown to reduce perinatal mortality. While these conclusions are not directly applicable today, they give cause to question the interventionist policies for the management of suspected 'fetal distress', which have become accepted practice without being subjected to randomized evaluation.

8 Conclusions

Amniotic fluid that is sparse or contains meconium is associated with an increased risk of perinatal mortality and morbidity. The status of the liquor when the membranes have ruptured spontaneously should be assessed early in labor, and the presence of meconium or low liquor volume should prompt more intensive fetal surveillance. Whether or not routine amnioscopy or artificial rupture of the membranes to assess the liquor is justified is not clear from the available evidence.

In the majority of pregnancies, intrapartum death is prevented equally effectively by intermittent auscultation and by continuous electronic fetal heart-rate monitoring, provided that intrapartum fetal heart-rate abnormalities are promptly recognized and followed by an appropriate clinical response, whatever the monitoring policy. The use of electronic fetal monitoring with fetal scalp sampling is associated with a lower rate of neonatal seizures, but not with a lower rate of serious long-term neurological disability.

Continuous electronic monitoring results in an increase in cesarean section rates and postpartum morbidity for the mother, with no compensating benefits to the baby except a decreased incidence of neonatal seizures. Whether or not it should be used will depend on the importance attached to the prevention of seizures. Selective use of electronic fetal monitoring could be based on assessment of risk by clinical history, and possibly by early intrapartum assessment.

Despite its practical problems, fetal acid-base assessment is, on the basis of current evidence, an essential adjunct to fetal heart-rate monitoring and should be much more widely used, during the second stage as well as during the first stage of labor. When electronic monitoring is used, both false-positives (false alarms) and false-negatives (a misplaced sense of confidence in the baby's welfare) are reduced by the use of fetal blood sampling as an adjunct.

Intrapartum amnio-infusion is an effective treatment for cord compression abnormalities noted in the presence of oligohydraminios. Prophylactic amnio-infusion for women with oligohydramnios but without signs of cord compression should not be used. The use of betamimetics for 'fetal distress' in labor may be a useful means of 'buying time' to permit definitive management of the situation.

A number of lessons can be learned from the trials of intrapartum electronic fetal heart-rate monitoring. First, 'more information' is not necessarily beneficial and can have harmful effects. Second, if a test result is predictive of an adverse outcome, it should not be taken as self-evident that intervention based on the results of that test will prevent or ameliorate that outcome. Third, the relationship between measures in the neonatal period and long-term outcome is not straightforward, and measures in the neonatal period may not be accurate surrogates of long-term outcome. Fourth, death and serious childhood morbidity are (thankfully) rare and very large numbers of labors must be studied if the evaluation is to be reliable. Fifth, there should be a healthy scepticism about new methods of intrapartum surveillance such that, when their development has reached the point that they are considered ready for use in clinical practice, they are introduced into clinical practice only in the context of large-scale randomized controlled trials.

Sources

Effective care in pregnancy and childbirth

Bryce, R., Stanley, F. and Blair, E., The effects of intrapartum care on the risk of impairments in childhood.

Grant, A., Monitoring the fetus during labour.

Cochrane Library

Hofmeyr, G.J., Prophylactic intravenous preloading for regional analgesia in labour.

Amnio-infusion for umbilical cord compression in labour.

Amnio-infusion for meconium-stained liquor in labour.

Prophylactice versus therapeutic amnio-infusion for oligohydramnios in labour.

Piracetam for fetal distress in labour.

Operative versus conservative management for 'fetal distress' in labour.

Maternal oxygen administration for fetal distress.

Kulier, R. and Hofmeyr, G.J., Tocolytics for suspected intrapartum fetal distress.

Mistry, R.T. and Neilson, J.P., Fetal electrocardiogram plus heart rate recording for fetal monitoring during labour.

Thacker, S.B. and Stroup, D.F., Continuous electronic heart rate monitoring versus intermittent auscultation for assessment during labour.

Other sources

Herbst, A. and Ingemarsson, I. (1994) Intermittent versus continuous electronic monitoring in labour: a randomised study. *Br. J. Obstet. Gynaecol.*, **101**, 663–8.

Mahomed, K., Nyoni, R., Mulambo, T., Kasule, J. and Jacobus, E. (1994). Randomised controlled trial of intrapartum fetal heart rate monitoring. *BMJ*, **308**, 497–500.

Westgate, J., Harris, M., Curnow, J.S. and Greene, K.R. (1993). Plymouth randomized trial of cardiotocogram only versus ST waveform plus cardiotocogram for intrapartum monitoring in 2400 cases. *Am. J. Obstet. Gynecol.*, **169**, 1151–60.

CHAPTER 31

Monitoring the progress of labor

1 Introduction

Labor is a special time, both emotionally and physically, for each woman. It is a time of intense physical activity, stress, and pain, and it may prove to be a time of overt or hidden danger. The care that a woman receives during labor should not only help her to cope with the effort, stress, and pain; it should minimize or remove the danger as well.

The purpose of monitoring the progress of labor is to recognize incipient problems, so that their progression to serious problems may be prevented. Prolonged labor can lead to adverse outcomes for both mother and baby, including maternal exhaustion, perinatal asphyxia, and even death. Inefficient uterine action can be recognized and corrected, and some adverse outcomes can be prevented. The progress of labor must be monitored with thought and consideration, rather than as an unthinking routine or a Procrustean attempt to make all women fit predetermined criteria of so-called normality (see Chapter 35).

2 Recognizing the onset of labor

Women usually make a diagnosis of labor by themselves, usually on the basis of painful, regular contractions. Sometimes they make the diagnosis after a show of mucus or blood, or after rupture of the membranes. Whether antenatal education for self-diagnosis of the onset of active labor decreases the need for intrapartum interventions and reduces other adverse outcomes is unknown.

On admission to hospital the woman's self-diagnosis of labor may, or may not, be confirmed by the professional staff. True labor must be differentiated from false labor. Whether or not true labor has started is one of the most important decisions to be made in labor care. Labor is, by definition, the presence of regular uterine contractions, leading to progressive effacement and dilatation of the cervix, and ultimately to the birth of the baby. While there is no difficulty in confirming the presence of labor when it is strong and well-established, the diagnosis is not always as clear-cut as this definition would suggest. To confirm or deny the diagnosis of labor in a woman self-admitted as 'in labor' is difficult when the cervix is uneffaced and closed. The problem may be ameliorated by the use of early-labor assessment, or triage areas, in which women who believe that they are in labor can be assessed or observed, rather than admitted (see Chapter 29). In one trial, the use of strict criteria by caregivers for the diagnosis of active labor in term pregnancy favorably affected labor outcomes by reducing the need for intrapartum oxytocics and analgesia, and the women reported greater feelings of control during labor and birth.

The time of onset of labor often is not precisely known. The most convenient and most used marker of the onset of labor for women giving birth in hospital (although an arbitrary rather than a biologically correct starting point), is the time when the woman is admitted in labor. For women who plan to give birth at home, the time at which the midwife arrives (having been called by the woman) may similarly be used. This serves as a semi-objective surrogate index of the onset of labor, and is a practical starting point from which subsequent progress can be monitored.

The point in labor at which a woman presents herself for admission to hospital, or asks her caregiver to attend, will vary from woman to woman. Several factors may influence this decision, including the way she feels, her expectations of labor, her experience in previous pregnancies, her anxiety about arriving too early or too late, and any complications that may have arisen. It will depend also on the advice that she has been given as to how and when she should recognize herself to be in labor and when to come to the hospital, which in turn will depend on the admission policy of each maternity unit. All of these factors will affect when a woman is first seen in labor and hence, the apparent length of her labor.

The timing of hospital admission may have important consequences for the progress of labor. Studies show that women who come to hospital early have more diagnoses of 'difficult labor' recorded, receive more intrapartum interventions, and more cesarean sections.

It is unlikely that any universal 'best' time will be determined for asking the midwife to attend at home or for hospital admission in labor. For most women, the 'best' time may be when they feel that they would be happier or more comfortable in hospital or with the midwife in attendance.

3 Condition of the mother

The physical and mental state, and the comfort and well-being of the woman must be just as carefully monitored during labor as the progress of contractions or the state of the cervix. The possible causes of symptoms such as nausea, dyspnea, or dizziness, should be fully assessed and treatment provided if necessary. The intensity of pain the woman experiences will determine her need for, and the timing of, pain relief. Every effort should be made to ensure that all women in labor receive continuous intrapartum support, not only from close companions, but also from caregivers specially trained to give support (see Chapter 28).

Adequate attention must be paid to the woman's physical condition. In most circumstances this will include, at least, initial assessment of her blood pressure, pulse, and temperature. Although such assessments have become traditional, there is little agreement as to how frequently they should be performed. The value, if any, of routinely repeated assessments of pulse and blood pressure in apparently normal labor is unknown. It is likely to be so small as to serve no useful purpose. In the presence of known or suspected abnormality (such as antepartum or intrapartum hemorrhage, or pre-eclampsia), such assessments should be made as frequently as necessary, or even continuously, rather than being dictated by a rigid schedule that is applied to all women.

4 Uterine contractions

Labor is initiated, and progress maintained, by contractions of the uterus. Almost always the woman herself is aware of the contractions, their frequency, duration, and strength. These parameters can be confirmed by abdominal palpation. Self-report by the woman, supplemented by abdominal examination when required, is quite sufficient to monitor the contractions in most situations.

Abdominal palpation cannot, however, accurately measure the changes in uterine pressure resulting from the contraction, and this constraint also applies to the record of uterine contractions made by an external tocodynamometer. It may provide an accurate record of the frequency and, to a lesser extent, of the duration of contractions, but not of their intensity.

The limited information available from controlled trials shows no advantage to be gained from the use of an intra-uterine pressure catheter, either in the monitoring the progress of labor or in the treatment of delays in labor progress.

5 Cervical dilatation

The rate of dilatation of the cervix is the most exact measure of the progress of labor. Cervical dilatation is usually estimated in centimetres, from 0 cm when the cervix is closed, to 10 cm at full dilatation. Assessment of cervical dilatation is not, however, as precise as one would like to believe. To our knowledge, no studies of either inter-observer or intra-observer variation have been reported, but personal experience has shown substantial variations in estimates of dilatation by different observers in the same situation, and even by the same observer on repeat examination. There is no clear guidance from the literature as to the best time to assess the dilatation in relation to a contraction, but consistent timing of observation is probably important when assessing progress.

Cervical dilatation and effacement can be assessed directly by vaginal examination or indirectly by rectal examination. Rectal examinations were advocated toward the end of the nineteenth century in the belief that, unlike vaginal examinations, they did not cause contamination of the genital tract. Several studies comparing vaginal and rectal examinations were made in the United States in the mid-1950s to 1960s; all showed a similar incidence of puerperal infection, whether rectal or vaginal examinations were employed during labor. Women's preference for vaginal rather than rectal examinations was clearly demonstrated in a randomized clinical trial. The available evidence suggests that rectal examinations have no place in monitoring the progress of labor.

There is no evidence that masks should be worn when vaginal examinations are performed. Masks have not been shown to be of value during vaginal surgery or in the delivery room, so it is highly unlikely that any infections are prevented by this practice.

The recommended frequency of vaginal examinations to assess the progress of cervical dilatation varies greatly among units and in the literature. This variation illustrates the lack of consensus for the optimal timing of vaginal examinations in labor. Like all assessments in labor, it would seem most sensible that care should be individualized. The number and timing of vaginal examinations should be frequent enough to permit adequate assessment of progress and to detect any problems promptly, but not more frequently than necessary to accomplish this end.

6 Descent of the presenting part

If the head is presenting, its relationship to the brim of the pelvis can be determined by abdominal or vaginal examination. Descent can be estimated abdominally by assessing the amount of the baby's head that is still above the pelvic brim. Abdominal assessment avoids the need for vaginal examination and is not influenced by the presence of a caput succedaneum or moulding.

On vaginal examination, the level of the presenting part can be related to the ischial spines. Moulding of the fetal head, an important observation in following the progress of labor if cephalopelvic disproportion is suspected, can also be determined by vaginal examination. Given the complementary information that can be obtained, both abdominal and vaginal examination should be carried out before any operative delivery is undertaken (see Chapter 35).

7 Normal progress in labor

Normal labor can be defined either in terms of the total length of labor or as a rate of progress of cervical dilatation (usually expressed in cm per hour); the latter measure is clinically more useful, as the total length of labor can only be known in retrospect.

A rate of 1 cm/hour in the active phase of labor is often accepted as the cut-off between normal and abnormal labor. The validity of this cut-off point can certainly be challenged. Many women who show slower rates of cervical dilatation proceed to normal birth. A rate of 0.5 cm/hour may be more appropriate as a lower limit for defining normal progress, but this too should be interpreted with discretion, in the context of the woman's total well-being.

8 Recording the progress of labor

When monitoring the progress of labor, recording the findings is almost as important as making the assessments. The primary reasons for doing so are to make the degree of progress readily apparent, so that problems will be recognized early, and to facilitate transfer of information to other caregivers. Several methods of recording measures of progress are in current use.

A time-based diary of events permits a detailed documentation of all important maternal and fetal assessments, but the recording and inspection of such a record can be tedious. It is often difficult to follow, particularly when labor is prolonged or when there is a change of staff. A more structured representation of events and progress can facilitate early recognition of potentially correctable problems.

The partogram, a structured graphical representation of the progress of labor, has been adopted in many units throughout the world and is considered by many as a necessary tool in the management of labor. In addition to the graph depicting cervical dilatation and descent of the presenting part in relation to time, space can be provided for notes on the frequency of contractions, degree of moulding, medications, the fetal heart rate, and other important events. With the use of a partogram, the progress of labor can be seen at a glance on one sheet of paper, failure to progress can be recognized readily, and the writing of lengthy descriptions can be avoided. It is simple to use, a practical teaching aid, and is an efficient means of exchange of technical information about labor progress between teams of caregivers. On the other hand, too much reliance on partograms, and especially on strict protocols of action related to partogram patterns, can be an agent for regimenting labor rather than for caring for the woman in labor.

Observational studies have reported improved pregnancy outcomes with the use of a partogram, with reduced risk of perinatal death and prolonged labor. Only recently has there been any controlled evaluation of the use of the partogram during labor. In a large multicenter trial in SE Asia, conducted by the World Health Organization, the use of the partogram with an agreed labor-management protocol reduced the incidence of prolonged labor, the proportion of labors requiring augmentation, the intrapartum stillbirth rate, and the emergency cesarean section rate.

9 Conclusions

The well-being of both the mother and the fetus must be carefully monitored during labor. This monitoring does not necessarily require the use of special equipment, but it always requires careful and individualized observation.

Monitoring the progress of labor requires more than the assessment of uterine contractions and dilatation of the cervix. The rate of progress must be considered in the context of the woman's total well-being, rather than simply as a physical phenomenon. A dilatation rate of 1 cm/h in a woman who is having strong contractions and is in severe distress, is far more worrying than a rate of 0.3 cm/hour in a woman who is comfortable, walking around, drinking cups of tea, and chatting with her companions (see Chapter 35).

Vaginal rather than rectal examination should be used to assess the progress of labor, but no more often than deemed necessary. Slow progress should alert caregivers to the possibility of abnormal labor, but should not automatically result in intervention. The use of a partogram to graphically represent the progress of labor is beneficial.

Sources

Effective care in pregnancy and childbirth

Crowther, C., Enkin, M.W., Keirse, M.J.N.C. and Brown, I., Monitoring the progress of labour.

Cochrane Library

Buchmann, E.J., Gulmezoglu, A.M. and Nikodem, V.C., Partogram for assessing the progress of labour [protocol].

Hodnett, E., Caregiver support for women during childbirth.

Lauzon, L. and Hodnett, E., Antenatal education for self-diagnosis of the onset of active labour at term.

Caregivers' use of strict criteria for diagnosing active labour in term pregnancy.

Other sources

World Health Organization Maternal Health and Safe Motherhood Program (1994). World Health Organization partograph in the management of labour. *Lancet*, 343, 1399–404.

The second stage of labor

1 Introduction

During the second stage of labor, the whole tempo and nature of activities surrounding labor tend to change. Although the principles of care throughout labor remain as a continuum, at this time women often become more vulnerable and dependent on the influence of those who assist them. Discussion about alternatives and choices is not easy at this time, and this leaves the caregiver with even more than usual responsibility to safeguard the interests of the mother and baby.

2 Diagnosis of the onset of the second stage of labor

By definition, the second stage of labor, which ends with the birth of the baby, begins when the cervix is fully dilated. This 'anatomical' onset may or may not coincide with the onset of the expulsion phase, when the mother begins to feel the urge to bear down. Some women feel the urge to bear down before the cervix is fully dilated; others may not feel this urge until well after full cervical dilatation is achieved.

The mother herself may signal the transition into the expulsive phase in words, by action, by a change in the expression on her face, or in the way she squeezes her companion's hand. If the presenting part is visible at the introitus, full cervical dilatation can be assumed. If the mother feels that she wishes to start pushing when the progress of labor gives reason to believe that the cervix may not be fully dilated, cervical dilatation should be checked by vaginal examination. If the cervix is less than 8 cm dilated, the woman should be asked to find the position in which she feels most comfortable and try to resist the urge to push by trying alternatives such as breathing techniques; epidural analgesia may be given if necessary. If there is only a rim of cervix left and the woman has an irresistible urge to push, she may feel better doing so; it is unlikely that any harm will come from this spontaneous pushing before full dilatation, as long as she does not exhaust herself.

When epidural analgesia has been administered for pain relief in labor, the urge to bear down may be reduced, delayed, or abolished. Abdominal palpation is a satisfactory way of gauging descent of the presenting part. Full dilatation can be tentatively diagnosed in this way and confirmed either by the appearance of the presenting part at the vulva or by vaginal examination.

3 Pushing during the second stage of labor

In a study of healthy nulliparous women who had received no formal childbirth education and were allowed to push spontaneously without any directions from those caring for them, three to five relatively brief (4–6 seconds) bearing-down efforts were made with each contraction. The number of bearing-down efforts per contraction increased as the second stage progressed and most were accompanied by the release of air. The minority of bearing-down efforts that were not accompanied by the release of air, were accompanied by very brief periods of breath holding (lasting less than 6 seconds). Despite this pattern of breathing, the average length of the second stage of labor was 45 minutes, and did not exceed 95 minutes for any of the 31 women studied.

The duration of breath holding (less than 6 seconds) in the women who spontaneously used this technique contrasts with the 10–30 seconds duration that is widely advocated for sustained, directed, bearing-down efforts. Although sustained bearing-down efforts accompanied by breath holding result in shorter second stages of labor, the wisdom of the commonly given advice to make these efforts can be questioned. In addition to respiratory-induced alterations in heart rate and stroke volume, maternal bearing-down efforts, particularly when the mother is lying flat on her back, are associated with compression of the distal aorta and reduced blood flow to the uterus and lower extremities. In combination with sustained maternal breath holding, these effects may compromise fetal oxygenation.

In the published controlled trials comparing different approaches to bearing down in which cord umbilical arterial pH assessments were available, mean cord umbilical arterial pH was lower (more acidotic) in the group in which sustained or early bearing down had been encouraged. Sustained bearing-down efforts also appear to predispose to abnormalities of the fetal heart rate and depressed Apgar score. When bearing down is delayed, the fetal condition should be monitored and the supine position avoided.

In women with epidural analgesia, both the first and second stages of labor are longer, and oxytocin use, malrotation and cesarean sections are more frequent. If the analgesia has not worn off before the second stage of labor, rotational forceps or vacuum deliveries are more commonly used, particularly among women who have been encouraged to bear down relatively early. There is no evidence that a policy of early bearing down has any compensating advantages for either the mother or the baby.

4 Position during the second stage of labor

The use of upright positions such as standing, kneeling, sitting on a specially designed chair, or squatting for delivery is common in many cultures. Despite this, in many hospitals women have been expected to adopt recumbent positions for childbirth. Constraining women to adopt positions that they find awkward or uncomfortable can only be justified if there is good evidence that the policy has important advantages for the health of either the mother or her baby.

Upright posture has been compared with the recumbent position during childbirth in several controlled trials. In most of these, either specially designed obstetric chairs or a back rest, wedge, or birth cushion were used to support the upright position. These studies showed that with upright postures the second stage of labor is shorter, and episodes of severe pain less frequent.

The type of support used influenced the effects of upright posture on perineal trauma and blood loss. In trials of the birth chair or stool, episiotomies were reduced but second degree perineal tears increased, as did estimated blood loss. With the birth cushion, second-degree tears and assisted deliveries were reduced, while episiotomies and post-partum hemorrhage were similar. The increased tendency to post-partum hemorrhage seen in women using birth chairs is probably due to perineal trauma, exacerbated by obstructed venous return. Excessive perineal edema and hemorrhoids have been observed in women who are upright in birth chairs for extended periods of time.

Abnormal fetal heart-rate patterns were observed less frequently among women who used an upright position. This reduction in abnormal fetal heart-rate patterns may be due to the avoidance of the aortocaval compression associated with lying down. In two trials, which compared the supine position to a 15 degree left lateral tilt, babies whose mothers were lying flat on their backs had lower umbilical cord arterial pH values.

Although some birth attendants report that upright positions sometimes caused them inconvenience, there has been a consistently positive response from the women who have used an upright position for birth.

The squatting position is not commonly used for excretion, resting, or other reasons in industrialized societies, and many people find it uncomfortable to maintain for long periods of time. The relative merits and possible disadvantages of the squatting position for birth have not yet been adequately explored. Women should be encouraged to give birth in the position they find most comfortable, with the exception that the untilted supine position should be avoided.

5 Duration of the second stage of labor

The second stage of labor has long been considered to be a time of particular risk to the fetus. Echoes of this view exist today in the widespread policies of imposing arbitrary limits on the length of the second stage.

Statistical associations have been demonstrated between prolonged second stage of labor and obviously undesirable outcomes, such as perinatal mortality, postpartum hemorrhage, puerperal febrile morbidity, and neonatal seizures, as well as with outcomes of less certain significance relating to the acid-base status of the baby at birth. On their own, these associations are not sufficient justification for concluding that the length of the second stage of labor *per se* is the crucial variable. Curtailing the length of the second stage of labor by active pushing or operative delivery can modify the decline in fetal pH that tends to occur over the course of labor. However, without some evidence that this policy has a beneficial effect on important infant outcomes, the maternal trauma and occasional fetal trauma resulting from the increased surgical interference can hardly be justified. One trial, available in abstract form only, found a shortened duration of second stage and decreased operative delivery rate with the use of an inflatable abdominal girdle during the second stage.

Decisions about curtailing the second stage of labor should be based on the same principles of monitoring the well-being of mother and baby that apply during the first stage of labor. If the mother's condition is satisfactory, the baby's condition is satisfactory, and there is evidence that progress is occurring with descent of the presenting part, there are no grounds for intervention. A single trial has assessed the use of prophylactic betamimetics with the aim of reducing fetal distress during the second stage; no positive effects were found.

Maternal exhaustion can occur at any time during labor but is more likely to occur during the second stage when the extra effort of pushing is added to the stress of the contractions. If the mother is not unduly distressed and is not actively pushing (particularly when she has epidural analgesia), there is no reason to think that the second stage is any more likely to cause exhaustion than the first stage.

Monitoring the fetal heart using intermittent auscultation may on occasions pose difficulties, as it is sometimes hard to find the fetal heart when the baby moves down into the pelvis. It can be frustrating and uncomfortable for a woman to have people continually trying to listen to her baby's heart, or to have to change her position in order to facilitate fetal auscultation. In these circumstances, electronic fetal monitoring is often more comfortable and less disruptive for the woman.

Failure of the presenting part to descend may be due to inadequate or incoordinate uterine contractions; to malposition or malpresentation of the baby; or to cephalopelvic disproportion. The cause of this failure to progress must be diagnosed and appropriately treated. Malpresentation, or minor degrees of cephalopelvic disproportion, may sometimes be overcome by encouraging the mother to vary her position. Intravenous oxytocin can be used if contractions are inadequate. Instrumental or manual manipulation, or sometimes cesarean section, may be necessary.

6 Care of the perineum

Reducing the risk of perineal trauma is important, because the consequent discomfort can dominate the experience of early motherhood and result in significant disability during the months and years that follow. This risk can be minimized by intervening to expedite delivery only on the basis of clear maternal or fetal indications, rather than 'because of the clock', and by the use of the vacuum extractor, rather than forceps when instrumental delivery is required (see Chapter 41).

Perineal damage may occur either from spontaneous lacerations or from episiotomy. Although some individual accoucheurs appear to be particularly skilful in assisting birth in a way that minimizes perineal trauma, in most hospitals at least two-thirds of all women giving birth for the first time sustain trauma sufficient to require suturing.

6.1 Guarding and massaging the perineum

The widespread practice of guarding the perineum, with the birth attendant's fingers held against the perineum during contractions, is based on the belief that this practice supports the tissues sufficiently to reduce the risk of spontaneous trauma. This is a reasonable hypothesis, especially if combined with gentle pressure applied to the fetal head to control the speed of crowning, as this is the time that the perineal tissues are most at risk of spontaneous damage. Others believe that a hands-off policy is better (except when necessary). These contrasting policies have been compared in a well-conducted randomized trial of over 5000 women. The primary outcome was perineal pain around the 10th day postpartum, and it was slightly, but significantly, less in the 'hands-on' group. The incidence of perineal trauma was similar in the two groups, as was the condition of the infant.

'Ironing out' (massaging) the perineum as the second stage of labor advances, sometimes with an emollient such as olive oil or the application of a hot pad, is designed to stretch the tissues and reduce the risk of trauma. These techniques have enthusiastic advocates, as well as detractors. The latter suggest that touch may be a disruptive distraction, and that the increase in vascularity and edema in tissues that are already at risk of trauma is counterproductive. In the only controlled comparison (released only as an abstract to date) no difference was found in the overall risk of perineal trauma, although fewer women in the perineal massage group had a third- or fourth-degree tear.

6.2 Episiotomy

If monitoring during the second stage of labor suggests that either the fetus or the mother has become distressed, or that progress has ceased, it may be necessary to hasten delivery, by episiotomy, instrumental delivery, or both. More controversial is the question of routine, or liberal use of episiotomy for less overriding indications.

Although episiotomy has become one of the most commonly performed surgical procedures in the world, it was introduced without strong scientific evidence of its effectiveness. The suggested beneficial effects of episiotomy are: a reduction in the likelihood of third-degree tears; preservation of the pelvic floor and perineal muscle leading to improved sexual function and a reduced risk of fecal and/or urinary incontinence; reduced risk of shoulder dystocia; easier repair and better healing of a straight, clean incision rather than a laceration; for the baby, reduced asphyxia, cranial trauma, cerebral hemorrhage, and mental retardation. On the other hand, a number of adverse effects of episiotomy have been suggested. These include: the cutting of, or extension into, the anal sphincter or rectum; unsatisfactory anatomic results, such as skin tags, asymmetry, or excessive narrowing of the introitus; vaginal prolapse, rectovaginal or anal fistulas; increased blood loss and hematoma; pain and edema; infection and dehiscence; and sexual dysfunction.

Liberal use of an operation with the risks described above could only be justified by evidence that such use confers worthwhile benefits. There is no evidence to support the postulated benefits of liberal use of episiotomy. Controlled trials show that restricted use of episiotomy results in less risk of posterior perineal trauma, less need for suturing perineal trauma, fewer healing complications, and no differences in the risk of severe vaginal or perineal trauma, postpartum perineal pain, dyspareunia, or urinary incontinence. The only disadvantage shown in the restrictive use of episiotomy is an increased risk of anterior perineal trauma. These results are similar for both mediolateral and midline episiotomy.

There is no evidence to support the suggestion that liberal use of episiotomy minimizes trauma to the fetal head. Data from the randomized trials show similar distributions of Apgar scores and rates of admission to the special care nursery.

Liberal and restricted use of episiotomy are associated with contrasting patterns of trauma: liberal use is associated with a lower frequency of anterior vaginal and labial tears. This raises the possibility that episiotomy may have a more specific protective effect on the tissues around the bladder neck. There is no good evidence, however, that more liberal use of episiotomy is protective against urinary incontinence. In the 3-year follow-up of a comparison of liberal with restricted use of episiotomy, rates and severity of incontinence were similar in the two trial groups.

6.3 Technique of episiotomy

Episiotomies are sometimes performed using scissors, sometimes with a scalpel. Those who favor scissors maintain that they are less likely to damage the presenting part of the baby and more likely to promote hemostasis in the wound edges because of their crushing as well as cutting action. Those who favor the scalpel say that it minimizes trauma and is thus followed by better healing of the perineal wound. There are no data on which to base any judgements about the validity of these claims.

The question of whether midline episiotomy results in a better outcome than mediolateral episiotomy has not been satisfactorily answered. The suggested advantages of performing a midline episiotomy are: better healing with improved appearance of the scar, and better future sexual function. Those not favoring the use of the midline method point out that it is associated with higher rates of extension of the episiotomy and consequently an increased risk of serious perineal trauma. In one trial, midline episiotomy was associated with less bruising, more third-degree perineal lacerations, and earlier resumption of sexual intercourse, but neither this nor a subsequent trial was methodologically sound enough to draw reliable conclusions. Well-controlled research to assess the short- and long-term advantages and disadvantages of midline and mediolateral episiotomies is long overdue.

7 Birth

Women may choose from a variety of positions for giving birth, and may change position frequently, if they are encouraged to discover for themselves which position is most comfortable for them. There is no justification for requiring, or actively encouraging, a supine or lithotomy position during childbirth; these positions are often especially painful and disruptive at this point. Women who choose to lie down for delivery often find a lateral position more comfortable.

A woman will often depend on the midwife or doctor's guidance to moderate her pushing effort, to allow an unhurried, gentle delivery of the head. This can be achieved by interspersing short pushing efforts with periods of panting, thus giving the tissues time to relax and stretch under pressure. Using this approach, several contractions may occur before the head crowns and is delivered.

After delivery of the head, the shoulders rotate internally. If the umbilical cord is tightly wound around the baby's neck, it may be possible to loosen it, then loop it over the baby's head. If necessary, it can be clamped and severed. Once rotation is complete, the shoulders are delivered one at a time to reduce the risk of perineal trauma. When the mother is in the semi-recumbent position, the anterior shoulder may deliver first; in the squatting or kneeling position, the posterior shoulder may be released first. The mother may then wish to grasp her baby and complete the rest of the delivery herself.

Difficulty with delivery of the shoulders is rare following spontaneous birth of the head. Delivery of the shoulders should not be attempted until they have rotated into the anteroposterior axis. Posterior traction on the head, combined with the mother's expulsive efforts, is usually sufficient to effect delivery of the anterior shoulder. The accoucheur should be aware of techniques to overcome the problem of shoulder dystocia on the rare occasions in which it does occur. These include wide abduction of the mother's thighs and complete flexion of her hips; manual rotation of the posterior shoulder anteriorly; and sustained pressure exerted by an assistant directly above the pubic bone.

8 Conclusions

There are no data to support a policy of directed pushing during the second stage of labor, and some evidence to suggest that it may be harmful. The practice should be abandoned.

Similarly, there is no evidence to justify forcing women to lie flat during the second stage of labor. With some reservations, the data tend to support the use of upright positions. There is a tendency for recumbency to lengthen the second stage of labor, to reduce the incidence of spontaneous births, to increase the incidence of abnormal fetal heart-rate patterns, and to reduce umbilical cord blood pH. On the other hand, at least some of the birthing chairs that have been introduced during recent years appear to predispose to perineal edema and venous engorgement which, in conjunction with perineal trauma, can result in increased loss of blood. Use of a birthing chair is not, however, the only way of adopting an upright position during labor. The mother should be encouraged to use the position that she prefers.

There is no evidence to suggest that, when the second stage of labor is progressing and the condition of both mother and fetus is satisfactory, the imposition of any upper arbitrary limit on its duration is justified. Such limits should be discarded.

There is some evidence to support the practices of guarding the perineum, but none to support claims that liberal use of episiotomy reduces the risk of severe perineal trauma, improves perineal healing, prevents fetal trauma, or reduces the risk of urinary stress incontinence after delivery. Episiotomy should be used only to relieve fetal or maternal distress, or to achieve adequate progress when it is the perineum that is responsible for lack of progress.

Sources

Effective care in pregnancy and childbirth

Sleep, J., Roberts, J. and Chalmers, I., Care during the second stage of labour.

Cochrane Library

Carroli, G., Belizan, J. and Stamp, G., Episiotomy for vaginal birth.

Hofmeyr, G.J., Tocolysis for preventing fetal distress in second stage of labour.

Howell, C.J., Epidural versus non-epidural analgesia for pain relief in labour.

Nikodem, V.C., Immersion in water during pregnancy, labour and birth.

Bearing down methods during the second stage of labour [protocol].

Pre-Cochrane reviews

Hay-Smith, J. and Renfrew, M.J., Insufflatable abdominal girdle in second stage labour. Review no. 07656.

Johanson, R., Forceps vs spontaneous vaginal delivery. Review no. 07087.

Nikodem, C., Early vs late pushing with epidural anaesthesia in 2nd stage of labour. Review no. 03403.

Sustained (valsalva) vs exhalatory bearing down in 2nd stage of labour. Review no. 03336.

Lateral tilt vs dorsal position for second stage. Review no. 03402.

Renfrew, M.J., Vacuum extraction compared to normal delivery. Review no. 06517.

Other sources

Homsi, R., Daikoku, N.H., Littlejohn, J. and Wheeless, C.R. Jr (1994). Episiotomy: risks of dehiscence and rectovaginal fistula. *Obstet. Gynecol. Surv.*, 49, 803–8.

Lede, R., Belizan, J.M. and Carroli G. (1996). Is routine use of episiotomy justified? *Am. J. Obstet. Gynecol.*, 174, 1399–402.

Mascarenhas, T., Eliot, B.W. and Mackenzie, I.Z. (1992). A comparison of perinatal outcome, antenatal and intrapartum care between England and Wales, and France. *Br. J. Obstet. Gynaecol.*, 99, 955–8.

McCandlish, R., Bowler, U., van Asten, H., Berridge, G., Winter, C., Sames, L. *et al.* (1998). A randomised controlled trial of care of the perineum during second stage of normal labour. *Br. J. Obstet. Gynaecol.*, 105, 1262–72.

Shiono, P., Klebanoff, M.A. and Carey, J.C. (1990). Midline episiotomies: more harm than good? *Obstet. Gynecol.*, 75, 765–70.

The third stage of labor

1 Introduction

After the climactic experience of giving birth to a baby, the delivery of the placenta (the third stage of labor) may seem tame and rather dull. This period is, however, a time of great potential hazard. Postpartum hemorrhage remains an important cause of maternal morbidity and mortality, particularly in developing countries. Retained placenta can necessitate manual removal; inversion of the uterus is a rare but frightening and life-threatening complication. The effects of care during this period can have important consequences. The aim of care during the third stage should be to minimize serious adverse effects, such as blood loss and retained placenta, while interfering as little as possible with physiological processes and interaction between mother and baby.

Routine or prophylactic care during the third stage involves a number of choices. The first is whether to adopt an 'expectant' (physiological) approach and manage complications only when they arise, or to take a more active, pre-emptive approach using one or more of the components of 'active management'.

Expectant management involves watchful waiting, with no use of prophylactic drugs, cord traction, or fundal pressure. Maternal effort aided by gravity suffices for delivery of the placenta, and the umbilical cord is clamped and divided after the placenta is delivered. The components of 'active management' include: prophylactic use of oxytocic drugs (either oxytocin and/or ergometrine or prostaglandins); early clamping and division of the umbilical cord; and controlled cord traction for delivery of the placenta. Some caregivers may also apply fundal pressure.

In practice the two approaches are not always as different as they may appear to be at first. Those who adopt an active approach may differ among themselves in the components they use, as may those who adopt a mainly expectant approach. As a result of this overlap, evaluation of these packages of care is difficult and the results are not always easy to interpret.

2 Components of care during the third stage

2.1 Routine prophylactic use of oxytocics
While few would dispute the valuable contribution of oxytocic drugs in the *treatment* of postpartum hemorrhage, the routine prophylactic administration of these drugs to reduce the risk of postpartum hemorrhage has not been so universally accepted.

A large number of trials, including over 8500 women, have compared those who did or did not receive prophylactic oxytocic preparations (usually in combination with other, variable, components of active management). The available data suggest that routine administration of oxytocics cuts the risk of postpartum hemorrhage in half, and reduces the therapeutic use of oxytocics by 70%.

The effect of prophylactic oxytocics on retention of the placenta is still not clear. There is some suggestion that routine administration of oxytocics increases the risk of retained placenta, but this finding may reflect selective reporting of outcome data, or may be the result of chance.

Less than half the studies provided information about hypertension as a potential side-effect of oxytocic use; those that did showed a statistically significant hypertensive effect of oxytocics. More general data on blood pressure from other studies also suggest that the prophylactic use of oxytocics, particularly ergometrine, leads to a rise in blood pressure.

The advantage of prophylactic oxytocics in terms of reduced risk of postpartum hemorrhage must be weighed against the rare but serious morbidity that has sometimes been associated with their administration. Maternal deaths from cardiac arrest and intracerebral hemorrhage have been attributed to ergometrine, as have non-fatal instances of cardiac arrest, myocardial infarction, postpartum eclampsia, and pulmonary edema. Serious morbidity related to prophylactic oxytocin is much less than with ergometrine. Because these events are so rare, the available randomized trials cannot provide meaningful estimates of the extent to which they may be attributed to oxytocic administration. Other rare adverse consequences of routine oxytocic administration include intra-uterine asphyxia of an undiagnozed second twin.

In theory, randomized trials should be able to provide useful information about more common, albeit less serious adverse effects, such as nausea and vomiting, and headaches. Unfortunately, little usable information on these is available from the trials. Apart from registering hypertensive effects, there have been few systematic attempts to quantify side-effects of oxytocic use. Ergometrine is known to lower serum prolactin levels, but few of the trials have investigated whether or not it interferes with breastfeeding. The two trials in which this was examined found no difference in breastfeeding at discharge from hospital.

Prostaglandins also have a powerful effect in stimulating uterine contractions. The injectable preparations are well established for treatment of severe or intractable postpartum hemorrhage. Their role for prophylaxis during the third stage, however, is less clear. They are expensive, and would need to be substantially better than oxytocics in order to be a cost-effective alternative. One small trial has compared intramuscular prostaglandin with placebo. This study suggests that prostaglandins may reduce the risk of postpartum hemorrhage and the need for therapeutic oxytocics, but the data are insufficient for any firm conclusions. Oral preparations are more promising, and these are discussed below.

2.2 Comparisons of different oxytocics
From the trials in which oxytocin has been compared with ergot alkaloids, usually ergometrine, the use of oxytocin was associated with a trend towards less postpartum hemorrhage, less delay in placental delivery, and fewer rises in blood pressure, although none of these differences achieved statistical significance.

Syntometrine, (a combination of ergometrine and oxytocin which was devised to take advantage of the more rapid onset effect of oxytocin and the more sustained effect of ergometrine) has a similar effect to ergot alkaloids used alone on the rate of postpartum hemorrhage. Syntometrine appears somewhat less likely than ergot alkaloids alone to be associated with a prolonged third stage. Only one small trial considered effects on blood pressure, with insufficient evidence to draw any firm conclusions.

Syntometrine reduces the risk of postpartum hemorrhage by 20% over oxytocin alone. This has been demonstrated by six trials, involving over 10 000 women. There was no apparent difference between the two drugs in the need for manual removal of the placenta or blood transfusion. Only half the studies reported possible side-effects, but in those that did Syntometrine was associated with a much higher risk of vomiting and raised blood pressure. These disadvantages may have been exaggerated by selective reporting. The few trials reporting Apgar scores, neonatal jaundice, and breastfeeding at discharge from hospital suggested no difference between the two agents on these outcomes.

Six trials with 1200 women have compared prostaglandins (intramuscular or rectal) with oxytocics. Because of the rarity of the outcome, these studies have been too small to assess whether prostaglandins are better or worse than oxytocics for minimizing the risk of postpartum hemorrhage, but they do suggest that intravenous prostaglandins may have more side-effects, such as vomiting, abdominal pain, and diarrhea. As injectable prostaglandins are also expensive, there seems little justification for further trials, particularly in developing countries. However, misoprostol, a prostaglandin analog, seems more promising. It has the advantages of being cheap, and can be used orally or rectally. A further potential benefit for developing countries is that, unlike oxytocics, it is stable at ambient temperature in tropical climates. Misoprostol is being evaluated in several ongoing trials, the largest of which is a comparison with oxytocin. The results of these studies will indicate whether misoprostol has any important advantages over oxytocics, but until these studies are complete misoprostol cannot be recommended for clinical use.

2.3 Clamping and division of the umbilical cord

Active management of the third stage of labor usually entails clamping and dividing the umbilical cord relatively early, before beginning controlled cord traction. Pre-empting physiological equilibration of the blood volume within the fetoplacental unit in this way may predispose to retained placenta, postpartum hemorrhage, fetomaternal transfusion, and a variety of unwanted effects in the neonate, respiratory distress in particular. Delayed cord clamping results in a placental transfusion to the baby, amounting to between 20% and 50% of the baby's blood volume, depending on when the cord is clamped, at what level the baby is held before clamping, and whether or not oxytocics have been administered.

Several trials have compared different timings for cord clamping. They are difficult to interpret, however, as they used varying definitions of 'early' and 'late', reported different outcomes, and some of them were methodologically weak. Earlier cord clamping leads to higher residual placental blood volumes and heavier placentas, but these observations have no clinical relevance. The trials are too small for any reliable conclusions about possible effects of the timing of cord clamping on the frequency of postpartum hemorrhage.

Early cord clamping results in lower hemoglobin values and hematocrits in the newborn, but these effects are minimal at 6 weeks of age and undetectable by 6 months after birth. Neonatal bilirubin levels are lower in the babies after early cord clamping. This seems to be reflected in more clinical jaundice following delayed clamping, but this difference is not statistically significant.

This issue is of special interest in the care of preterm babies, where early clamping is often carried out to facilitate resuscitation. Theoretical considerations suggest that a delay of as little as 30 seconds may have important clinical benefits for these babies. This suggestion is supported by results from three small trials.

Allowing free bleeding from the placental end of the cord reduces the risk of fetomaternal transfusion, which may be important with regard to blood group iso-immunization.

2.4 Controlled cord traction

Controlled cord traction involves traction on the cord, while maintaining counter-pressure upwards on the lower segment of the uterus using a hand placed on the lower abdomen. There have been two trials in which controlled cord traction was compared with less active approaches, one of which sometimes entailed the use of fundal pressure. Controlled cord traction was associated with a lower mean blood loss and shorter third stage, but the trials provide insufficient data to warrant firm conclusions about its effects on either postpartum hemorrhage or manual removal of the placenta. One of the investigators noted that the umbilical cord had ruptured in 3% of the women managed with controlled cord traction, and that women were more likely to find fundal pressure uncomfortable.

2.5 Intra-umbilical vein injection

Injection of oxytocin into the intra-umbilical vein at, or shortly after, cord clamping has been suggested as a way of encouraging placental separation, thereby speeding delivery of the placenta and reducing postpartum hemorrhage. The theory is that oxytocin stimulates contraction of uterine muscle, and/or the increased blood volume in the placenta encourages sheering from the uterine wall. The few trials evaluating intra-umbilical injection of either oxytocin or saline alone have been too small to assess the effects of these interventions on clinically important outcomes.

Intra-umbilical vein injection of oxytocin has also been compared with intramuscular oxytocin, but again these trials are too small for any firm conclusions.

2.6 Nipple stimulation

Immediate suckling after delivery to aid uterine contraction has been practised for many years, and may be used either in addition to various components of active management, or as part of expectant management. Stimulating the nipple in this way may increase release of oxytocin which may then stimulate uterine contractions, encouraging placental separation and reducing postpartum hemorrhage. A randomized trial of a policy of encouraging early suckling at deliveries attended by traditional birth attendants failed to demonstrate any reduction in postpartum hemorrhage. Alternative approaches include manual stimulation of the nipple by the woman, and breast pumps. These simple strategies for reducing the hazards of the third stage of labor merit further evaluation, particularly in developing country settings.

3 Active versus expectant management of the third stage

The effects of prophylactic oxytocics, early clamping of the cord, and controlled cord traction were considered separately in the controlled trials from which the above conclusions were drawn. If these three components are interdependent, as has been suggested, the conclusions of these trials must be viewed with caution.

Active management of the third stage (including all three of those elements) has also been directly compared to a policy of expectant, or physiological, management (which includes no prophylactic oxytocics, cord clamping after placental delivery, and no cord traction). Four out of the five trials comparing active with expectant management were carried out in centers where active management was the normal practice. The fifth was conducted in a setting where both expectant and active managements were in regular use.

In all of these trials, active management of the third stage of labor was found to be associated with important reductions (more than a halving) in the risk of postpartum hemorrhage, low hemoglobin levels postpartum, and use of blood transfusion. It was also associated with a shorter third stage and a reduction in the use of therapeutic oxytocics.

Some adverse effects have been observed. Active management results in an increase in nausea and vomiting, headache, and hypertension postpartum. Overall, manual removal of the placenta was more frequent with active management, but this effect was not statistically significant and was not observed in all trials. There was no clear effect on the risk of subsequent retained products requiring surgical removal. There was a trend towards less jaundice and fewer admissions to the special care nursery after active management, but the differences were not statistically significant and these outcomes were not reported for all trials. No effects on Apgar score at 5 min were detected. In the two trials that assessed breastfeeding, there were no differences either on discharge from hospital, or six weeks later.

Where the views of mothers have been sought, more seem to favour active management.

4 Complications of the third stage

4.1 Postpartum hemorrhage

The care for a woman with postpartum hemorrhage depends on a rapid but careful assessment of the cause, and prompt arrest of the bleeding before the situation becomes critical. If the source of the bleeding is traumatic, this will require surgical repair; if it is due to uterine atony, contraction of the uterus must be achieved by ensuring that the uterus is empty and well contracted.

Oxytocin and ergometrine have been the traditional first line approaches for achieving contraction of the uterus when the hemorrhage is due to uterine atony. Prostaglandins and prostaglandin analogs have also been used. Although the effectiveness of prostaglandins and their analogs for arresting postpartum hemorrhage due to uterine atony has not been demonstrated in controlled trials, their dramatic effect when all other measures have failed shows that these drugs are worthwhile. Injection of prostaglandins into the myometrium may obviate the need for uterine packing, internal iliac artery ligation, or even hysterectomy. Serious maternal side-effects have been reported following intramyometrial prostaglandin injection. The advantages must be weighed against the risks, and special attention paid to the doses used. More recently, rectal administration of a large dose of misoprostol (1000 mg) has been described for the management of postpartum hemorrhage. Thus far, there is little information on its effectiveness.

4.2 Retained placenta
The conventional treatment for retained placenta is manual removal following digital separation of the placenta from the uterine wall, usually under either general anesthesia, epidural, or spinal block. In areas where anesthesia is not available, analgesia with either an intravenous injection of pethidine and diazepam or paracervical block have been suggested as alternatives.

Other methods for encouraging separation of the placenta have also been proposed. The available evidence suggests that injection of oxytocin solution into the umbilical vein reduces the need for manual removal of the placenta, in comparison to either injection of saline alone or expectant management. It does not appear to affect the risk of postpartum hemorrhage. No evidence of any adverse effects of the oxytocin solution have been reported, although manual removal following oxytocin may be more difficult than usual because of a firmly contracted uterus. Trials have also evaluated the use of saline alone injected into the cord; no effect was found on the incidence of manual removal of the placenta. One trial has evaluated the injection of a prostaglandin solution into the cord, but it was too small for any conclusions to be drawn.

4.3 Inversion of the uterus
Inversion of the uterus is now very rare. It may occur as a result of excessive cord traction in the presence of a relaxed uterus, vigorous fundal pressure, or exceptionally high intra-abdominal pressure as a result of coughing or vomiting. Inappropriate cord traction without

counter-pressure to prevent fundal descent is said to result in the occasional case of uterine inversion. Treatment involves prompt replacement of the inversion, often facilitated by general anesthesia and/or tocolysis. Hemorrhage or retained placenta should then be managed as outlined above.

5 Conclusions

The routine use of oxytocic drugs in the third stage of labor will result in a reduced risk of postpartum hemorrhage, when compared with other techniques (including some components of active management) without a prophylactic oxytocic drug.

The evidence available provides no support for the prophylactic use of injectable prostaglandins or ergometrine alone. The use of Syntometrine (ergometrine + oxytocin) rather than oxytocin (10 units) is associated with a small (20%) reduction in the risk of postpartum hemorrhage, but at the cost of increased hypertension and vomiting. Prophylactic syntometrine is probably best avoided for women with pre-existing hypertension or pre-eclampsia. Otherwise, the choice of agent will depend on a balance between assessment of the woman's risk, the values attached to these competing risks, and her personal preferences.

Oral prostaglandin analogs, such as misoprostol, are promising for prophylaxis during the third stage, but cannot as yet be recommended for clinical practice. A large ongoing trial is comparing misoprostol with oxytocin.

The available evidence does not reveal any effect of early cord clamping upon blood loss or postpartum hemorrhage. Early cord clamping should be avoided in Rh-negative women, unless the placental end of the cord is allowed to bleed freely, because it increases the risk of fetomaternal transfusion. More information is needed about the effects of the timing of cord clamping for preterm babies. Simple strategies such as early suckling and nipple stimulation also merit further evaluation.

As a package, active management of the third stage has been clearly shown to have a significant protective effect against postpartum hemorrhage when compared to components of expectant management. The implications for practice depend on the relative weight placed on the different outcomes considered, and the personal preferences of the woman. In terms of postpartum blood loss, active management is clearly better. Depending on the oxytocic preparation used, however, there is an increased risk of nausea, vomiting, and hypertension. In settings where postpartum hemorrhage is particularly hazardous, active management has potentially life saving advantages. In addition to oxytocin and ergometrine, prostaglandins or a prostaglandin analog (when available) should be used for the treatment of severe intractable postpartum hemorrhage. Which preparation, dose, or route of administration is most effective has not yet been established.

Sources

Effective care in pregnancy and childbirth

Prendiville, W. and Elbourne, D., Care during the third stage of labour.

Cochrane Library

Carroli, G. and Bergel, E., Umbilical vein injection for management of retained placenta.

Gulmezoglu, A.M., Prostaglandins for prevention of postpartum haemorrhage.

McDonald, S., Prendiville, W.J. and Elbourne, D., Prophylactic syntometrine versus oxytocin for delivery of the placenta.

Prendiville, W.J., Elbourne, D. and McDonald, S., Active versus expectant management of the third stage of labour.

Other sources

Bullough, C.H., Msuku, R.S. and Karonde, L. (1989). Early suckling and postpartum haemorrhage: controlled trial in deliveries by traditional birth attendants. *Lancet*, 2, 522–5.

Irons, D.W., Sriskandabalan, P. and Bullough, C.H. (1994). A simple alternative to parenteral oxytocics for the third stage of labor. *Int. J. Gynaecol. Obstet.*, 46, 15–8.

Kinmond, S., Aitchison, T.C., Holland, B.M., Jones, J.G., Turner, T.L. and Wardrop, C.A. (1993). Umbilical cord clamping and preterm infants: a randomised trial. *BMJ*, 306, 172–5.

Nordstrom, L., Fogelstam, K., Fridman, G., Larsson, A. and Rydhstroem, H. (1997). Routine oxytocin in the third stage of labour: a placebo controlled randomised trial. *Br. J. Obstet. Gynaecol.*, 104, 781–6.

Problems during childbirth

Control of pain in labor

1 Introduction

Women experience a wide range of pain in labor, and an equally wide range of responses to it. A woman's reactions to labor pain may be modified by the environment in which she gives birth and the support she receives from her caregivers and companions (see Chapter 28), as well as by the methods of pain relief she uses. She will require accurate information to choose what is best for her, and reinforcement of her choice.

Caregivers should ask each woman, preferably before labor begins or at least before it is well advanced, what she hopes for and expects in terms of pharmacologic pain relief. Making it easier for her to achieve her wishes is an important factor in helping her to feel good about her childbirth experience. There are a great many options, both pharmacological and non-pharmacological, from which she may choose. Although epidural analgesia is the most effective method of pain control, and is the most popular method of pain control in many countries, a number of women prefer to avoid pharmacologic methods if possible. The wish to maintain personal control during labor and birth, the desire to participate fully in the experience, and concerns about untoward effects of medications during labor, are among the factors that influence their attitudes. Because they may be helpful to all women, particularly in the early stages of labor before pharmacologic options may be appropriate, we are presenting non-pharmacological options first in this chapter.

2 Non-pharmacological methods

The study of pain transmission and its modulation have produced many exciting findings, which have been applied in a variety of non-pharmacological approaches to relieving the pain of childbirth. Some of these approaches are a revival of traditional methods, while others have been newly developed. They can be usefully classified as: techniques that reduce painful stimuli; techniques that activate peripheral sensory receptors; and techniques that enhance descending inhibitory neural pathways. Many of these techniques are taught in antenatal childbirth preparation classes (see Chapter 4).

2.1 Techniques that reduce painful stimuli
The most obvious solution to the problem of pain is to avoid or reduce the stimuli that cause it. In labor, the painful stimuli arise from the

uterine contractions or from pressure exerted on the cervix, vagina, and pelvic joints by the presenting part of the fetus. They cannot be avoided but techniques to reduce these painful stimuli are at least theoretically possible. This is the intended purpose of various maternal positions, movement, counter-pressure, and abdominal decompression.

2.1.1 Maternal movement and position changes

Laboring women find that they experience less pain in some positions than in others. If left to their own devices, they will usually select the positions that are most comfortable to them. Many laboring women today are restricted to bed, either because of cultural expectations or because of obstetrical practices, such as electronic fetal monitoring, intravenous hydration, and medications that render movement out of bed difficult or unsafe.

Despite these constraints, women seem to prefer freedom of movement when it is allowed. Given encouragement to assume any position in or out of bed during the course of their labor, laboring women spontaneously adopt upright postures, such as sitting, standing, and walking, often returning to a lying-down position in advanced labor.

When the mother changes position, she alters the relationships between gravity, uterine contractions, the fetus, and her pelvis. This may enhance the progress of labor and reduce pain. For example, pressure of the fetal head against the sacroiliac joint may be relieved if the mother moves from a semi-recumbent to other postures, including 'hands and knees', lying on her side, or various upright positions. The effects of maternal position on pain are influenced by a number of factors, including the fetal size and position, the relationship between the fetal head and the maternal pelvis, and the strength of the uterine contractions. Knowing this, experienced caregivers try not to restrict women, but encourage them to seek comfortable positions, suggest possible positions, and trust the woman's judgement.

Few data from controlled trials are available about the effects of ambulation on pain relief. No effects have been demonstrated on the use of analgesia or anesthesia. A malpositioned fetal head may result in severe back pain during labor and is associated with slow progress and increased risk of operative delivery. While there are no controlled trials of their effectiveness in labor, positions which make use of gravity and/or maximize the width of the pelvis, such as hands/knees and lunging, may help to rotate the fetal head.

2.1.2 Counter-pressure

Counter-pressure consists of steady, strong force, applied to a spot on the low back during contractions, using one's fist, 'heel' of the hand, or a firm object, or of pressure on the side of each hip, using both hands. While there are no controlled trials of its effectiveness, counter-pressure appears to alleviate back pain in some laboring woman. It seems to be most effective when a woman suffers extreme back pain, often related to an occiput posterior position.

2.1.3 Abdominal decompression

Abdominal decompression (see Chapter 16) was introduced in the mid-1950s as a non-pharmacological method for shortening labor and reducing labor pain. Although anecdotal reports were positive, it has now largely disappeared from use, partly because of the lack of good evidence that it is beneficial, but also because some women found the decompression apparatus to be cumbersome, constrictive, noisy, and uncomfortable.

2.2 Techniques that activate peripheral sensory receptors

2.2.1 Superficial heat and cold

Superficial heat is generated from hot or warm objects, such as hot water bottles, hot moist towels, electric heating pads, heated silica gel packs, warm blankets, baths, and showers. Superficial cold can come from ice bags, blocks of ice, frozen silica gel packs, and towels soaked in cool or ice water.

In addition to possible direct effects on pain perception, several physiological responses elicited by heat and cold may indirectly result in pain relief. The therapeutic uses of heat and cold have not been evaluated in randomized, controlled trials. Observational evidence suggests that they may both be effective. The use of hot compresses applied to the low abdomen, groin or perineum, a warm blanket over the entire body, or ice packs on the low back, anus or perineum, relieves pain in labor for some women. As comfort measures, heat and cold are widely accepted, if not fully understood.

2.2.2 Immersion in water during labor and birth

The healing and pain-relieving properties of water – hot or cold, flowing or still, sprayed or poured – have been hailed for centuries. In recent years, immersion in water during labor and birth has aroused interest in many countries, in response to women's requests for this form of comfort. Practice varies widely and includes the use of showers, tubs, whirlpools, and specially designed 'birth pools'. Women at home may use either their own household tub or a birth pool. Some hospitals allow women to bring in a birth pool, and an increasing number of hospitals are installing tubs, pools, and/or showers. There is no consistency in the criteria developed to guide practice. Guidelines may exclude some women from using a pool because of conditions such as raised blood pressure or the need for electronic fetal monitoring. They may specify a minimum cervical dilatation before entering the water, the temperature of the water, and whether or not women are allowed to stay in the water for second stage, delivery, or third stage. These guidelines have been derived from experience and theoretical considerations, as there is currently little or no evidence on which to base them.

Advocates stress the relaxing effect of water, which may reduce the need for pharmacological methods of pain relief. Some suggest that immersion in water may accelerate labor, decrease blood pressure, increase the mother's control over the birth environment, result in less perineal trauma and intervention in general, and introduce the baby into the world gently. Critics maintain that there may be an increased risk of infection for both mother and baby, possible inhibitions of effective contractions, increased risk of perineal trauma, postpartum hemorrhage, water embolus, and trauma to the baby from a labor and/or birth in water. Caregivers, too, may be at risk from infection and back injury.

Recent case reports raise two other possible problems. The use of very hot water over several hours of labor has been linked to hyperthermia, possibly causing brain damage or death of the baby. A few baby deaths have been reported, when the baby was held under the water after birth, presumably in the belief that a slow transition from the water into air would result in a gentle introduction to life. Large well-controlled trials are needed to determine the safety and efficacy of immersion in water during birth, particularly in regard to potential neonatal complications. In the meantime, it would seem sensible to restrict the temperature of the water to body temperature or lower, and to bring the baby to the surface as soon as it is born.

Immersion in water during labor but not during birth has been assessed in four randomized trials involving more than 1400 women. No clear benefits or complications to mothers or babies were identified, although in the most recent Canadian trial, women who used the tub reported less pain after immersion, and over 80% stated that they would use the tub in subsequent labors.

2.2.3 Touch and massage

The use of touch in various forms can convey pain-reducing messages, depending on the nature and circumstances of the touch. A hand placed on a painful spot, a pat of reassurance, stroking hair or a cheek in an affectionate gesture, a tight embrace, or more formal purposeful massage of the hand or other parts of the body – all communicate to the recipient a message of caring, of wanting to be with her and help her.

The objective of massage is to make people feel better, or to relieve pain and facilitate relaxation. Massage takes the form of light or firm stroking, vibration, kneading, deep circular pressure, continual steady pressure, and joint manipulation. One may use fingertips, entire hands, or various devices, that roll, vibrate, or apply pressure. In theory, the various forms of massage stimulate different sensory receptors. When they are discontinued, the woman's awareness of her pain increases. In addition, the phenomenon of adaptation may diminish the pain-relieving effects of massage over a period of time. Therefore, use of intermittent massage, or variation in the type of stroke and location of the touch may prolong the pain-reducing effects.

None of the touch or massage techniques has been subjected to careful scientific evaluation, but the intervention seems to be harmless and is well-received by many laboring women. It can be easily discontinued if the woman wishes.

2.2.4 Acupuncture and acupressure

Acupuncture consists of the insertion of strategically placed needles in any of more than 365 points along the 12 'meridians' of the body. It is usually combined with an electrical current, which is believed to augment the pain-relieving effect. Practitioners vary in their choice of points, size of needle, and method of insertion. Acupuncture appears to block both sensory and emotional components of pain, but the mechanism is poorly understood.

No controlled trials of acupuncture during labor have been published, despite suggestions that it might provide good analgesia. The techniques involved are complex and time-consuming, and the use of multiple needles attached to electrical stimulators is inconvenient and may immobilize the woman.

Acupressure has been called 'acupuncture without needles'. The technique involves the application of pressure or deep massage to the traditional acupuncture points, with thumb, fingertip, fingernail or palm of hand. There are no published reports of its effects, either anecdotal or scientific. Acupressure can be learned and applied by a non-professional companion of the laboring woman. Well-controlled evaluation of its effectiveness would be worthwhile to establish its place (if any) as a comfort measure for labor.

2.2.5 Transcutaneous electrical nerve stimulation (TENS)

Transcutaneous electrical nerve stimulation (TENS) is a non-invasive and easy to use method, which can be discontinued quickly if necessary. Used originally for the relief of chronic pain, trauma, and post-surgical pain, transcutaneous electrical nerve stimulation has also been introduced for pain relief in labor.

The TENS unit consists of a portable, hand-held box containing a battery-powered generator of electrical impulses. A low-voltage electric current is transmitted to the skin using surface electrodes, and this results in a 'buzzing' or tingling sensation. The laboring woman may vary the intensity, pulse frequency, and patterns of stimulation, so that she can increase, decrease, or pulse the sensations as she wishes.

Safety concerns have focused on theoretically possible effects of high-intensity transcutaneous electrical nerve stimulation on the fetus' heart function, especially when electrodes are placed on the low abdomen close to the fetus. A further concern is that it may interfere with signals of electronic fetal monitors. Though no untoward effects on the fetus have been reported, there has been only one investigation of the fetal safety aspects of TENS. In 15 births, the investigators established a limit or maximum current density level at 0.5 mA/mm^2 when TENS was used in the suprapubic region. No adverse fetal effects were detected. Less concern has been raised when electrodes are placed only on the back, which is where they have been placed in most studies.

Transcutaneous electrical nerve stimulation for childbirth pain has been subjected to more controlled trials than any of the other modalities of non-pharmacological pain relief. Unfortunately, the results of the trials still remain inconclusive. In some studies, TENS has been reported to increase, rather than decrease, the incidence of intense pain, yet it was favorably assessed by the women who used it. Direct comparison of TENS and pethidine (meperidine) failed to demonstrate any differential effect on pain experienced, and the use of TENS has no obvious effect on the use of other forms of analgesia.

2.2.6 Intradermal injection of sterile water

Controlled trials have demonstrated a dramatic analgesic effect on low-back pain in labor from intradermal injection of small amounts (0.1 ml) of sterile water at four spots in the low-back area, approximately corresponding to the borders of the sacrum. This simple measure deserves further evaluation, but even on the basis of presently available data would seem worth trying.

2.2.7 Aromatherapy

Aromatherapy has been used increasingly in recent years. The term refers to the use of essential oils such as lavender, rose, camomile, and clary sage. These can be administered in a variety of ways, including in oil during a massage, in hot water as a bath or footbath, directly on a taper or a drop on the palm or forehead of the laboring woman, or applied with a hot face cloth. Oils are considered to have a number of specific properties. For example, camomile is said to be calming, and clary sage to strengthen contractions by dissipating stress and tension. Aromatherapy may also reduce stress and tension among caregivers and labor companions.

There are no trials of the use of these oils in labor, although there are reports that women find them comforting and effective. Randomized trials are needed to clarify the possible benefits and risks. For example, it would be helpful to have assessments of the effects on uterine action, on the use of other forms of pain relief, and possible adverse side-effects including allergic reactions, and (because laboring women may be acutely sensitive to smell) nausea, vomiting, and headache.

2.3 Techniques that enhance descending inhibitory pathways

2.3.1 Attention focusing and distraction

Many methods for coping with pain involve the conscious participation of the individual in attention focusing or mind-diverting activities, designed to 'take one's mind off the pain.'

Attention focusing may be accomplished by deliberate intentional activities on the part of the laboring woman. Examples include attention to verbal coaching, visualization and self-hypnosis, performing familiar tasks (such as grooming and eating), concentration on a visual, auditory, tactile, or other stimulus, and patterned breathing. While patterned breathing continues to be taught in many childbirth education programs, no controlled studies have evaluated its effectiveness. The results of a small study of patterned breathing suggest that it may increase the mother's fatigue if begun too early in labor, and should be restricted to active labor.

Distraction may be a more passive form of attention focusing, with stimuli from the environment (television or a walk out of doors) or from other people drawing a woman's attention away from her pain. It does not require as much mental concentration as deliberate attention-focusing measures, and is probably ineffective when pain is severe. Attention focusing and distraction are usually used in combination with other strategies.

2.3.2 Hypnosis

Hypnosis was introduced into obstetrics in the early nineteenth century and has been used in various ways ever since. It is defined as 'a temporarily altered state of consciousness, in which the individual has increased suggestibility'. Under hypnosis, a person demonstrates physical and mental relaxation, increased focus of concentration, ability to modify perception, and ability to control normally uncontrollable physiological responses, such as blood pressure, blood flow, and heart rate.

Hypnosis is used in two ways to control pain perception in childbirth: self-hypnosis and post-hypnotic suggestion. Most hypnotherapists teach self-hypnosis, so that women may enter a trance during labor and reduce awareness of painful sensations. Among the techniques used are: relaxation; visualization (helping the woman imagine a pleasant, safe scene and placing herself there, symbolizing her pain as an object that can be discarded, or picturing herself as in control or free of pain); distraction (focusing on something other than the pain); and glove anesthesia (through suggestion, creating a feeling of numbness in one of her hands, and then spreading that numbness wherever she wishes by placing her numb hand on the desired places of her body). The woman is taught to induce these techniques herself; only rarely do hypnotherapists accompany their clients in labor.

Other therapists rely almost completely on post-hypnotic suggestion. These hypnotherapists do not teach their clients to enter a hypnotic state routinely during labor, because they will not need to. Most women, they claim, will be comfortable as a result of the effectiveness of the post-hypnotic suggestions. Exceptions to this are circumstances such as forceps delivery or episiotomy and repair, for which it would be necessary to go into a trance.

To date, only one randomized trial of hypnosis in labor has been reported. There was no difference in analgesia use between the experimental and control groups. The mean duration of pregnancy and the mean duration of labor were both statistically significantly longer in the hypnosis group.

Hypnosis had lost its popularity among obstetricians by the early 1970s, probably due to the development of better methods of anesthesia and to the amount of time required for adequate hypnosis preparation.

2.3.3 Music and audio-analgesia

Music and audio-analgesia are used to control pain in numerous situations, including dental work, post-operative pain, treatment of burns, and occasionally in childbirth. Many childbirth educators use music in antenatal classes to create a peaceful and relaxing environment, and also advocate it for use during labor as an aid to relaxation.

Audio-analgesia for pain relief in obstetrics consists of the use of soothing music between contractions combined with 'white sound', the volume of which is controlled by the laboring woman, during contractions. The only published placebo-controlled trial of audio-analgesia noted a trend towards better pain relief in the audio-analgesia group, but the effect was confined to primigravidae, and was not statistically significant. As the 'placebo' consisted of a lower intensity of white sound, which might have had pain-relieving qualities in itself, a true benefit of the audio-analgesia might have been masked. A number of other investigators reported a decreased use of analgesic medication and less pain with the use of audio-analgesia in non-randomized cohort studies. These results, though equivocal, merit further better controlled trials.

The pleasing qualities of music may offer an added dimension beyond the distraction brought about by white sound. Music creates a pleasant and relaxing ambience, and music transmitted through earphones can block out disturbing, distracting, or unpleasant sounds. When carefully chosen, music may be used to reinforce rhythmic breathing patterns and massage strokes, or to facilitate visualizations and induction of hypnosis. Thus, music may have the potential to reduce stress and to enhance other pain-relieving measures. Music may also elicit more relaxed and positive behavior from the staff and from the woman's chosen companions.

The few small studies of the pain-relieving effects of music in labor have found positive effects. These small studies of childbirth pain, when combined with findings of the effects of music or auditory stimulation on other types of pain (e.g. postoperative pain, dental pain, pain associated with burn therapy), suggest that music has the capacity to reduce pain, at least in some circumstances. Given that there are no known risks associated with the use of music during labor, and that music preferences vary widely, women who believe some form of music may be helpful should be encouraged to try it.

2.3.4 Biofeedback

Trials of electromyographic biofeedback taught during prenatal classes failed to demonstrate any significant effect on the use of pharmacological analgesia or other interventions during childbirth.

3 Pharmacological control of pain in labor

Pharmacological control of pain in childbirth has a long history. The use of opiates was mentioned in early Chinese writings; the drinking of wine was noted in the Persian literature; and wine, beer, and brandy were commonly self-administered in Europe during the Middle Ages. Various concoctions and potions have been used over time, some inhaled, some swallowed, and some applied to the laboring woman's skin.

There have been more clinical trials of pharmacological pain relief during labor and childbirth than of any other intervention in the perinatal field. The benefits of pain relief are obvious, but the possible adverse effects on the mother or infant have received little attention in this research. The clinically important question is 'what method will achieve an acceptable degree of pain relief while least compromising the health of the mother and child?'

3.1 Regional analgesia and anesthesia

Over the past 20 years, techniques of regional analgesia have emerged as the major approach to pain relief in obstetrics, not only for labor, but for operative vaginal deliveries and for cesarean section as well. There are many reasons for the popularity of regional analgesia. The most important are that it is more effective in relieving pain than other agents, and that the mother remains conscious.

3.1.1. Epidural analgesia

The 'gold standard' for pain control in labor is analgesia or anesthesia via the epidural route. Regional anesthetic agents (bupivicaine, xylocaine, etc.) and opioid analgesics (fentanyl, sufentanyl, etc.) may be administered alone or in combination via the epidural route. When complete or partial motor blockade is the desired goal, local anesthetics are administered. When analgesia without total motor blockade is the goal, lower doses of local anesthetics are administered, sometimes preceded by, or in combination with, opioids.

Eleven randomized controlled trials have compared epidural analgesia with other forms of analgesia during labor and birth. Epidural analgesia provides better and more lasting pain relief in the first stage of labor, although a few women fail to obtain adequate relief. Adverse effects of epidural analgesia suggested by these rather small trials include increased length of first and second stage labor, increased use of oxytocin to augment labor, and greater likelihood of fetal malposition and instrumental vaginal delivery. The meta-analysis also shows a strong trend toward increased cesarean delivery with epidural analgesia.

The timing of epidural analgesia may be important, as the increase in operative delivery rates in these trials were found only in women who had epidural analgesia in early labor. Further study is required to confirm or refute this, since there are as yet no randomized studies to address this important question. The increased risk of instrumental delivery associated with epidural analgesia may be reduced by careful timing of top-up doses and a liberal attitude to length of the second stage of labor. Comparisons of early versus delayed pushing in second stage under epidural analgesia suggest that delaying pushing until the fetal head is visible at the introitus will lower the risk of operative delivery.

A number of complications of epidural analgesia have been reported, including inadvertent dural puncture, hypotension with associated nausea and vomiting, localized short-term backache, shivering, and prolonged labor, as well as increased use of operative vaginal delivery and cesarean section. Rare complications include neurological sequelae, toxic drug reactions, respiratory insufficiency, and maternal death. As yet unproven, but possible complications are bladder dysfunction, chronic headache, long-term backache, tingling and numbness, and 'sensory confusion'. Randomized comparisons will be needed to confirm or refute these observations.

Inadvertent puncture of the dura during the placement of an epidural block may result in severe, often incapacitating, headache. The use of a prophylactic epidural blood patch is highly effective in reducing the incidence of post-dural puncture headache. Unfortunately, no data about possible long-term effects are available. Patient characteristics such as HIV status or sepsis may contra-indicate the use of a blood patch. Epidural saline or dextran are alternatives when epidural blood patch is unsuccessful or contra-indicated. Epidural morphine has been suggested as an alternative to epidural blood patch for primary therapy, with blood patch reserved as a second-line modality. Other drugs that appear to be effective include oral or intravenous caffeine, theophyllin, and sumatriptan. While there are numerous observational studies and case reports, there are few controlled trials of the various suggested treatments. Little is known about the effects of epidural analgesia on the fetus and newborn. The fetus may suffer complications as a result of maternal effects (e.g. hypotension) or direct drug toxicity, although it may benefit from increased placental blood flow. No differential effects on fetal heart-rate abnormalities or passage of meconium during labor were detected in the few trials in which these outcomes were reported. One trial compared epidural analgesia with paracervical block, and found that babies born to mothers who received the epidural analgesia were more likely to experience hypoglycemia. Further trials are need to confirm or refute this observed effect.

The dose of local anesthetic used for epidurals may vary significantly among hospitals. Numerous trials, usually involving small numbers of women, have compared dose regimens of various anesthetic agents. The effort spent on these trials is disproportionate to their value, in view of the importance of clarifying the safety and efficacy of the method itself as compared to the effects of specific drugs or dose regimens. Some caregivers believe that low dose epidural analgesia will reduce the need for operative delivery by promoting freedom of movement during labor and birth, and by avoiding relaxation of pelvic musculature. To date, several trials comparing low dose with standard epidural analgesia have failed to find differences in operative delivery rates. However, while women were permitted to ambulate in the trials, they spent little time out of bed.

Epidural analgesia can be administered either by continuous administration with an infusion device or by intermittent 'top-up' doses, by way of an indwelling catheter. In either case, care must be taken to ensure that the height of the block is carefully monitored. When used as a top-up technique, regularly scheduled top-ups provide better pain relief than top-ups on maternal demand.

In healthy women, there is evidence from one controlled trial that preloading with intravenous fluids is an effective means of reducing the incidence and extent of the hypotension that so commonly occurs with epidural analgesia in labor. The relative risks and benefits of fluid preloading before epidural anesthesia in the presence of pregnancy complications, such as pre-eclampsia and cardiac disease, require further evaluation.

Epidural administration of opioids appears to potentiate the analgesic effect of the local anesthetic. Unwanted effects of epidural opioids include pruritus, urinary retention, and delayed respiratory depression in the mother.

Almost no data from randomized trials are available to explore the possible long-term effects of epidural analgesia on either mother or baby. Observational studies of long-term maternal problems have suggested that epidural analgesia may increase the likelihood of chronic backache, headache, bladder problems, tingling and numbness, and sensory confusion, but these effects have not been investigated in the randomized trials. A single report of neurobehavioral assessments of 18-month-old children failed to detect differences between the epidural and non-epidural groups at this age.

In summary, epidural analgesia is a more effective form of pain relief than alternative forms of analgesia, but it increases the likelihood of operative delivery. Little more can be deduced with confidence about its effects from currently available information. It is particularly worrying that there are so few experimentally-derived data available to assess its effects on infants or its long-term effects on the mother. Hospitals that have 24-hour epidural analgesia services have very low rates of narcotic analgesia usage in labor, but one cannot infer from this that epidural is, on balance, superior to other forms of pharmacologic pain relief.

Where resources permit the various pain-relief options to be available, women's informed preferences should guide decisions about what and how much to use. Women should be made aware that one form of care with no known risks (continuous labor support), reduces the likelihood that they will need pharmacologic pain relief in labor (see Chapter 28).

3.1.2 Other routes of regional analgesia

Combined spinal/epidural techniques (intrathecal opiates in the first stage of labor, followed by epidural bupivicaine later in labor) have become popular in some hospitals. As with epidural opiates, mothers may develop side-effects of pruritus, nausea and vomiting, and urinary retention, with respiratory depression in the early postpartum period.

There has been a recent upswing in interest in the use of spinal anesthesia due to the introduction of new, smaller gauge needles, which are reported to result in fewer dural puncture headaches.

Caudal block is rarely used today for labor analgesia. It requires a larger dose of the anesthetic agent, results in more blocked neural segments, and the spread of the anesthetic is less easily controlled than with the usual form of epidural analgesia. Failures occur in 5–10% of women due to variation in sacral anatomy. The only advantage of the caudal approach over the lumbar epidural technique is the decreased likelihood of dural puncture. There may be some useful applications for caudal block for perineal analgesia, but these have yet to be evaluated.

Paracervical block provides adequate analgesia and has the advantage that it can be administered by the obstetrician, thus avoiding the need for anesthetic personnel. This form of analgesia was popular in the 1950s and 1960s, but has fallen out of favor because of reports of fetal bradycardia, acidosis, and fetal death associated with its use.

3.2 Systemic agents

3.2.1 Opioids

Systemic opioids (such as pethidine) can provide some pain relief, but can have unwanted side-effects. As these effects are dose-related, the amount of analgesia achievable is limited by the side-effects of the drug. Maternal side-effects include orthostatic hypotension, nausea, vomiting, dizziness, and delayed stomach emptying. Opioids cross the placenta and this may cause respiratory depression in the baby. Trial data have shown lower Apgar scores and more neonatal behavioral abnormalities in babies of mothers who received narcotic analgesia in labor than in babies of mothers who received a placebo.

There have been 16 trials comparing different opioids and different doses of opioids. Because of methodological problems and lack of consistency in reporting outcomes, it is not possible to draw conclusions about the superiority of any one drug or any dose.

Self-administered intravenous pethidine results in better pain relief and a lower total dose of narcotic, than intramuscular pethidine administered by a caregiver. This suggests that self-administration may be preferable, at least for women who are already receiving an intravenous infusion.

Narcotic antagonists (Naloxone, nalorphine, or levallorphan) have been administered to counteract the depressant effects of opioids, either with each dose of narcotic, or 10–15 min before delivery. The rationale was to provide analgesia with minimal respiratory depression, but narcotic antagonists also reverse the analgesic effects of the narcotics. After birth, there is a role for administration of narcotic antagonists (Naloxone in particular) to neonates depressed by narcotics.

3.2.2 Sedatives and tranquilizers

While once a popular choice of clinicians, in the belief that they reduced anxiety and promoted sleep in early labor, sedatives and tranquilizers are rarely prescribed during labor today. The barbiturates (secobarbital, pentobarbital, and amobarbital) are no longer popular for use in obstetrics because they have no analgesic properties, and because they may have a profound depressant effect on the newborn. They are still used for their sedative effect in some countries in the early latent phase of labor. Diazepam (a benzodiazepine) can cause neonatal respiratory depression, hypotonia and lethargy, and hypothermia.

3.3 Inhalation analgesia

Once popular in many countries, the use of inhalation analgesia in labor has been decreasing in recent years, primarily because it does not provide reliable or complete pain relief. Side-effects of nausea and vomiting, as well as the possibility of aspiration of gastric contents in cases of accidental overdose, further decrease the usefulness of the method. It is no longer available in many settings because of concerns about possible long-term effects of exposure to inhalation agents on the medical and nursing staff.

The advantages of inhalation analgesia are that the mother remains awake and in control of the analgesia; that neither uterine activity nor 'bearing down' during the second stage is affected; that the duration of effect is short, which allows better control; and that no clinically important side-effects on the mother or fetus have been noted.

The most commonly used inhalation analgesia agent is nitrous oxide, usually in a 50% concentration with 50% oxygen. Trials comparing 50% with 70% nitrous oxide administration showed no significant differences in pain relief in normal labors. Other inhalation analgesic agents (methoxyflurane, enflurane, isoflurane, trichloroethylene) have also been employed, but their use has been curtailed or eliminated because of the difficulty of providing adequate analgesia without inducing general anesthesia, with its inherent dangers in labor.

4 Conclusions

Satisfaction in childbirth is not contingent upon the absence of pain. Many women are willing to experience some pain in childbirth, but they do not want the pain to overwhelm them. For women whose goals for childbirth include the use of measures to manage pain with minimal drug use, and for those who have little or no access to pharmacological methods of pain relief, the non-pharmacological methods of analgesia in childbirth, in combination with continuous support, are useful alternatives. They cannot match epidural analgesia for analgesic effectiveness, but they seem to help some women and are not likely to have harmful side-effects.

Systemic opioids can reduce pain in labor, although they do not provide as effective pain relief as epidural analgesia. Their use in effective doses is limited by their side-effects of maternal drowsiness, nausea and vomiting, and neonatal respiratory depression. These effects, plus their effect in delaying stomach emptying, must be kept in mind, particularly if general anesthesia might be required for delivery. Self-administered intravenous opioids appear to give better pain relief with lower doses than does intermittent use, although the lack of availability of suitable infusion devices may limit widespread use.

Barbiturates have no analgesic effect. Diazepam can result in neonatal respiratory depression, hypotonia and hypothermia. Inhalation agents, such as 50% nitrous oxide in oxygen, are only moderately effective analgesics, but are simple to use, have a short duration of action, and are under the control of the mother. No major side effects have been noted.

Remarkably little is known about the short-term and long-term effects of epidural analgesia during labor, on women and their babies. All that can be concluded with confidence is that epidural analgesia is likely to provide more effective pain-relief during labor than alternative methods, but may result in a substantial increase in operative delivery. We need better designed trials of epidural analgesia, which examine important questions about both short- and long-term effects on the mother and baby. In view of the many important unanswered questions about the effects of epidural analgesia during labor, more randomized comparisons with alternative methods of pain relief are required.

Consideration of the needs of each individual laboring woman, along with knowledge of the analgesic effectiveness and the adverse side-effects of each form of analgesia, will help the woman to make an informed choice among the alternatives available to her.

Sources

Effective care in pregnancy and childbirth

Dickersin, K., Pharmacological control of pain during labour.

Simkin, P., Non-pharmacological methods of pain relief during labour.

Cochrane Library

Elbourne, D. and Wiseman, R.A., Types of intra-muscular opioids for maternal pain relief in labour.

Hodnett, E.D., Caregiver support for women during childbirth.

Hofmeyr, G.J., Prophylactic intravenous preloading for regional analgesia in labour.

Howell, C.J., Epidural versus non-epidural analgesia for pain relief in labour.

Nikodem, C., Immersion in water during pregnancy, labour, and birth.

White, G.E., Diazepam for pain relief in labour [protocol].

Other sources

Carroll, D., Tramer, M., McQuay, H., Nye, B. and Moore, A. (1997). Transcutaneous electrical nerve stimulation in labour pain: a systematic review. *Br. J. Obstet. Gynaecol.*, 104, 169–75.

Choi, A., Laurito, C.E. and Cunningham, F.E. (1996). Pharmacologic management of postdural puncture headache. *Ann. Pharmacother.*, 30, 831–9.

Christensen-Szalanski, J. (1984). Discount functions and the measurement of patients' values. Women's decisions during childbirth. *Med. Decis. Making.*, 4, 47–58.

Maresh, M., Choong, K. and Beard, R.W. (1983). Delayed pushing with lumbar epidural analgesia in labour. *Br. J. Obstet. Gynaecol.*, 90, 623–7.

Russell, R. and Reynolds, F. (1996). Epidural infusion of low-dose bupivicaine and opioid in labour. Does reducing motor block increase the spontaneous delivery rate? *Anaesthesia*, 51, 266–73.

Simkin, P. (1995). Reducing pain and enhancing progress in labor: a guide to nonpharmacologic methods for maternity caregivers. *Birth*, 22, 161–71.

Vause, S., Congdon, H.M. and Thornton, J.G. (1998). Immediate and delayed pushing in the second stage of labour for nulliparous women with epidural analgesia: a randomised controlled trial. *Br. J. Obstet. Gynaecol.*, **105**, 186–8.

Prolonged labor

1 Introduction

Slow progress in the first stage of labor can occur in either the latent or active phase. It does not necessarily mean abnormal labor or the presence of a problem. It should, however, draw attention to the possibility of a problem and be an indication for further assessment, including the possible need for intervention.

Attention devoted to the prevention of prolonged labor is at least as worthwhile as the attention that is usually devoted to its cure. Friendly support and allowing women to move about as they please have been demonstrated to be effective. Both of these measures may be seen as characteristics of a welcoming environment, rather than as specific interventions. (see Chapter 28).

2 Prolonged labor

2.1 Prolonged latent phase
The latent phase of labor, from the start of uterine contractions until progressive dilatation of the cervix commences (usually from about

4-cm dilatation onwards), is poorly understood. As this phase usually starts before the woman is admitted to hospital, its precise time of onset is often difficult to determine. The duration of the latent phase varies so widely from woman to woman that a normal range is difficult to define. According to some studies, a prolonged latent phase is not associated with increased perinatal morbidity, mortality, or other adverse outcome. Other studies have shown a significantly higher incidence of cesarean section and lower 5-min Apgar scores, in both primigravidae and multigravidae, with a prolonged latent phase. Whether these adverse effects were due to the underlying condition or the result of injudicious treatment is uncertain.

Differentiating between a prolonged latent phase and false labor is often difficult. This distinction can only be made in retrospect. There is an urgent need for controlled studies about this common, distressing, and poorly understood problem in labor, its etiology, its significance, and the best policy of care.

2.2 The diagnosis of the active phase of labor

When active labor is mistakenly diagnosed, failure of the cervix to dilate within a prescribed period of time results in the erroneous diagnosis of dystocia. Mothers may feel inadequate because of not achieving the expected progress, and may lose confidence in their caregivers when a diagnosis of active labor is made in error. Interventions to stimulate labor and cesarean sections for dystocia are sometimes performed before the establishment of true labor (see Chapter 31).

2.3 Prolonged active phase

Slow progress or failure to progress in the active phase of labor can be defined either as an overall measurement (e.g. longer than 'x' hours), or as a rate-related measurement (e.g. a rate of cervical dilatation of less than 'y' cm/hour). The commonly cited 12-hour duration of the active phase is roughly equivalent to a rate of 0.5 cm/hour, half as fast as the 1 cm/hour that is also commonly used. The diagnosis of slow progress depends on careful documentation of the labor progress, preferably by plotting changes in cervical dilatation and descent of the head on a labor graph.

Deviation from this arbitrarily defined 'normal' rate of dilatation should be an indication for evaluation rather than for intervention. While there is certainly an association between prolonged labor and adverse outcome, the extent to which the relationship is causal is by no means certain.

Cephalopelvic disproportion must be considered when progress in labor is slow. Intrapartum x-ray pelvimetry has not proven to be useful for women with the fetus in a cephalic presentation. The available controlled trials show a significant increase in cesarean section or symphisiotomy rates with the use of intrapartum x-ray pelvimetry, but no significant benefits in terms of reduced neonatal morbidity. The diagnosis of cephalopelvic disproportion is made by excluding functional causes (uterine hypotonia) for slow progress in labor. Uterine contractions of adequate intensity must be assured, by stimulation if necessary, before this diagnosis can be made. If gross cephalopelvic disproportion, possibly suggested by marked moulding of the fetal skull, is present, a cesarean section is necessary.

Epidural analgesia may be associated with an increase in the length of the first and second stage of labor, the need for oxytocin, the incidence of fetal malposition, the use of instrumental delivery if the block is maintained beyond the first stage of labor, and the need for cesarean section for failure to progress.

3 Prevention and treatment of prolonged labor

Protracted labor has been recognized as a problem for centuries, and a bewildering variety of treatments has been proposed to correct the condition. The assumption underlying all these treatments is that, in some way, 'inadequate' progress is bad and that 'something should be done about it'. In the past, proposed remedies have included homeopathic medications, various spasmolytic drugs, sparteine sulphate, estrogens, relaxin, caulophyllum, dimenhydrate, nipple stimulation, intracervical injections of hyaluronidase, vibration of the cervix, and acupuncture. The most commonly used measures today are amniotomy (artificial rupture of the membranes) and intravenous oxytocin infusion.

Many factors can influence uterine contractions and the progress of labor. Consideration of these factors suggests a number of measures that can help to prevent prolonged labor and obviate much of the need for augmentation. The presence of a supportive companion and ambulation during labor have been shown to result in shorter labors and a lesser use of oxytocics.

When more active intervention is required, this may consist of measures to increase the power of the uterine contractions, or to reduce the degree of resistance to cervical dilatation and descent of the presenting part.

3.1 Increasing uterine contractility

There is a close relationship between low levels of uterine contractility and slow progress in labor. Treatments to increase uterine contractility may be based either on increasing the endogenous production of prostaglandins by amniotomy or the administration of uterine stimulants, such as exogenous oxytocin or prostaglandins.

3.1.1. Amniotomy

A policy of early amniotomy leads to a reduction, on average, of between 60 and 120 minutes in the duration of labor, and also to a reduction in the incidence of dystocia (defined as a mean rate of dilatation less than 0.5 cm/hour). In one trial, the reduction in labor duration was limited to primiparous women. Oxytocin augmentation is used less frequently after early amniotomy. No effects of early amniotomy have been noted on the use of analgesia or rates of instrumental vaginal delivery. Early amniotomy was associated with a trend to increased use of cesarean section, possibly related to increased diagnosis of fetal distress. In a recent trial, early amniotomy was associated with an increased rate of fetal heart-rate abnormalities.

The effects of early amniotomy on the baby are also open to interpretation. Meta-analysis of the controlled trials shows that early amniotomy is associated with fewer low 5-minute Apgar scores but has no effect on the incidence of low arterial cord pH. There is a non-significant trend toward an increase in the frequency of cephalhematoma and meconium aspiration. A variety of adverse effects have been postulated but they have not been confirmed by controlled studies. The studies that purported to show these harmful effects of amniotomy on the fetus and neonate were all subject to considerable selection bias, precluding an adequate assessment of the effects of amniotomy.

In HIV-infected women, observational studies indicate that ruptured membranes for more than 4 hours before delivery increases the risk of neonatal infection. On this basis, amniotomy may be dangerous for the babies of these women.

In the studies that assessed mothers' views of the policy of membrane management, there was no evidence that the differences in policy affected the mothers' opinions. However, a policy of early amniotomy is associated with a statistically significant reduction in the risk of experiencing 'horrible or excruciating' pain at some time in labor.

None of the reported studies specifically addressed the question of whether or not amniotomy is effective in augmenting slow or prolonged labor. Given the evidence that is available from the controlled trials in spontaneous labor, and from the data on induction of labor, it is highly likely that amniotomy would enhance progress in prolonged labor as well.

3.1.2 Oxytocin

Intravenous infusion of synthetic oxytocin, usually after either spontaneous or artificial rupture of the membranes, is the most widely used treatment to expedite labor when progress is deemed to be inadequate. Despite this, there is remarkably little evidence about the effects of oxytocin from controlled trials.

The effect of oxytocin stimulation on duration of labor is still not clear. Of three earlier trials that provide data on the length of labor when intravenous oxytocin infusion was used in cases of poor progress, only one showed a shorter mean duration in women allocated to early oxytocin augmentation compared with controls. In one trial in which women in the control group were encouraged to get up and to move around, stand, or sit as they wished, the mean duration of labor was slightly shorter in the control group than in the augmented group. A recent small trial showed improved labor progress with oxytocin.

There is no evidence from these trials that a policy of early oxytocin use influences the method of delivery.

Neither Apgar scores nor the incidence of admission to a special care nursery were detectably different between oxytocin augmentation and control groups in the trials that reported on these outcomes. No other categorical data on infant outcomes are available from controlled trials.

In one study, over half of the women asked about their opinion on the oxytocin treatment said that it was unpleasant and indicated that they would like to try without the drug when next giving birth. Over 80% felt that it had increased the amount of pain that they had experienced, whereas less than 20% of the women in the ambulant group felt that walking about had increased their pain. Conversely, in a recent trial women expressed a preference for active management when poor progress of labor was diagnosed.

From the data available thus far, it is not clear that liberal use of oxytocin augmentation in labor is of benefit to the women and babies so treated. This does not imply that there is no place for oxytocin augmentation in slow progress of labor. In the earlier controlled trials, a high proportion of the women assigned to be controls ultimately received oxytocin for subsequent failure to show adequate progress in labor (as defined by the authors). These studies thus indicate that many women who are not treated early with oxytocin for inadequate progress, will still receive an oxytocin infusion before delivery. It does suggest, however, that other simple measures, such as allowing the woman freedom to move around and to eat and drink as she pleases, may be at least as effective and certainly more pleasant for a sizeable proportion of women considered to be in need of augmentation of labor.

Situations will undoubtedly remain in which pharmacological augmentation will be necessary to correct inadequate uterine activity, in order to prevent maternal exhaustion, and risks of fetal and maternal infection. Logic would dictate that, in such circumstances, the smallest effective drug dose be given, in the most effective manner. As individual sensitivity to oxytocin varies greatly from woman to woman, oxytocin titration by means of an intravenous infusion is the treatment of choice. It is less clear, however, what the initial dose should be, how large the increments should be, and at what interval they should be implemented. Little data are available to answer these questions.

Two principles should guide the clinician when using oxytocin to augment labor: first, to avoid hyperstimulation; second, that the therapeutic trial should be sufficient to minimize the risk of a false diagnosis of cephalopelvic disproportion. Insufficient doses will take an unacceptably long time to achieve an adequate response, while excessive doses will result in hyperstimulation.

Slow progress in cervical dilatation is not necessarily due to subnormal levels of uterine activity. The level of activity that is needed both to ensure adequate progress and to avoid hyperstimulation has not yet been established. A major additional factor in the rate of progress of labor is the amount of resistance that must be overcome.

3.1.3 Active management of labor

The term 'active management of labor' was introduced to describe a comprehensive program of care in labor, the key elements of which include, in addition to strict diagnostic criteria for labor, early amniotomy, early use of oxytocin, and continuous professional support.

Uncontrolled studies have suggested that liberal use of both amniotomy and oxytocin augmentation may be instrumental in achieving low cesarean-section rates. This may well prove to be the case but it has not been demonstrated by the results of the published controlled trials. Two published trials showed a small and statistically insignificant reduction in the cesarean-section rate; the others showed no effect. The results for other outcomes (use of epidural, neonatal morbidity) also showed no effects of the policy. Unfortunately, the total number of women included in these trials is too small to give a clear indication of the effect of active management of labor on the rates of cesarean section or operative vaginal delivery. Analysis of studies of the various components of 'active management of labor' has found evidence of improved outcome for labor support but not for the other two main components of active management: early amniotomy and oxytocin use.

3.2 Influencing resistance

Between a third and a half of the women with slow progress in labor have levels of uterine activity usually judged to be adequate. One care alternative for these women would be the use of high doses of oxytocin, to augment uterine activity to levels well in excess of those encountered during normal spontaneous labor. A more logical approach would be to reduce cervical resistance.

Three methods to influence resistance in order to accelerate cervical dilatation have been tested in controlled trials: the use of intravenous or intramuscular porcine relaxin; local cervical injections of hyaluronidase; and cervical vibration. The trials did not demonstrate any advantage from the use of these modalities. Observational studies, however, have suggested that vibration may be useful when cervical dilatation is not achieved despite satisfactory uterine activity in the absence of cephalopelvic disproportion, and that the procedure appears to be safe. Evaluation awaits a controlled trial of adequate size.

Despite the fact that their use would seem reasonable, measures to reduce soft tissue resistance have not been adequately explored.

4 Conclusions

Slow progress or lack of progress in the first stage of labor usually, but not necessarily, results from a lower level of uterine contractility than that seen in normally progressing labors. It may be due to a higher resistance in the soft parts of the birth canal or to cephalopelvic disproportion. It will often be necessary to ensure that adequate uterine contractility exists, if necessary by oxytocic stimulation, in order to differentiate these dissimilar mechanisms. Every effort should be made to correct uterine hypotonia before resorting to cesarean section for dystocia.

It is too early to recommend active management of labor on the basis of currently available evidence. Approximately half of the women judged to have slow labor or poor progress in cervical dilatation will progress equally well whether or not oxytocic drugs are administered. When augmentation becomes necessary, the first approach should be to rupture the membranes. The data that are available suggest that amniotomy will shorten the length of spontaneous labor and that it may forestall the need for oxytocin infusion in some of these women. Moreover, the combination of amniotomy with oxytocin may provide a better stimulation of labor than oxytocin alone. A possible exception is HIV-infected women, because of the possible increased risk of neonatal infection.

There is no evidence that high and rapidly escalating doses of oxytocin confer any advantage over a more moderate approach in which small doses are increased at half-hourly intervals in response to uterine contractility. The risks of hyperstimulation and increased pain are greater with larger doses of oxytocin.

Other methods for augmenting uterine activity, including the use of prostaglandins, are certainly worth considering, but they have been inadequately explored up to the present time.

In view of the importance of labor progress and the amount of discomfort that slow progress can provoke in the woman, the fetus, and the caregivers, it is important that the many suggested guidelines for care be substantiated by solid research evidence.

Sources

Effective care in pregnancy and childbirth

Crowther, C., Keirse, M.J.N.C. and Brown, I., Monitoring the progress of labour.

Keirse, M.J.NC., Augmentation of labour.

Cochrane Library

Fraser, W.D., Krauss, I., Brisson-Carrol, G., Thornton, J. and Breart, G., Amniotomy for shortening spontaneous labour.

Hodnett, E.D., Caregiver support for women during childbirth.

Howell, C.J., Epidural versus non-epidural analgesia for pain relief in labour.

Lauzon, L., Hodnett, E., Caregivers' use of strict criteria for diagnosing active labour in term pregnancy.

Antenatal education for self-diagnosis of the onset of active labour at term.

Pattinson, R.C., Pelvimetry for fetal cephalic presentations at term.

Pre-Cochrane reviews

Fraser, W.D., Early oxytocin to shorten spontaneous labour. Review no. 04136.

Relaxin to shorten spontaneous labour. Review no. 04132.

Cervical vibration to shorten spontaneous labour. Review no. 04133.

Other sources

Blanch, G., Lavender, T., Walkinshaw, S. and Alfirevic, Z. (1998). Dysfunctional labour: a randomised trial. *Br. J. Obstet. Gynaecol.*, 105, 117–20.

Johnson, N., Lilford, R., Guthrie, K., Thornton, J., Barker, M. and Kelly, M. (1997). Randomised trial comparing a policy of early with selective amniotomy in uncomplicated labour at term. *Br. J. Obstet. Gynaecol.*, 104, 340–6.

Rogers, R., Gilson, G.J., Miller, A.C., Izquierdo, L.E., Curet, L.B. and Qualls, C.R. (1997). Active management of labor: does it make a difference? *Am. J. Obstet. Gynecol.*, 177, 599–605.

Thornton, J.G. and Lilford, R.J. (1994). Active management of labour: current knowledge and research issues. *BMJ*, 309, 366–9.

Zhang, J., Bernasko, J.W., Leybovich, E., Fahs, M. and Hatch, M.C. (1996). Continuous labor support from labor attendants for primiparous women: a meta-analysis. *Obstet. Gynecol.*, 88, 739–44.

Repair of perineal trauma

1 Introduction

One-third to nearly all women in some countries in the developed world are likely to require repair of perineal trauma after vaginal birth (70% in the UK). The majority of these women experience perineal pain or discomfort in the immediate postpartum period. Even 3 months later, as many as 20% still have problems such as pain during intercourse, which can be related to perineal trauma and its repair. This can lead to major physical, psychological, and social problems, and can affect the woman's ability to care for her newborn infant and other members of her family. It has been linked with marital breakdown. There is much postpartum maternal morbidity that women never report to health professionals.

2 Technique of perineal repair

Perineal trauma is most commonly repaired in layers. The vagina may be repaired with a continuous suture or (less commonly) with interrupted sutures. In theory, a continuous stitch might 'concertina' the vagina and for this reason, a locking stitch is usually recommended.

The deeper perineal tissues are usually closed with interrupted sutures but sometimes continuous 'running' sutures are used. The skin may be closed with interrupted transcutaneous sutures or a continuous subcuticular suture, using an absorbable material, may be used. A technique using loose continuous sutures throughout has been described. Another approach, to simply appose the deeper tissues with no separate suturing of the skin, has been found to result in satisfactory healing with less pain and dyspareunia at 3 months than alternative suturing techniques.

In addition to the nature and extent of the trauma, the technique of repair and the choice of suture material will have a bearing on the extent of morbidity associated with perineal trauma. A variety of techniques and suture materials are in current use, and there is little consensus as to which are best.

The evidence from randomized trials is that women allocated to perineal repair with continuous subcuticular sutures, experienced less pain and used less analgesia in the immediate postpartum period than those repaired with interrupted sutures. No substantial differences between the two techniques were found with respect to long-term pain or pain during intercourse. Midwives and students are usually taught to suture using the interrupted technique because it is considered easier to learn and less liable to cause problems in the hands of inexperienced or novice operators.

3 Choice of suture material

Trials comparing the use of absorbable sutures (Dexon) with non-absorbable skin sutures (silk, nylon, or Supramid), show that the groups repaired with absorbable sutures generally had less pain and used less analgesia in the first few days after delivery. They were also less likely to require resuturing. No clear differences were noted on other longer term morbidity, although women commonly reported the need for removal of some absorbable material in the 3 months after delivery.

The absorbable materials most commonly used for perineal closure are polyglycolic acid (Dexon, Vicryl) and chromic catgut. The use of polyglycolic acid sutures results in less short-term pain and less use of analgesia than chromic catgut. In the one trial that included an adequate follow-up after discharge from hospital, both perineal pain and pain during intercourse were equally common in the two groups 3 months after delivery. There was less dyspareunia at 1 year in the polyglycolic acid group.

Removal of some suture material was reported more frequently after the use of polyglycolic acid sutures than with chromic catgut sutures. This was particularly marked in the first 10 days but persisted up to

3 months postpartum. The commonest reasons given were 'irritation' and 'tightness'. The number of women requiring resuturing was small but this occurred more frequently after suturing with chromic catgut than with polyglycolic acid.

In summary, the evidence suggests that polyglycolic acid sutures cause less pain than chromic catgut in the immediate postpartum period but may cause irritation sufficient to lead to the removal of some suture material in an important minority of women. Catgut is reported to cause an inflammatory response in the tissues, due to the fact that it is broken down by proteolytic enzymes and phagocytosis. Polyglycolic acid sutures cause less tissue reaction. This may explain why their use is associated with less pain in the immediate postpartum period. Another suggested explanation for the trial findings is that they reflect differences in the tightness of the stitches rather than differences in the materials *per se*.

Glycerol-impregnated catgut has also been compared with chromic catgut, both materials being used for all layers. In the better conducted trial, the use of glycerol-impregnated catgut was associated with more pain 10 days after delivery and with a higher frequency of pain during intercourse 3 months postpartum. The increased prevalence of pain during intercourse persisted and was reported nearly twice as commonly 3 years after delivery by women sutured with glycerol-impregnated catgut. On the basis of these findings, glycerol-impregnated catgut sutures should not be used for repair of perineal trauma.

Of the non-absorbable materials, polyamide sutures, such as nylon or Supramid, would be expected to cause less pain than silk because they cause less tissue reaction and pass more easily through the tissues. Handling and knotting polyamides is less easy, however. They tend to be stiff and have a 'memory', and they thus require three or four throws in a knot. The handling properties of silk, on the other hand, are probably the best of all suture materials; it knots easily and securely. These latter characteristics almost certainly explain silk's continuing popularity for perineal repair, despite the fact that it results in increased discomfort.

A tissue adhesive, Histoacryl, has been compared to chromic catgut sutures in one trial. It suggested excellent results in terms of reduced pain and analgesic use in the 48 hours after delivery. This approach is a promising development but there is no information about long-term outcome and the single trial does not provide adequate evidence to introduce Histoacryl into practice.

4 Who should perform the repair?

It is likely that the skills of the operator are as important, if not more important, than the materials and techniques used. There is, however, little research evidence on the effects of skill on symptoms associated with perineal repair. Experience does not necessarily result in a better outcome – the same mistakes may be made with increasing confidence. There is an urgent need for this to be clarified in respect of the repair of perineal trauma.

Perineal repairs are often delegated to a junior or trainee obstetrician, or midwife. Training is likely to have an important effect on the outcome of perineal repair and is often considered inadequate. The approach often is 'see three, do three, and now you are on your own!' Video recordings have been introduced in some units to supplement this, and apparatuses on which to practice suturing are becoming available. Ideally, the usefulness of these developments should be carefully assessed before they are introduced widely.

5 Episiotomy breakdown

Episiotomy breakdown is a rare but unpleasant complication. One trial has compared a policy of primary resuturing plus antibiotic cover with wound cleansing and expectant treatment. Women managed with primary resuturing spent less time in hospital and made fewer visits to the hospital as outpatients. They resumed sexual intercourse sooner and intercourse was more likely to be pain-free. In the resutured group, 4 women out of 20 had a 'superficial rupture' but none suffered serious wound breakdown.

The results of this single trial are not definitive but they suggest that serious consideration should be given to primary resuturing (with antibiotic cover) following rupture of perineal trauma during the puerperium.

6 Conclusions

A continuous subcuticular stitch is preferable to interrupted transcutaneous sutures for episiotomy skin closure because it results in less short-term pain, without any clear difference in the long term. On balance, absorbable sutures are preferable to non-absorbable material for skin closure.

On the basis of currently available evidence, polyglycolic acid sutures (Dexon or Vicryl) should be chosen for both the deep layers and the skin. Questions still remain about the long-term effects of polyglycolic sutures but the available evidence is reassuring. The relatively frequent need to remove polyglycolic acid material in the puerperium because of irritation indicates either that this material is not ideal or that the stitches were tied too tightly. The option of a two-layer approach, leaving the skin unsutured, looks promising but needs further evidence from good-quality trials before it is widely adopted. Whichever material is chosen for the skin, polyglycolic acid currently appears to be the material of choice for the deeper tissues. However, in under-resourced settings, cost may be a barrier to its use.

Further research is required to evaluate the differential long-term effects of various suture materials and techniques, and to confirm or refute the suggested benefits of primary repair as opposed to conservative management when perineal trauma ruptures during the puerperium.

Sources

Effective care in pregnancy and childbirth

Grant, A.M., Repair of perineal trauma after childbirth.

Cochrane Library

Kettle, C. and Johanson, R.B., Continuous versus interrupted sutures for perineal repair.

Absorbable synthetic versus catgut suture material for perineal repair.

Pre-Cochrane reviews

Grant, A.M., Glycerol-impregnated catgut vs chromic catgut for perineal repair. Review no. 03694.

Polyglycolic acid vs nylon for perineal repair. Review no. 03693.

Polyglycolic acid vs silk for perineal repair. Review no. 03794.

Povidone iodine prior to perineal suturing. Review no. 05574.

Primary resuturing vs expectancy for ruptured episiotomy. Review no. 07017.

Histoacryl vs chromic catgut for perineal skin closure. Review no. 07056.

Other sources

Fleming, N. (1990). Can the suturing method make a difference in postpartum perineal pain? *J. Nurse Midwif.*, 35, 19–25.

Glazener, C.M. (1997). Sexual function after childbirth: women's experiences, persistent morbidity and lack of professional recognition. *Br. J. Obstet. Gynaecol.*, 104, 330–5.

Glazener, C.M., Abdalla, M., Stroud, P., Naji, S., Templeton, A. and Russell, I.T. (1995). Postnatal maternal morbidity: extent, causes, prevention and treatment. *Br. J. Obstet. Gynaecol.*, 102, 286–7.

Grant, A.M. (1989). The choice of suture materials and techniques for repair of perineal trauma: an overview of the evidence from controlled trials. *Br. J. Obstet. Gynaecol.*, 96, 1281–9.

Preterm birth

1 Introduction

Preterm birth is the most important single determinant of adverse infant outcome, in terms of both probability of survival and quality of life.

The likelihood of preterm birth increases with increasing gestational age up to the internationally defined cut-off point of 37 weeks. Less than a quarter of preterm births occur before 32 weeks. The birth of a very preterm infant (gestational age of less than 32 completed weeks), or of an extremely preterm infant (gestational age of less than 28 completed weeks), presents the greatest challenges. There is no specific gestational age or estimated fetal weight above and below which a hands-off approach suddenly changes from being appropriate to being negligent.

Preterm birth may occur as a result of spontaneous preterm labor or as a planned intervention. In comparison to birth at term, it is more frequently associated with other conditions, such as inadequate fetal growth, pre-eclampsia, prelabor rupture of the membranes, multiple pregnancy, placenta praevia, placental abruption, fetal congenital malformations, abnormal fetal lie, and severe disease of the mother, all of which add their own hazards to the baby.

Only a few decades ago the prognosis for survival of very preterm infants was considered to be too poor to warrant special care for their birth. This is no longer the case, as modern neonatal care has improved the prognosis for these tiny infants in many parts of the world. Now care decisions for birth are dominated by considerations of the likelihood of survival and of disability-free survival, at particular gestational ages.

Measures that have been clearly demonstrated to be beneficial for the infant and safe for the mother, such as corticosteroid administration (see Chapter 25), can be applied with greater confidence at very low gestational ages than other measures, such as cesarean section, the value of which has yet to be established.

2 Estimated weight or gestational age as basis for care options

Although a wealth of information is available on short- and long-term outcomes of infants weighing less than 1000 g, less than 1500 g, or less than 2500 g, experienced clinicians are aware of the pitfalls of using birthweight-specific data as a basis for their care options. These data often refer to infants transferred to neonatal units after all of the selection processes that occur between the onset of labor and arrival in a neonatal unit. They also include data on infants whose intra-uterine growth was restricted and who were, therefore, born at a more mature gestational age than would be expected from their birthweight.

Estimates of what the actual weight of the baby will be at birth remain notoriously inaccurate. Clinical estimates are often far off the mark, while the accuracy of fetal-weight estimation by ultrasound is still far from satisfactory. This applies in particular to the lower weight ranges.

Even if birthweight could be estimated more accurately, it remains inferior to gestational age as a determinant of infant outcome and care options. For very preterm and extremely preterm infants, organ maturity is more important than organ weight. For these infants, estimated gestational age is a better predictor of both mortality and morbidity than birthweight.

Estimation of gestational age during pregnancy from a carefully taken menstrual history and from an early ultrasound examination, if available, will be more helpful than estimation of fetal weight as the basis for care decisions.

3 Types of preterm birth

Reported outcomes of preterm birth vary widely, depending largely on the vantage point of those who accumulate the data. Neonatal data often do not include stillbirths or grossly malformed infants, and they rarely refer to the significant pathology that may be present in mother or fetus before birth. Such data pertain to the outcome for liveborn infants who have received modern intensive neonatal care, rather than to the fetuses for whom the obstetrician must make a decision.

Preterm births may be associated with antepartum fetal death or lethal malformations. Many ensue, causally or incidentally, from pathological processes in the mother, such as hypertension, antepartum hemorrhage, or in the baby, such as inadequate fetal growth. Others occur as a result of a planned decision to end the pregnancy because of a clinical judgement that continuation would pose a greater danger to either mother or baby.

3.1 Antepartum death and lethal malformations

For between 10 and 15% of all preterm births, the form of care cannot influence the outcome for the baby, because the infant has died before the onset of labor or admission, or has malformations that are incompatible with life. These babies account for over 50% of the total perinatal mortality associated with preterm birth. Although the prognosis for the baby is already determined, the care chosen can have a profound effect on the mother's well-being. The objectives of care in these cases should be directed at maternal rather than at fetal or neonatal interests.

The frequency with which preterm birth is associated with a dead or malformed fetus mandates an ultrasound of fetal morphology before undertaking any form of care that carries a substantial risk of morbidity to the mother.

3.2 Multiple pregnancy

Nearly half of all multiple births occur preterm, and multiple births are 15 times more frequent among preterm births than among births at term. Babies from multiple pregnancies make up 20% of all liveborn preterm infants (see Chapter 17).

3.3 Elective delivery

Preterm birth as a result of a planned obstetric decision to end the pregnancy constitutes an entirely different obstetric problem from that of preterm birth following the spontaneous onset of labor. The issue of how best to achieve birth is secondary to that of whether or not one should attempt to achieve delivery at that time.

The prognosis for the baby, if elective delivery is undertaken, will not necessarily be similar to that after preterm birth following the spontaneous onset of labor. Data on survival, morbidity, and follow-up of low birthweight (<2500 g), very low birthweight (<1500 g), and extremely low birthweight (<1000 g) infants, may not be relevant to the outcome for the subgroups of electively delivered infants of comparable weight or maturity.

3.4 Maternal and fetal pathology

Preterm birth may relate to pathological processes such as pre-eclampsia, antepartum hemorrhage, or intra-uterine growth restriction. Spontaneous preterm labor in these circumstances is often interpreted as demonstrating that nature is trying to remove the fetus from a 'hostile intra-uterine environment'. Whether or not this interpretation is correct in any individual situation may be difficult to ascertain, but it can profoundly influence the type of care offered or provided.

4 Place of and preparations for birth

4.1 Place of birth

Whenever possible, a very preterm infant should be born in a perinatal center with adequate facilities and equipment, persons capable of managing and handling the equipment, sufficient manpower to ensure 24-hour utilization of its resources, and professionals in various disciplines ready and willing to collaborate in the care of the mother and baby.

It is particularly dangerous for a preterm baby to be born is in a hospital with caregivers who believe that they have, but do not really have, the equipment and skills necessary to care effectively for these tiny babies before and after birth. Misplaced self-confidence can result in failure of timely referral to institutions where such facilities are available.

4.2 Preparations for birth

The woman at imminent risk of preterm delivery requires an immediate assessment as to whether transfer to a perinatal center would be appropriate. The decision will depend on the gestational age of the fetus, on the facilities that are available (which may, for example, be sufficient for a baby born at 36 but not at 31 weeks), and on the imminence of the expected birth.

If the woman is in labor, it is wise to inhibit labor with drugs in order to postpone delivery at least until she arrives at the perinatal center. Administration of corticosteroids should be commenced before transfer, unless gestational age has advanced beyond the stage at which respiratory distress syndrome is likely to be a problem.

Given the frequency with which preterm birth is associated with maternal disease, the institutions where preterm delivery is undertaken should be able to draw on the expertise not only of neonatologists or perinatologists, but on that of other professionals who may be needed to provide counseling or advice. Ultrasonography should be available for every preterm labor or birth. Full laboratory facilities should be available at all times. Resuscitation equipment should be available in the labor ward, and the presence and proper working order of this equipment should be verified before each birth.

Fetal assessment before birth should identify multiple pregnancy, assess whether or not the fetus is alive and well, differentiate the normally formed from the malformed fetus, and determine the fetal presentation. As mentioned earlier, careful review of the gestational data is necessary. All of these are prerequisites for proper care for preterm birth. A professional who is skilled in resuscitation, and who can devote all her or his attention to the infant, should be in attendance at all preterm births.

4.3 Prevention of intraventricular hemorrhage

Intraventricular hemorrhage is an important cause of mortality and morbidity in the very preterm infant. The risk of hemorrhage is inversely related to gestational age, ranging from more than 70% for babies born under 26 weeks, to less than 10% for those born after 33 weeks. More than 90% of the hemorrhages occur in infants below 35 weeks of gestation.

The use of prenatal corticosteroids for women in preterm labor reduces the risk of intraventricular hemorrhage (see Chapter 25).

Trials have addressed the question of whether the incidence of intraventicular hemorrhage in preterm infants can be reduced by the administration of either phenobarbital or vitamin K to the women before delivery. Initial reports were encouraging but in later, better quality trials, neither of these approaches were shown to be effective.

5 Route of delivery

One of the main decisions about care for preterm birth, and certainly the most controversial one, is the choice between vaginal birth and cesarean section. From the volume of literature that has been published, one would expect a wealth of evidence to be available for selecting the best approach. This is not the case. Calls have been made repeatedly for clinical trials to provide unbiased comparisons between vaginal and abdominal routes of delivery, yet there have been very few attempts to conduct such trials. Those that have been attempted were abandoned either before or soon after they started. To date, insufficient unbiased information is available to shed light on the question of when a cesarean section might add sufficient benefits to the infant to warrant the operation.

Breech presentation is far more common among preterm infants than among term infants, and breech presentation at birth carries a higher risk for the preterm infant than does cephalic presentation. This increased risk has paved the way for 'prophylactic cesarean section' being hailed as a safer method of delivery for the preterm baby presenting as a breech. In some centers, the supposed but unproven benefits of this approach have been extended to all preterm babies, without adequate evidence that the assumed gain in safety is indeed a gain and not a loss.

Observational studies have usually reported higher survival rates after cesarean section than after vaginal birth. Unfortunately, even when genuine attempts were made to control for as many confounding factors as possible, these studies may not have compared like with like. Infants born vaginally are more likely to be those who are considered to be too small, too early, or too sick to receive sufficient benefit from cesarean section. They may be those whose mothers arrived too late in second stage labor to have a cesarean section. They are more likely to have foregone the benefits of prenatal corticosteroid treatment, because they were born too quickly for these drugs to be administered or to have their full effect. Infants born vaginally are more likely to have been born in the absence of a senior obstetrician and neonatologist.

In contrast, infants born by cesarean section are more likely to be those for whom delivery could be planned in advance. They are more likely to be born as the result of a planned decision to end the pregnancy. Birth is more likely to have been preceded by thorough assessment of the fetal condition, the use of prenatal corticosteroids, and after full preparations were made for neonatal care. These infants are likely to be more mature and to have higher birthweights than those born vaginally.

As infants born vaginally or by cesarean section vary in so many other ways, in addition to the mode of delivery, observational or descriptive studies provide little useful information. Properly controlled studies are the only reliable way to provide answers to this important question.

5.1 Cesarean section

Although cesarean section is considered to be one of the safest of the major surgical procedures, it still carries an important risk of mortality and morbidity. Some special considerations apply to a preterm cesarean section.

A careful ultrasound examination is essential before cesarean delivery of a preterm infant. First, it is important to determine whether or not the fetus is normally formed; a cesarean to deliver a fetus with an undetected, lethal abnormality is a double tragedy. Second, an exact diagnosis of the fetal presentation may allow correction of a malpresentation before the uterus is incised. This may reduce the likelihood of a traumatic extraction of a malpositioned infant through a poorly formed and thick lower uterine segment. Third, it is useful to know whether or not the placenta will be in the way. Trauma to the aftercoming head will not easily be avoided, for example, if a relatively large head must be delivered through a small incision in a thick uterine segment, with the placenta as well as the body of the baby bulging through it.

At cesarean section, particularly when it is performed for breech presentation, it is important to assess whether the lower uterine segment is sufficiently wide to permit easy delivery of the head. Often, and particularly in elective, preterm, cesarean birth, there will be little lower uterine segment, and the incision is made through the body of the uterus. Some authors recommend a vertical rather than a transverse incision, but no controlled trials have been conducted to evaluate the relative merits of these alternative policies.

If the presentation is not longitudinal it should be corrected before the uterine incision is made, preferably to a vertex presentation. This is usually not too difficult, especially when there is a normal volume of amniotic fluid. It is just as important to strive for easy and gentle delivery of the fetal head at cesarean delivery as it is at a vaginal birth.

5.2 Vaginal delivery

The head of the preterm baby, with its soft bones and wide skull sutures, is more vulnerable than that of the term baby to compression by the maternal pelvic tissues, and to sudden decompression when the baby emerges from the birth canal. Several measures have been proposed to minimize the occurrence of these changes in intracranial pressure. These include liberal use of epidural analgesia to lower resistance in the birth canal; routine use of 'prophylactic forceps' delivery to counteract both compression before and decompression after birth; and routine use of early episiotomy to remove the resistance of rigid perineal tissues. There is little, if any, evidence to support the use of any of these measures.

Vacuum extraction should not be carried out on the very small baby, because of the softness of the skull bones (see Chapter 41).

5.2.1 Epidural and other analgesia

Adequate analgesia is as important for women giving birth preterm as for women delivering at term. The main difference may be that a woman in preterm labor may be less well-prepared for birth, and may be overcome by the suddenness of it all and the increased risk of giving birth preterm. It is important to respond to her anxiety and discomfort in ways that do not disadvantage the baby. When, as is often the case, pharmacological analgesia is required, an epidural block is probably safer than narcotics, although there have been no controlled studies to substantiate this recommendation.

The routine use of epidural, particularly for the preterm breech, has been suggested as a means of reducing the urge to push before the cervix is fully dilated, and to reduce the resistance of the pelvic musculature, most relevant for primiparous women. These are reasonable hypotheses, but as yet there is no controlled evidence to support them. Similar or greater protection might be gained by close communication with, and careful instructions to, the woman.

5.2.2 Elective forceps delivery

Prophylactic forceps have become accepted practice for preterm vaginal delivery in many places, but there have been few attempts to assess the value, if any, of this practice. The postulated protection of the baby's head can be questioned on theoretical grounds. Forceps are effective levers, and any compression applied at the handles is transmitted directly to the blades and hence to the fetal head. In addition, a substantial part of the traction force during delivery is transmitted as compression force to the fetal head. This may be particularly damaging to a preterm baby with soft skull bones and wide skull sutures. There is at present no unbiased evidence to suggest that routine use of forceps to deliver the preterm baby confers more benefit than harm.

5.2.3 Routine use of early episiotomy

The few unbiased data on the question of whether or not routine use of early episiotomy for birth of the preterm baby improves neonatal outcome do not support a policy of routine episiotomy for preterm birth.

6 Immediate care at birth

The physiological consequences of early versus late cord clamping have not been studied as well in the preterm infant as they have been at term. In the preterm infant, delayed cord clamping is associated with a 50% increase in red cell volume and over half of this placental transfusion occurs within the first minute after birth. Proponents of early clamping suggest that the large transfusion may encourage pulmonary edema and increase the risk of intracranial hemorrhage and hyperbilirubinemia. Those who advocate delayed clamping point out that the placental transfusion may expand the pulmonary bed and prevent respiratory distress, hypovolemia, hypotension and periventricular hemorrhage, and increase hemoglobin concentrations, packed cell volume, and total body iron stores.

It remains unknown whether alternative policies of cord clamping following preterm birth will have a significant impact on neonatal outcome. The available evidence from the few trials that have been reported show that delayed clamping reduces the duration of supplemental oxygen dependence and red cell transfusion requirements, but no clear effect is demonstrated on other outcomes. From the available evidence there seems to be no justification for rushing to clamp the cord unless urgent pediatric attention is required (see Chapter 33).

A pediatrician should be present at all preterm births. For the very preterm and extremely preterm infant, the pediatrician should be an experienced neonatologist. Decisions with regard to resuscitation and ventilation should be her or his prerogative, taken in consultation with the parents and the obstetrician, ideally after discussion before the birth.

The simple measure of providing adequate heat in the delivery room can contribute significantly to neonatal well-being (see Chapter 44).

It is as important for the mother of a preterm infant to see and, if possible, touch her baby, as for the mother of a baby born at term. Every possible step should be taken to facilitate mother–infant contact and bonding.

7 Conclusions

The expression 'preterm birth' encompasses a variety of different clinical presentations. In some the risk is little different from that of birth at term; in others the utmost sophistication of facilities and skills is necessary to give the infant even a remote hope of intact survival. Many of these small babies are already compromised by other factors, such as congenital malformations, poor intra-uterine growth, multiple pregnancy, or complicating maternal illness. Care for preterm birth must, therefore, be carefully individualized, taking all these factors into consideration.

The plan of care for birth of a preterm baby should be governed by consideration of gestational age rather than of estimated weight, because gestational age is a better indicator of prognosis.

The baby should be born in an institution that has all the necessary facilities and skilled personnel readily available. Transfer of the baby after birth is not as effective as birth in a center that is adequately equipped and staffed to ensure that the fetus is alive and well, rule out congenital malformation, establish fetal presentation before birth, and perform the skilled resuscitation that may be necessary at the moment of birth. Even for the woman in active labor, labor may be inhibited to delay birth long enough to permit transfer of the mother to such a perinatal center. The choice between vaginal birth or cesarean section is not always easy. Observational data on the differential effects of abdominal and vaginal delivery are subject to major biases. In the absence of guidance from controlled trials, cesarean section, with its known risks to the women, should be the exception rather than the rule. This applies to the fetus presenting as a breech, as well as to that presenting as a vertex.

Assessment of fetal morphology by ultrasound is essential before cesarean delivery of a preterm infant to exclude identifiable, lethal, congenital malformations, to determine fetal presentation and allow correction if necessary before the uterus is incised, and to determine the position of the placenta, which may interfere with the extraction of the baby. The uterine incision must be adequate in size, even though this is sometimes difficult with the poorly developed lower segment characteristic of the preterm uterus.

The head of the preterm baby is more vulnerable to injury, either from compression or sudden expansion, than that of the baby at term. There is no evidence to suggest that either elective forceps delivery or performing an episiotomy reduces this risk. The routine use of both these procedures should be abandoned, except in the context of controlled trials.

As the evidence in favour of early or late clamping of the umbilical cord is conflicting, decisions about when to clamp the cord should be based on the urgency of the need for resuscitation.

A pediatrician should be in attendance at all preterm births, and an experienced neonatologist capable of making the decisions and performing the skilled resuscitation that may be necessary, should be present at the births of very preterm or extremely preterm infants.

Meticulous attention to the features that should be present for all births, such as a warm environment and careful consideration, is even more important for the preterm baby than for the infant born at term without complications.

Sources

Effective care in pregnancy and childbirth
Keirse, M.J.N.C., Preterm delivery.

Cochrane Library

Carroli, G., Bellizan, J. and Stamp, G., Episiotomy for vaginal birth.

Crowther, C.A. and Henderson-Smart, D., Vitamin K prior to preterm birth for the prevention of periventricular haemorrhage.

Phenobarbital prior to preterm birth for the prevention of neonatal periventricular haemorrhage (PVH).

Crowley, P., Prophylactic corticosteroids for preterm delivery.

Grant, A., Elective versus selective Cesarean section for delivery of the small baby.

Pre-Cochrane reviews

Elbourne, D.R., Early cord clamping in preterm infants. Review no. 05944.

Other sources

Hofmeyr, G.J., Gobetz, L., Bex, P.J., Van-der-Griendt, M., Nikodem, C., Skapinker, R.et al. (1993). Periventricular/intraventricular hemorrhage following early and delayed umbilical cord clamping. A randomized controlled trial. *Online J. Curr. Clin. Trials*,110, 26.

Kinmond, S., Aitchison, T.C., Holland, B.M., Jones, J.G., Turner, T.L. and Wardrop, C.A. (1993). Umbilical cord clamping and preterm infants: a randomised trial. *BMJ*, **306**, 172–5.

CHAPTER 38

Labor and birth after previous cesarean section

1 Introduction

Policies of routine repeat cesarean section for all women with a scarred uterus were never widely practised in Europe, and now the dogma is being questioned in North America as well. The catchy aphorism 'once a cesarean always a cesarean' came from a paper published in 1916, entitled 'Conservatism in obstetrics'. It was neither a prescription nor a recommendation, but rather an observation and a caution to avoid a primary cesarean if at all possible, because it might doom the women to surgical delivery in future pregnancies. The warning was given when the cesarean rate was under 2%, sections were usually done for severe cephalopelvic disproportion, and the classical (vertical) incision in the muscular body of the uterus was almost universally used. It is hardly apropos today.

Two general propositions underlie the practice of repeat cesarean section: that planned vaginal birth after cesarean, with its inherent risk of uterine rupture, represents a significant hazard to the well-being of mother and baby; and that planned repeat cesarean operations are almost completely free of risk. Are these underlying premises true?

2 Results of a planned vaginal birth after cesarean

The proportion of women with previous cesarean section who are allowed a trial of labor varies from country to country and from center to center. Among individual units, there appears to be no significant correlation between the proportions of women allowed to labor and the rate of successful vaginal birth.

No randomized, controlled trials have compared the results of routine repeat cesarean section with those of planned vaginal birth for women who have had a previous cesarean section. In the absence of such trials, the best available data on the relative safety of a planned vaginal birth after cesarean come from observational prospective cohort studies. In these studies, in which the proportion of women who undertook a planned vaginal birth after previous cesarean varied from 20 to 80%, successful vaginal births occurred in from 67 to 84%, averaging about 80% of the women who made the attempt. In the series for which total data are available for both women who had elective cesareans and those who had a planned vaginal birth after cesarean section, well over half of all women with a previous cesarean gave birth vaginally.

Overall, attempted vaginal birth for women with a single previous low transverse cesarean section is associated with a lower risk of complications for both mother and baby than routine repeat cesarean section. The morbidity associated with successful vaginal birth is about one-fifth that of elective cesarean. Failed trials of labor, with subsequent cesarean section, involve almost twice the morbidity of elective section, but the lower morbidity in the 80% of women who successfully give birth vaginally means that overall women who opt for a planned vaginal birth after cesarean suffer only half the morbidity of women who undergo an elective cesarean section.

Maternal mortality and serious morbidity are fortunately very rare, and for this reason estimates of their frequency are imprecise. A large meta-analysis showed maternal mortality of 2.8 per 10 000 for women undergoing trials of labor, and 2.4 per 10 000 for women having an elective cesarean. Uterine dehiscence (asymptomatic separations of the uterine scar) or ruptures occur in less than 2% of trials of labor, the same proportion as is seen among women who have routine repeat cesareans. Most of these are asymptomatic and of no clinical importance.

Obstetricians' fear of uterine rupture has had a major influence on clinical practice. This fear may be justified in developing countries in which pelvic contraction and cephalopelvic disproportion are common, and access to clinical facilities often difficult. In these circumstances, when obstructed labor occurs after a previous cesarean section, dehiscence of the wound may extend into a rupture of other parts of the uterus and become a threat to the life of both mother and baby.

These are not, however, the conditions in 'developed' countries in which the cesarean section rates are highest. In these countries, dehiscences that are encountered are usually slight, often representing so-called 'windows' in the uterus, and do not result in any health problems. Indeed, the prospective observational studies found evidence of dehiscence in 0.5–2.0% of women undergoing planned cesarean section before labor had even started. The corresponding figure for women undergoing a trial of vaginal birth (successful or unsuccessful) was little different (0.5–3.3%), although, because of lack of randomization, the two figures are not directly comparable. The important point is that serious wound dehiscence is a rare complication during labor after previous cesarean section.

Perinatal mortality and morbidity rates were similar with planned vaginal birth after cesarean and elective repeat cesarean section in the studies that report these data. Such comparisons, however, are of little value, because the groups compared are not equivalent. In the absence of randomized trials, both patient choice and physician choice are involved. The decision to perform a repeat cesarean section or to permit a planned vaginal birth after cesarean may be made on the basis of whether or not the fetus is alive, dead, anomalous, or immature. In one large meta-analysis, the perinatal mortality was 18 per 1000 births in the planned vaginal birth after cesarean group and 10 per 1000 in the elective cesarean groups. However, when antenatal deaths (which could not be affected by the mode of birth) and deaths of immature babies weighing less than 750 g (when elective cesarean would be unlikely) were excluded, the perinatal mortality rates were similar, at 3 per 1000 for planned vaginal birth after cesarean and 4 per 1000 with elective cesarean.

3 Risks of cesarean section

3.1 Risks to the mother

Large series of cesarean sections have been reported with no associated maternal mortality. One should not be lulled into a false sense of security by this; no operation is without risk. The risk of a mother dying with cesarean section is small, but is still considerably higher than with vaginal birth.

The rate of maternal death associated with cesarean section (approximately 4 per 10 000 births) is four times that associated with all types of vaginal birth (1 per 10 000 births). The maternal death rate associated with elective repeat cesarean section (around 2 per 10 000 births), although lower than that associated with cesarean sections overall, is still twice the rate associated with all vaginal deliveries, and nearly four times the mortality rate associated with normal vaginal birth (0.5 per 10 000 births).

Most forms of maternal morbidity are higher with cesarean section than with vaginal birth. In addition to the risks of anesthesia attendant on all surgery, there are risks of operative injury, infection, postpartum pain, effects on subsequent fertility, and of psychological morbidity as well. The prolonged hospitalization and increased costs of cesarean section compared to vaginal birth, may also be considered as a form of maternal morbidity.

3.2 Risks to the baby

The major hazards of cesarean section for the baby relate to the risks of respiratory distress contingent on either the cesarean birth itself or on preterm birth as a result of miscalculation of dates. Babies born by cesarean section have a higher risk of respiratory distress syndrome than babies born vaginally at the same gestational age.

The availability of more accurate and readily available dating with ultrasound should decrease the risk of unexpected preterm birth. Nevertheless, it is unlikely that errors in dating can ever be completely eliminated.

4 Factors to consider in the decision about a planned vaginal birth after cesarean

A mathematical, utilitarian approach, comparing the balance of risks and benefits of planned vaginal birth after cesarean with those of planned cesarean section, will not always be the best way to choose a course of action. Such an approach can, however, provide important data that may be helpful in arriving at the best decision.

The technique of decision analysis has been used to determine the optimal birth policy after previous cesarean section. The probabilities and utilities of a number of possible outcomes, including the need for hysterectomy, uterine rupture, iatrogenic preterm birth, need for future repeat cesarean sections, prolonged hospitalization and recovery, additional cost, failed trial of labor, discomfort of labor, and inconvenience of awaiting labor, were put into a mathematical model comparing different policies. Over a wide range of probabilities and utilities, which included all reasonable values, planned vaginal birth after cesarean proved to be the safer choice.

The choice of the woman concerned plays an important role in the decision, and her informed choice should be the major deciding factor. When given the option, from 30 to 50% of women choose to undergo repeat cesarean delivery. Women's preferences and expectations regarding the birth method are based not only on their assessment of medical risks, but are also influenced by personal and attitudinal factors. In a randomized, controlled trial of a prenatal 'vaginal birth after cesarean' (VBAC) education and support program, the most frequent reasons reported for choosing elective repeat cesarean section were the fear of failed trial of labor, concerns about the dangers of vaginal birth, the fear of pain, and the convenience of scheduling.

4.1 More than one previous cesarean section

Data on the results of trials of labor in women who have had more than one previous cesarean section tend to be buried in studies of planned vaginal birth after previous cesarean section as a whole. Now that vaginal birth after one cesarean section has received widespread acceptance, reports specifically about series of trials of labor in women who have had two or more cesareans are appearing in the literature. The available data show that among these women the overall vaginal birth rate is little different from that seen in women who have had only one previous cesarean section. Successful trials of labor have been carried out on women who have had three or more previous cesarean sections.

The rate of uterine dehiscence in women who have had more than one previous cesarean section is slightly higher than the dehiscence rate in women with only one previous cesarean, but dehiscences in the reported series tend to be asymptomatic and without serious sequelae. No data have been reported on other maternal or infant morbidity specifically associated with multiple previous cesarean sections.

While the number of cases reported is still small, the available evidence does not suggest that a woman who has had more than one previous cesarean section should be treated any differently from the woman who has had only one cesarean section.

4.2 Reason for the primary cesarean section

The greatest likelihood of vaginal birth following previous section is seen when the first cesarean section was done because of breech presentation; vaginal birth rates are lowest when the initial indication was failure to progress in labor, dystocia, or cephalopelvic disproportion. Even when the indication for the first cesarean section was disproportion, dystocia, or failure to progress, successful vaginal birth was achieved in more than 50% of the women in most published series, and the rate was over 75% in the largest series reported. It is clear that a history of cesarean section for dystocia is not a contra-indication to a planned vaginal birth after cesarean. It has only a small effect on the chances of vaginal birth when a trial of labor after previous cesarean is permitted.

4.3 Previous vaginal birth

Mothers who have had a previous vaginal birth in addition to their previous cesarean sections are more likely to give birth vaginally than mothers with no previous vaginal births. This advantage is increased even further in those mothers whose previous vaginal birth occurred after, rather than before, the original cesarean section.

4.4 Type of previous incision in the uterus

Modern experience with operative approaches other than the lower segment operation for cesarean section is limited. There is, however, a growing trend towards the use of vertical incisions in preterm cesarean sections. This, and the inverted T incision sometimes necessary to allow delivery through a poorly formed lower segment, show that consideration of the type of uterine scar is still relevant.

The majority of dehiscences after lower segment transverse incisions are 'silent', 'incomplete', or incidentally discovered at the time of repeat cesarean section. The potential dangers of uterine rupture are related to the rapid 'explosive' rupture, which is most likely to be seen in women who have a classical midline scar. Rupture of the scar after a classical cesarean section is not only more serious than rupture of a lower segment scar, it is also more likely to occur. Rupture may occur suddenly during the course of pregnancy, prior to labor, and before a repeat cesarean section can be scheduled. A review of the literature at a time when classical cesarean section was still common, showed a 2.2% rate of uterine rupture with previous classical cesarean sections and a rate of 0.5% with previous lower segment cesarean sections. That is, the scar of the classical operation was more than four times more likely to rupture in a subsequent pregnancy than that of the lower segment incision.

Unfortunately, even in the older literature, there are very few data on the risk of uterine rupture of a vertical scar in the lower segment. One 1966 study reported an incidence of rupture of 2.2% in classical incision scars, 1.3% in vertical incision lower segment scars, and 0.7% in transverse incision lower segment scars. The distinction between the risk of rupture of vertical and transverse lower segment scars may be related to extension of the vertical incision from the lower segment into the upper segment of the uterus.

The uncertain denominators in the reported series make it difficult to quantify the risk of rupture with a previous classical or vertical incision lower segment scar. It is clear, however, that the risk that rupture may occur, that it may occur prior to the onset of labor, and that it may have serious sequelae, are considerably greater with such scars than with transverse incision lower segment scars. It would seem reasonable that women who have had a hysterotomy, a vertical uterine incision, or an 'inverted T' incision, be treated in subsequent pregnancies in the same manner as women who have had a classical cesarean section, and that trial of labor, if permitted at all, should be carried out with great caution, and with acute awareness of the increased risks that are likely to exist.

4.5 Gestational age at previous cesarean section

During the past decade, improved neonatal care has increased the survival rate of preterm babies. This in turn has led to a reduction in the stage of gestation at which obstetricians are prepared to perform cesarean sections for fetal indications. It has resulted in cesarean sections being used to deliver babies at, or even before, 26 weeks. At these early gestations, the lower segment is poorly formed and so-called 'lower segment' operations at this period of gestation are, in reality, transverse incisions in the body of the uterus. Whether or not such an incision confers any advantage over a classical incision remains in doubt. Indeed, some obstetricians now recommend performing a classical incision in these circumstances.

Whichever of these incisions is used at these early gestational ages, their consequences for subsequent pregnancies are currently unknown. It is quite possible, in theory at least, that they may result in a greater morbidity in future pregnancies than that associated with the lower segment operation at term.

5 Care during a planned vaginal birth after cesarean

5.1 Use of oxytocics

The use of oxytocin or prostaglandins for induction or augmentation of labor in women with a previous cesarean section has remained controversial, because of speculation that there might be an increased risk of uterine rupture or dehiscence. This view is not universally held, nor is it strongly supported by the available data. A number of series have been reported in which oxytocin or prostaglandins were used for the usual indications with no suggestion of increased hazard. Review of the reported case series shows that any increased risk of uterine rupture with the use of oxytocin or prostaglandins is likely to be extremely small. When dehiscenses occur they are more likely to occur in women who have received more than one oxytocic agent, rather than a single agent used in an appropriate manner.

Such comparisons, of course, are rendered invalid by the fact that the cohorts of women who received, or did not receive oxytocics, may have differed in many other respects in addition to the use of oxytocic agents. Nevertheless, the high vaginal birth rates and low dehiscence rates noted in these women suggest that oxytocics can be used for induction or augmentation of labor in women who have had a previous cesarean section, with the same precautions that should always attend the use of oxytocic agents.

5.2 Regional analgesia and anesthesia

The use of regional (caudal or epidural) analgesia in labor for the woman with a previous cesarean section has been questioned because of fears that it might mask pain or tenderness, which are considered to be early signs of rupture of the scar. The extent of the risk of masking a catastrophic uterine rupture is difficult to quantify. It must be minuscule, as only one case report of this having occurred was located. In a number of reported series, regional block is used whenever requested by the woman for pain relief, and no difficulties were encountered with this policy.

There does not appear to be any increased hazard from uterine rupture associated with the use of regional anesthesia for women who have had a previous cesarean section. It is sensible, safe, and justified, to use analgesia for the woman with a lower segment scar in the same manner as for the woman whose uterus is intact.

5.3 Manual exploration of the uterus

In many reported series of vaginal births after previous cesarean section, mention is made of the fact that the uterus was explored postpartum in all cases, in a search for uterine rupture or dehiscence without symptoms. The wisdom of this approach should be seriously challenged.

Manual exploration of a scarred uterus immediately after a vaginal birth is often inconclusive. It is difficult to be sure whether or not the thin, soft, lower segment is intact. In any case, in the absence of bleeding or systemic signs, a rupture without symptoms discovered postpartum does not require any treatment, so the question of diagnosis would be academic. In the absence of epidural or general anesthesia, it is also very painful to the woman.

No studies have shown any benefit from routine manual exploration of the uterus in women who have had a previous cesarean section. There is always a risk of introducing infection by the manual exploration, or of converting a dehiscence into a larger rupture. A reasonable compromise consists of increased vigilance in the hour after delivery of the placenta, reserving internal palpation of the lower segment for women with signs of abnormal bleeding.

6 Rupture of the scarred uterus in pregnancy and labor

In many reported series, true uterine rupture has not been distinguished from uterine scar dehiscence. Bloodless uterine scar dehiscence does not have negative consequences for mother or baby, whereas complete rupture of the uterus can be a life-threatening emergency. Fortunately, the true rupture is rare in modern obstetrics, despite the increase in cesarean section rates, and serious sequelae are even more rare. Although often considered to be the most common cause of uterine rupture, previous cesarean section is a factor in less than half the reported cases.

Excluding symptomless wound breakdown, the rate of reported uterine rupture has ranged from 0.09 to 0.8% for women with a singleton vertex presentation who underwent a planned vaginal birth after a previous transverse lower segment cesarean section. To put these rates into perspective, the probability of requiring an emergency cesarean section for acute other conditions (fetal distress, cord prolapse, or antepartum hemorrhage) in any woman giving birth, is approximately 2.7%, or up to 30 times as high as the risk of uterine rupture with a planned vaginal birth after cesarean. The extremely low level of the risk does not minimize the importance of this complication to the individual women who suffer it, but comparisons may help to put it in a more reasonable perspective.

Treatment of rupture of a lower segment scar does not require extraordinary facilities. Hospitals whose capabilities are so limited that they cannot deal promptly with problems associated with a planned vaginal birth after cesarean are also incapable of dealing appropriately with other obstetrical emergencies. Any obstetrical department that is prepared to look after women with much more frequently encountered conditions, such as placenta praevia, abruptio placentae, prolapsed cord, and acute fetal distress, should be able to manage a planned vaginal birth safely after a previous lower segment cesarean section.

7 Gap between evidence and practice

Obstetric practice has been slow to adopt the scientific evidence confirming the safety of vaginal birth after previous cesarean section. The degree of opposition to vaginal birth after cesarean section, in North America in particular, is difficult to explain, considering the strength of the evidence that vaginal birth after previous cesarean is, under proper circumstances, both safe and effective. Two national consensus statements and two national professional bodies, in Canada and the United States, have recommended policies of trial of labor after previous cesarean section. A randomized trial of different strategies to encourage implementation of these policies showed that local opinion leaders were more effective than either national promulgation of guidelines or audit and feedback to obstetricians.

Many women choose to attempt a vaginal birth after a cesarean section. Their earlier cesarean experience may have been emotionally or physically difficult. They may be unhappy because they were separated from their partners or from their babies. They may wonder if it was all necessary in the first place. They may be aware of the accumulated evidence on the relative safety and advantages of planned vaginal birth after cesarean and simply be looking for a better experience this time. Other women, of course, may prefer an elective repeat cesarean section.

In recent years, a number of consumer 'shared predicament' groups have appeared, with the expressed purposes of demythologizing cesarean section, of combating misinformation, and of disseminating both accurate information and their own point of view. Hospital and community-based prenatal VBAC education and support programs have been developed in many communities, but there is little evidence as to whether these programs increase rates of vaginal birth after cesarean section or improve women's perception of the quality of the birth experience. This has been assessed in one Canadian multicentered randomized trial involving over 1300 women, which compared the results for women who were given an individualized educational program with those for a control group who were only provided with a pamphlet documenting the benefits of a planned vaginal birth. Rates of vaginal birth were similar in the two groups (53 and 49%, respectively), as were the women's perception of control over the birth experience. It is difficult to know to what extent these results can be generalized to the broader population. Women with a high motivation for vaginal birth were much more likely to be successful, irrespective of the type of educational program that they received.

8 Conclusions

A planned vaginal birth after a previous cesarean section should be recommended for women whose first cesarean section was by lower segment transverse incision, and who have no other indication for cesarean section in the present pregnancy. The likelihood of vaginal birth is not significantly altered by the indication for the first cesarean section (including 'cephalopelvic disproportion' and 'failure to progress'), nor by a history of more than one previous cesarean section.

A history of classical, low vertical, or unknown uterine incision, or hysterotomy, carries with it an increased risk of uterine rupture, and in most cases is a contra-indication to trial of labor.

The care of a woman in labor after a previous lower segment cesarean section should be little different from that of any woman in labor. Oxytocin induction or stimulation, and epidural analgesia, may be used for the usual indications. Careful monitoring of the condition of the mother and fetus is required, as for all pregnancies. The hospital facilities required do not differ from those that should be available for all women giving birth, irrespective of their previous history.

Sources

Effective care in pregnancy and childbirth

Enkin, M., Labour and delivery following previous caesarean section.

Other sources

Cragin, E.B. (1916). Conservatism in obstetrics. *NY Med. J.*, CIV:1–3.

Fraser, W., Maunsell, E., Hodnett, E., Moutquin, J.M. and the Childbirth Alternatives Post-Cesarean Study Group (1997). Randomized controlled trial of a prenatal vaginal birth after cesarean section education and support program. *Am. J. Obstet. Gynecol.*, **176**, 419–25.

Lomas, J., Enkin, M., Anderson, G., Hannah, W., Vayda, E. and Singer, J. (1991). Opinion leaders vs audit and feedback to implement practice guidelines. Delivery after previous cesarean section. *JAMA*, **265**, 2202–7.

Paterson, C.M. and Saunders, N.J. (1991). Mode of delivery after one caesarean section: audit of current practice in a health region. *BMJ*, **303**, 818–21.

Rosen, M.G. and Dickinson, J.C. (1990). Vaginal birth after cesarean: a meta-analysis of indicators for success. *Obstet. Gynecol.*, **76**, 865–9.

Rosen, M.G., Dickinson, J.C. and Westhoff, C.L. (1991). Vaginal birth after cesarean: a meta-analysis of morbidity and mortality. *Obstet. Gynecol.*, **77**, 465–70.

Techniques of induction and operative delivery

CHAPTER 39

Preparing for induction of labor

1 Introduction

The decision to bring pregnancy to an end before the spontaneous onset of labor is one of the most drastic ways of intervening in the natural process of pregnancy and childbirth. The reasons given for elective delivery (which may be achieved either by inducing labor or by elective cesarean section) range from the life-saving to the trivial. There has been very little methodologically sound research on the indications for elective delivery; most of the research has been concerned with the methods to achieve it. Although comparisons of these methods are secondary to the more fundamental question of when or whether an elective delivery is required, once the decision for an elective delivery is made, the method chosen becomes important.

2 Assessing the cervix

The state of the cervix at the time of induction is one of the most important determinants of the subsequent course of events. An 'unripe' cervix (one which is not ready for induction of labor) fails to dilate adequately in response to uterine contractions. Attempted induction when the cervix is not ripe may result in high rates of induction failure, protracted and exhausting labors, a high cesarean-section rate, and other complications, such as intra-uterine infection when amniotomy is employed, as well as uterine hypertonus and other complications with the use of oxytocics.

Assessment of the state of the cervix is highly subjective and even experienced examiners may differ in their appraisal of cervical features. Several scoring systems have been developed in attempts to establish more comparable guidelines for cervical assessment. The best known of these is the score proposed by Bishop, which rates five different qualities: effacement, dilatation, and consistency of the cervix; position of the cervix relative to the axis of the pelvis; and descent of the fetal presenting part. Most other scoring systems use the same components, although with different weighting. There is some evidence that cervical dilatation alone is more predictive of subsequent progress than the composite score

As there is considerable overlap between the processes of cervical ripening and labor induction, this chapter should be read in conjunction with chapter 40 (methods of inducing labor).

3 Prostaglandins for cervical ripening

Doses of prostaglandins, which by themselves are insufficient to induce labor successfully, produce a marked softening of the uterine cervix. This softening results more from an effect on the cervical connective tissue than from uterine contractions.

Prostaglandins can effectively ripen the cervix and facilitate induction of labor. Labor commences before the start of induction (during the period allocated for cervical ripening) more often in women receiving prostaglandins for cervical ripening than in women who receive placebo or no specific treatment. Prostaglandin-ripening of the cervix increases the likelihood of a successful induction of labor, and of achieving vaginal birth within 12 or 24 hours.

The effect of prostaglandin-ripening on the pain experienced during labor is not clear. The few reports that provide data on the use of pharmacological or epidural analgesia show that epidural analgesia is less frequently used among prostaglandin-treated women than among women in the control groups, which at least suggests that these women may experience less pain.

'Uterine hypertonus' or 'uterine hyperstimulation' (excessive uterine contractility), either during the period of cervical ripening or during the subsequent induction of labor, occurs more often in prostaglandin-treated women than among women who receive placebo or no treatment prior to induction. Whether for this or for other reasons, fetal heart-rate abnormalities also tend to occur more frequently with prostaglandin treatment. Neither of these trends lead to an increased incidence of operative delivery. On the contrary, prostaglandin treatment reduces the rate of operative delivery with a modest but statistically significant decrease in the cesarean-section rate and a more marked decrease in the rate of instrumental vaginal delivery.

Few trials provide data on the incidence of postpartum hemorrhage and/or the use of blood transfusion. The available data do not suggest that these outcomes are influenced by the use of prostaglandins for cervical ripening, but the estimates are not precise.

None of the data available suggest any influence, good or bad, of cervical ripening on neonatal outcomes. There is a trend towards fewer low Apgar scores in babies born to mothers who received prostaglandins but few trials provide data on more substantive infant outcome measures, such as resuscitation of the newborn, admission to a special care nursery, and perinatal death.

3.1 Oral prostaglandins

Oral prostaglandin E_2 has been shown to be little or no better than either placebo or no treatment for cervical ripening. The synthetic prostaglandin E_1 analog misoprostol, administered orally, appears to be effective both for cervical ripening and induction of labor but there are inadequate data on its safety (see Chapter 40).

3.2 Vaginal prostaglandins

Vaginal administration of prostaglandins for cervical ripening has been studied more extensively than oral administration. The results show an increase in the frequency of labor onset during the ripening period, a decrease in the incidence of failed induction, and an increase in the likelihood of 'hypertonus' or 'hyperstimulation'. The rate of both instrumental vaginal delivery and cesarean section is decreased with the use of vaginal prostaglandins. No effect has been demonstrated on any infant outcomes.

Women receiving vaginal prostaglandins for cervical ripening are more likely to undergo cesarean section during the time interval allowed for cervical ripening than women receiving the control treatment. This higher incidence of cesarean section during cervical ripening is more than compensated for by a lower cesarean-section rate during induced labor.

Of the many preparations used for vaginal administration, the modern gel and pessary preparations are more effective than the tablet forms previously used. Vaginal administration of misoprostol is discussed in Chapter 40.

3.3 Endocervical prostaglandins

Evaluations of prostaglandins administered in a viscous gel in the cervical canal have been conducted mostly with 0.5 mg PGE_2, a dose that is much smaller than is used with either the oral or vaginal routes of administration. Endocervical prostaglandin administration is more likely than either placebo or no treatment to result in uterine activity, in the onset of labor, in a reduction of the need for formal induction of labor at the end of the ripening period, and in delivery during the ripening period. As with vaginal prostaglandins, more women undergo cesarean section during the ripening period, but this is again compensated for by a reduction in the rate of cesarean during labor. The likelihood of failed induction is reduced, as is the rate of operative delivery.

3.4 Extra-amniotic prostaglandins

Few placebo-controlled trials have evaluated extra-amniotic administration of a prostaglandin for cervical ripening. The few data available do not permit adequate judgement about the relative merits or hazards of this specific route of administration.

3.5 Direct comparisons between different routes

Controlled comparisons of endocervical with vaginal PGE_2 gel for cervical ripening suggest that the endocervical approach results in more women going into labor or delivering during ripening (if this is considered to be a desirable outcome). No statistically significant differences are found in any other outcomes. The choice between these approaches may be best determined by clinical preference.

Labor is more likely to occur during ripening with the use of extra-amniotic rather than vaginal or endocervical prostaglandins. No differential effects on other outcome measures have been found in the few controlled trials that have been conducted, but the trials were too small to detect modest differences.

4 Other methods for cervical ripening

4.1 Estrogens
The use of estrogens for cervical ripening has been suggested on the theoretical grounds that these agents might ripen the cervix without concomitant effects on uterine contractility. Data from controlled trials with a variety of estrogenic preparations, failed to show any beneficial effects.

4.2 Oxytocin
Oxytocin infusions for prolonged periods of time (as is usually the case when the aim is to ripen the cervix) are unpleasant, limit the woman's mobility, and may lead to water intoxication when administered in large doses. Oxytocin administration to ripen the cervix (rather than to induce labor) serves no useful purpose and should be abandoned.

4.3 Mechanical methods
Mechanical devices, such as catheters with or without extra-amniotic saline infusion, laminaria tents, and synthetic hydrophylic materials, have been shown to increase cervical ripeness scores and may increase the proportion of women going into labor. No effect has been shown on the incidence of operative delivery, puerperal fever, or low Apgar scores.

Several recent trials have shown little difference, if any, in effects between various mechanical methods and prostaglandins administered vaginally or intracervically, but all of these trials have been small. Factors to be taken into account when choosing a method of cervical ripening are, on the one hand, that mechanical methods are more uncomfortable to apply, while on the other hand, they are less expensive and less likely to cause uterine hyperstimulation than prostaglandins.

4.4 Relaxin
The use of porcine relaxin to soften the cervix and shorten labor had a brief vogue of popularity in the 1950s. Placebo-controlled trials failed to show any benefit.

Recent trials with a purer preparation and recombinant human relaxin have also failed to demonstrate any useful effects. Relaxin should not be adopted into clinical practice unless large, properly controlled trials show evidence of benefit.

4.5 Breast stimulation

In an attempt to explore 'natural' methods for ripening the cervix, two groups of investigators have evaluated the effects of breast stimulation. Both reported that women allocated to breast stimulation were more likely to go into labor during the intervention period than those allocated to the control group, but there was no suggestion as to whether this resulted in easier labor or delivery.

5 Prostaglandins versus other methods

A number of small trials have compared prostaglandins with alternative agents for cervical ripening, including oxytocin and estrogens. None of these trials were large enough to provide useful estimates of effect, either individually or by combining their data. The general conclusion derived from these studies suggests that prostaglandins are more effective than the other agents.

6 Hazards of cervical ripening

Increasing the readiness of the cervix for induction is not a trivial intervention. Depending on the method used, the risks of the ripening include a (small) danger of intra-uterine infection with mechanical procedures and extra-amniotic drug administration, an increased likelihood of uterine hypertonus and fetal heart-rate abnormalities, and a certain amount of discomfort and inconvenience for the mother. Some of these hazards, uterine hypertonus and fetal heart-rate abnormalities in particular, are ill-defined and of unclear significance but they have sometimes prompted cesarean sections during cervical ripening.

The risks of cervical ripening are not limited to those related to the intervention itself but include those associated with induction of labor. The greatest hazard is that the ease of cervical ripening may result in unnecessary induction of labor in women for whom an artificial ending of pregnancy would not otherwise have been contemplated.

7 Conclusions

No attempts should be made to ripen the cervix, unless there are valid grounds for ending pregnancy artificially. None of the successful methods of cervical ripening act exclusively on the cervix and all of them tend to increase myometrial contractility. When it is necessary to induce labor in the presence of an 'unripe' cervix, the method used should not only increase cervical readiness, but must also increase the likelihood of spontaneous vaginal birth of a healthy baby within a reasonable period of time and involve minimal inconvenience or discomfort for the mother.

Use of prostaglandins decreases the likelihood of 'failed induction', decreases the incidence of prolonged labor, and increases the chances of a spontaneous vaginal birth. There are still insufficient data to allow any confident conclusions about the effects on the baby.

Oral administration of prostaglandins, other than misoprostol, has no value for ripening the cervix. Extra-amniotic administration, if used at all, should be reserved for women with very 'unripe' cervices and for those who are unlikely to respond adequately to vaginal or endocervical administration.

Vaginal and endocervical administration of prostaglandin PGE_2 in gel or pessary form are the current methods of choice. The two forms of administration seem equally effective. The vaginal route has the advantage of ease of application.

Recent reports have demonstrated the effectiveness of mechanical methods, particularly those employing a catheter balloon, though the discomfort caused by insertion may limit the acceptability of these methods.

Sources

Effective care in pregnancy and childbirth

Chalmers, I. and Keirse, M.J.N.C., Evaluating elective delivery.

Keirse, M.J.N.C. and van Oppen, A.C., Preparing the cervix for induction of labour.

Cochrane Library

Alfirevic, Z., Howarth, G. and Gausmann, A., Oral misoprostol for induction of labour with a viable fetus.

Boulvain, M. and Irion, O., Stripping/sweeping the membranes for inducing labour or preventing post-term pregnancy.

Boulvain, M., Irion, O., Lohse, C. and Matonhodze, B., Mechanical methods for inducing labour [protocol].

Hofmeyr, G.J. and Gulmezoglu, A.M., Vaginal misoprostol for cervical ripening and labour induction in late pregnancy.

Lumbiganon, P., Laopaiboon, M., Kuchaisit, C. and Chinsuwan, A., Oral prostaglandins (excluding misoprostol) for cervical ripening and labour induction when the baby is alive [protocol].

Turnbull, D.A., Wilkinson, C.S. and Griffiths, E., Breast stimulation for cervical ripening in pregnancy [protocol].

Other sources

Brennand, J.E., Calder, A.A., Leitch, C.R., Greer, I.A., Chou, M.M. and MacKenzie, I.Z. (1997). Recombinant human relaxin as a cervical ripening agent. *Br. J. Obstet. Gynaecol.*, 104, 775–80.

Gilson, G.J., Russell, D.J., Izquierdo, L.A., Qualls, C.R. and Curet, L.B. (1996). A prospective randomized evaluation of a hygroscopic cervical dilator, Dilapan, in the preinduction ripening of patients undergoing induction of labor. *Am. J. Obstet. Gynecol.*, 175, 145–9.

Keirse, M.J.N.C. and de Koning Gans, H.J. (1995). Randomized comparison of the effects of endocervical and vaginal prostaglandin E₂ gel in women with various degrees of cervical ripeness. Dutch Collaborative Prostaglandin Trialists' Group. *Am. J. Obstet. Gynecol.*, 173, 1859–64.

Stempel, J.E., Prins, R.P. and Dean, S. (1997). Preinduction cervical ripening: a randomized prospective comparison of the efficacy and safety of intravaginal and intracervical prostaglandin E2 gel. *Am. J. Obstet. Gynecol.*, 176, 1305–9.

St. Onge, R.D. and Connors, G.T. (1995). Preinduction cervical ripening: a comparison of intracervical prostaglandin E2 gel versus the Foley catheter. *Am. J. Obstet. Gynecol.*, 172, 687–90.

Williams, M.C., Krammer, J. and O'Brien, W.F. (1997). The value of the cervical score in predicting successful outcome of labor induction. *Obstet. Gynecol.*, 90, 784–9.

Methods of inducing labor

1 Introduction

For practical purposes, modern obstetric practice uses only three broad approaches to the induction of labor: mechanical methods (such as sweeping of the membranes or use of a dilator); amniotomy (artificial rupture of the membranes); and oxytocic drugs (oxytocin or a prostaglandin). Other methods, although still occasionally reported, have generally been abandoned. Traditional practices, such as the use of castor oil, have not been formally evaluated.

Standardized 'scoring' of the cervix prior to labor induction has been recommended, although cervical dilation alone may more predictive of successful labor induction. Oxytocin has the disadvantages of a high failure rate when the cervix is unfavorable (low cervical score), and it requires monitoring of continuous intravenous infusion. Artificial rupture of membranes is also less effective or may not be possible when the cervix is unfavorable.

Unsuccessful labor induction is most likely when the cervix is unfavorable and, in this circumstance, prostaglandin preparations have proved to be beneficial. Uterine hyperstimulation has been identified as a potential problem during labor induction with prostaglandins; on occasion this has warranted treatment with tocolytics (see Chapter 39).

2 Mechanical methods

2.1 Sweeping (stripping) the membranes
Sweeping the membranes (digital separation of the fetal membranes from the lower uterine segment) has been used for many years to induce labor or to pre-empt formal induction of labor with either oxytocin, prostaglandins, or amniotomy. There are good theoretical reasons to suggest that it may be effective, in that it stimulates intrauterine prostaglandin synthesis. When the cervix is closed, a cervical massage has been proposed.

Studies have been conducted to evaluate stripping/sweeping of the membranes, either as a general policy in women at or near term to prevent post-term pregnancy or in a selected group of women thought to require labor induction. The available evidence suggests that sweeping of the membranes reduces the duration of pregnancy, and thus the proportion of women requiring formal labor induction for 'post-dates' pregnancy. For women thought to require induction of labor, a reduction in the use of more 'formal' methods of induction could be expected. However, no clear benefits on substantive outcomes (e.g. cesarean section) were reported.

Sweeping of the membranes is probably safe, provided that the intervention is avoided in pregnancies complicated by placenta praevia or when contra-indications for labor and/or vaginal birth are present. There is no evidence that sweeping the membranes increases the risk of maternal and neonatal infection. A trend towards an increased frequency of prelabor rupture of membranes was noted. Women's discomfort during the procedure, and 'minor' side-effects must be balanced with the expected benefits before submitting women to a sweeping of the membranes.

2.2 Other mechanical methods

Mechanical methods were the first methods developed to ripen the cervix or to induce labor. Devices that were used in this context include various type of catheters and laminaria tents, introduced into the cervical canal or through the cervix into the extra-amniotic space. Mechanical methods were never completely abandoned but during recent decades have been largely replaced by pharmacological methods. Potential advantages of mechanical methods over pharmacological ones may include simplicity of use, lower cost, and reduction of some of the side-effects. The goals of these interventions are to ripen the cervix through direct dilatation of the canal or, indirectly, by increasing prostaglandin and/or oxytocin secretion. In addition, these methods may lead to labor onset. The Foley catheter is currently used, as well as a specially developed 'Atad' double-balloon catheter. The catheter is introduced through the cervical canal to reach the extra-amniotic space. The balloon is then inflated to keep the catheter in place. Traction is sometimes applied to the catheter. In addition, some clinicians inject saline or prostaglandins in the extra-amniotic space, in an attempt to enhance the efficacy of the method.

Laminaria tents, made from sterile sea-weed or synthetic hydrophilic materials (e.g. Lamicel), are introduced into the cervical canal to achieve a gradual stretching of the cervix. In addition to the local effect, mechanisms that involve neuroendocrine reflexes (the Ferguson reflex) may promote the onset of contractions.

3 Amniotomy

3.1 Amniotomy used alone

Amniotomy (rupturing the membranes) can induce labor but its use implies a firm commitment to delivery; once the membranes have been ruptured, there is no turning back. The main disadvantage of amniotomy, when used alone for the induction of labor, is the unpredictable and, occasionally, long interval to the onset of uterine contractions and thus to delivery. It may increase the risk of infection if labor does not proceed promptly. Rupture of the membranes may also increase the vertical transmission of specific maternal infections, such as HIV.

3.2 Amniotomy with oxytocic drugs versus amniotomy alone

In order to shorten the interval between amniotomy and delivery, oxytocic drugs are usually used either at the time that the membranes are ruptured or after an interval of a few hours if labor has not started. Evidence from controlled trials shows that women who receive oxytocics from the time of amniotomy are more likely to be delivered within 12 and 24 hours, and less likely to give birth by cesarean section or forceps, than those who have had amniotomy alone.

Women who receive early oxytocin use less analgesia than those receiving oxytocin later. This does not necessarily mean that early oxytocin results in a less painful labor for these women; it may simply reflect the shorter interval between amniotomy and birth. The trials for which data are available also suggest a lower incidence of postpartum hemorrhage when amniotomy is combined with early oxytocin administration.

Low Apgar scores are seen less frequently with a policy of using oxytocin from the time of amniotomy. No other differential effects on the baby have been noted in controlled trials.

3.3 Amniotomy with oxytocic drugs versus oxytocic drugs alone

When compared with a policy in which the membranes are left intact, routine amniotomy at the time of starting oxytocic drugs to induce labor is more likely to result in established labor within hours of starting the induction. The limited number of controlled trials precludes firm conclusions on other outcome measures, such as the likelihood of birth within 24 hours, cesarean section, or perinatal morbidity and mortality.

Observational data derived from studies conducted in the 1960s, however, suggest that about a third of women in whom induction of labor is attempted with oxytocin administration but without concurrent amniotomy, will remain undelivered 2–3 days after the beginning of the induction attempt. Not surprisingly, in the light of these observations, amniotomy has come to be used routinely at the time that oxytocin is started to induce labor. Only with the development of prostaglandin preparations has the choice of leaving the membranes intact during induction of labor become a reasonable option.

3.4 Hazards of amniotomy

A number of undesirable consequences have been attributed to artificial rupture of the membranes. These include: pain and discomfort; intra-uterine infection (occasionally leading to septicemia); early decelerations in the fetal heart rate; umbilical cord prolapse; and bleeding, either from fetal vessels in the membranes, from the cervix, or from the placental site. Serious complications, fortunately, are rare.

Any instrument (or a finger) passing up the vagina in order to rupture the amniotic sac will carry some of the vaginal bacterial flora with it. The risk of clinically significant intra-uterine infection ensuing from these procedures depends largely on the interval between amniotomy and delivery.

The view that amniotomy predisposes to fetal heart-rate decelerations, is largely based on potential cord compression due to diminished amniotic fluid volume, but there is no evidence that this risk is important enough to be a main determinant in choosing a method for the induction of labor.

4 Oxytocin

4.1 Routes and methods of administration

No formal comparisons between the usual intravenous route and other routes of administration have been reported.

Intravenous oxytocin has been administered in different ways ranging from simple, manually adjusted, gravity-fed systems, through mechanically or electronically controlled infusion pumps, to fully automated closed-loop feedback systems in which the dose of oxytocin is regulated by the intensity of uterine contractions. Gravity-fed systems have the disadvantage that the amount of oxytocin infused may be difficult to regulate accurately and may vary with the position of the woman. A further disadvantage is that the amount of fluid administered intravenously may be large, and may thus increase the risk of water intoxication. Automatic oxytocin-infusion equipment, by contrast, delivers oxytocin at a well-regulated rate, in a small volume of fluid. In theory it should optimize efficacy and safety during oxytocin administration, but there is no evidence that these theoretical advantages confer any benefit in practice.

The only formal comparisons of different methods for administering oxytocin to induce labor consist of trials comparing automatic oxytocin-infusion systems with 'standard regimens'. These trials have been too small to detect differences in substantive outcomes. The merits and risks of automated infusion systems and alternative dose regimens must be more thoroughly evaluated before their place, if any, in clinical practice can be determined.

4.2 Hazards of oxytocin administration

The possible hazards of oxytocin *per se* must be distinguished from the hazards associated with any attempt to induce labor, and those associated with any artificial stimulation of uterine contractions.

The antidiuretic effect of oxytocin can result in water retention and hyponatremia, and may lead to coma, convulsions, and even maternal death. These risks are mainly associated with oxytocin infusions at early stages of pregnancy, when uterine sensitivity to oxytocin is far less than it is at term and when much larger doses are required to stimulate uterine contractions. In women with an already reduced urinary output, the danger of water intoxication is an important consideration at any stage of gestation.

Any agent that causes uterine contractions, whether it be a drug such as oxytocin or a prostaglandin, or a practice such as nipple stimulation, may also cause excessive uterine contractility. Excessively frequent or prolonged uterine contractions may affect blood flow from and to the placenta, which will in turn reduce fetal oxygenation. Uterine rupture is a further, though much rarer, consequence of excessive stimulation of uterine activity. The balance of evidence suggests that induction of labor with oxytocin increases the incidence of neonatal hyperbilirubinemia.

5 Prostaglandin E$_2$

5.1 Comparisons with placebo

Prostaglandins have been evaluated against placebo for the induction of labor. Not surprisingly, the rates of 'failed induction' and the proportions of women needing a second induction attempt are lower with prostaglandin administration (in various doses, formulations and routes) than with placebo treatments. There were fewer cesarean sections in the prostaglandin than in the placebo groups in the reported trials, but the rates of instrumental vaginal delivery rates were similar.

Most of the trials mentioned specifically that 'uterine hypertonus' and/or 'uterine hyperstimulation' were not observed, and several commented on the low incidence of gastro-intestinal side effects encountered. Very few infant outcomes were reported in any of these trials. Among those in which they were reported, none showed any differences between the prostaglandin and placebo groups.

For prelabor rupture of membranes at or near term, induction of labor by prostaglandins compared with expectant management, decreases the risk of maternal infection (chorio-amnionitis), neonatal antibiotic therapy, and admission to neonatal intensive care, without increasing the rate of cesarean section, although it is associated with a more frequent maternal diarrhea and use of anesthesia and/or analgesia. In the trials that systematically collected information on women's views, women were more likely to view their care positively if labor was induced with prostaglandins as opposed to expectant management.

5.2 Prostaglandin E$_2$ versus prostaglandin F

Both PGE$_2$ and PGF$_{2\alpha}$ (which are also naturally formed during spontaneous labor) have been used for the induction of labor.

In order to achieve a similar effect on uterine contractility, PGF$_{2\alpha}$ must be administered in a dose eight to ten times as large as that needed when PGE$_2$ is used. This difference in potency applies to the stimulating properties of these compounds on the myometrium. It does not apply, to the same extent, to their effects on other organ systems, such as the gastro-intestinal tract. Consequently, for a comparable uterotonic effect, the incidence of side-effects tends to be larger with PGF$_{2\alpha}$ than with PGE$_2$. Because of this, PGF$_{2\alpha}$ is no longer used and PGE$_2$ has become the only natural prostaglandin used for induction of labor.

5.3 Routes and methods of administration

Early studies of prostaglandins for the induction of labor used the intravenous route of administration. These studies showed few, if any, advantages of prostaglandins over other methods. Compared with oxytocin, they offered no real benefit and were considerably more expensive.

Oral administration of PGE$_2$ (in repeat doses increasing from 0.5 to 2 mg) became widely used as an alternative to intravenous infusions of prostaglandins for inducing labor, particularly when combined with amniotomy and in women with a favorable cervix. Gastro-intestinal side-effects were common and oral administration has been almost entirely replaced by vaginal administration, especially since the newer formulations using viscous gel became available.

Because intravenous, oral and, to some extent also, the vaginal administrations of prostaglandins, lead to high levels of these drugs in the blood, the gastro-intestinal tract, or both, intra-uterine (extra-amniotic) routes of administration have been used in attempts to reduce the side-effects associated with the other routes. Continuous or intermittent extra-amniotic infusion of a PGE_2 solution and extra-amniotic injection of a PGE_2 gel suspension have been used for this purpose.

There is a limited amount of controlled data comparing the extra-amniotic route with other routes of prostaglandin administration. Although the data are too limited for a precise estimate, they show no advantage for the more invasive extra-amniotic route, which is both cumbersome and inconvenient for the mother.

Another route of local administration, injection of PGE_2 in a viscous gel into the cervical canal, has been used mainly for ripening the cervix rather than for induction. The relative merits and hazards of endocervical versus vaginal administration have been assessed in a few trials. These have not indicated that either one of these approaches is clearly superior to the other, in terms of substantive outcome measures. The more complex and uncomfortable endocervical insertion procedure is, therefore, difficult to justify.

5.4 Hazards of prostaglandin E$_2$ administration

The specific hazards attributable to prostaglandins *per se* relate mainly to their effects on the gastro-intestinal tract (nausea, vomiting, and diarrhea). These effects are minimal when the drugs are administered vaginally, endocervically, or extra-amniotically, and maximal when routes of administration (intravenous, oral) that lead to high levels of the drugs in either the blood or the gastro-intestinal tract are used.

Fever may result from a direct effect of prostaglandins on thermoregulating centers in the brain. This is particularly a problem with systemic prostaglandin E$_2$ administration, and may give rise to concern that intra-uterine infection has supervened. This concern may be further fuelled by a rise in the leucocyte count, which can also be stimulated by prostaglandin administration. Fever is rarely observed with the newer vaginal and endocervical preparations.

More worrying than the specific hazards associated with prostaglandins, are concerns that the simplicity of their administration may encourage their use for trivial indications or without adequate surveillance of mother and fetus.

6 Prostaglandin E₂ versus oxytocin for inducing labor

The important question is whether prostaglandin E_2 is, on balance, superior to oxytocin for the induction of labor, particularly when the cervix is 'unripe'.

6.1 Effects on time and mode of delivery

The total amount of uterine work required to achieve delivery is lower with prostaglandin E_2 than with oxytocin, presumably because the former also influences connective tissue compliance (cervical 'ripening'), whereas the latter does not. The proportions of women who give birth within 12 hours after the start of induction are similar for women induced with prostaglandin E_2 and for those induced with oxytocin. By 24 hours, however, fewer women have not given birth after induction with prostaglandin E_2, and after 48 hours the proportion of women who have not given birth shows an even larger difference in favor of prostaglandins. When only women who give birth vaginally are considered, this advantage of prostaglandin E_2 becomes even more pronounced.

There is no clear evidence of a differential effect of prostaglandin E_2 and oxytocin on the cesarean-section rate. The rate of instrumental vaginal delivery is lower in the women induced with prostaglandins, as is the incidence of operative delivery overall. This may be due partly to prostaglandins' influence on connective tissue and partly to the greater freedom of movement allowed because it is not administered intravenously.

6.2 Effects on the mother

There are some major differences between the effects of oxytocin and prostaglandins on organ systems other than the uterus. More women experience gastro-intestinal side-effects, such as nausea, vomiting, and diarrhea, when prostaglandins rather than oxytocin are used for the induction of labor. Fever during labor is more likely to occur with prostaglandins than with oxytocin, although the differential effect is found only in the earlier studies of intravenous PGE_2.

Uterine hyperstimulation occurs more frequently with prostaglandin than with oxytocin administration. This complication is seen mainly in institutions with little experience in the use of prostaglandin and was not observed in many trials. A diagnosis of hyperstimulation may lead to a variety of interventions ranging from changes in position, through fetal scalp blood sampling, administration of betamimetic agents, and cesarean section. Thus hyperstimulation is important to the mother, irrespective of whether or not it directly jeopardizes her or the fetus.

Data on the incidence of retained placenta, of postpartum hemorrhage, and of fever during the puerperium, show no difference in the effects of prostaglandin E_2 and oxytocin.

Few data on mothers' views of induction have been reported but they are consistently in favor of prostaglandin E_2 administration, which is considered to be more agreeable, more natural, and less invasive than intravenous administration of oxytocin.

6.3 Effects on the infant

In view of the increased incidence of uterine hyperstimulation associated with induction using prostaglandin E_2, it is reassuring to note that the incidence of fetal heart-rate abnormalities is similar in labors induced with prostaglandin E_2 and among fetuses of women receiving oxytocin.

Unfortunately, few trials provide data on substantive infant outcomes, such as resuscitation of the newborn, admission to a special care nursery, or early neonatal convulsions. Even data on perinatal death are only available from half of the trials. From those trials that provide data, no differential effects of prostaglandin E_2 and oxytocin emerge, but the precision of these estimates is extremely low.

Somewhat more data are available on the incidence of low 1-min and 5-min Apgar scores, but these show no statistically significant differences between prostaglandin E_2 and oxytocin inductions.

The incidence of neonatal hyperbilirubinemia (jaundice) appears to be lower among infants born after induction of labor with prostaglandin E_2 than among those born after induction with oxytocin, but the difference found may have arisen by chance.

6.4 Prelabor rupture of membranes at or near term

Induction of labor with prostaglandin E_2 increases the number of vaginal examinations and the risk of maternal infection (chorioamnionitis).

It may also increase the risk of neonatal infection, but the harmful effect of induction of labor with prostaglandin E_2 on this outcome may be less than suggested by the Cochrane review. In only one trial was the search for, and determination of, neonatal infection conducted blind to the allocation group and duration of membrane rupture. Induction of labor with prostaglandins increases the rate of neonatal antibiotic therapy and admission to neonatal intensive care for more than 24 hours.

There is no evidence from high-quality trials that a policy of induction of labor with prostaglandin E_2 increases or decreases the rate of cesarean section, although it is associated with a less frequent use of epidural analgesia and internal fetal heart-rate monitoring.

7 Misoprostol

The prostaglandin preparations that have been registered for cervical ripening and labor induction are expensive and unstable, requiring refrigerated storage. Misoprostol (Cytotec, Searle) is a methyl ester of prostaglandin E_1 and is marketed for use in the prevention and treatment of peptic ulcer disease caused by prostaglandin-synthesis inhibitors. It is inexpensive, easily stored at room temperature, and has few systemic side-effects. It is rapidly absorbed orally and vaginally. Misoprostol has been used widely for obstetric and gynecological indications, despite the fact that it has not been registered for such use. It has, therefore, not undergone the extensive testing for appropriate dosage and safety required for registration. Third-trimester cervical ripening and labor induction with misoprostol have been reported using the oral, vaginal and rectal routes.

Results from several trials show that vaginal misoprostol (in dosages ranging from 25 micrograms 2–3-hourly, 50 micrograms 4-hourly (most studies), to 100 micrograms 6–12-hourly) appears to be more effective than oxytocin or dinoprostone in the usual recommended doses for induction of labor. It is associated, however, with increased rates of meconium-stained liquor and of uterine hyperstimulation, both with and without fetal heart-rate changes. The rates of cesarean section were inconsistent, tending to be reduced with misoprostol. No differences in perinatal or maternal outcome were shown. However, the trials were not sufficiently large to assess the likelihood of uncommon, serious adverse perinatal and maternal complications. The possibility of inadvertent bias because of the unblinded nature of these studies should be kept in mind.

A lower dosage regimen of misoprostol (25 micrograms 6-hourly) was less effective than a higher dose (25 micrograms 3-hourly), with possibly reduced rates of uterine hyperstimulation.

The finding of a significant increase in meconium-stained liquor with misoprostol is of interest. One study suggested the possibility of meconium passage in response to uterine hyperstimulation or a direct effect of absorbed misoprostol metabolites on the fetal gastro-intestinal tract.

Misoprostol administered orally is also an effective method of inducing labor, and has the advantage of convenience and avoidance of internal examinations. As for vaginal misoprostol, insufficient data have been produced to evaluate the safety of this approach.

Thus, though misoprostol shows promise as a highly effective, inexpensive, and convenient agent for labor induction, it cannot be recommended for routine use at this stage. It is also not registered for such use in many countries.

Because of the enormous economic and possible clinical advantages of misoprostol, there is the need for further trials to establish its safety.

8 Conclusions

The most important decision to be made when considering the induction of labor is whether or not the induction is justified, rather than how it is to be achieved. Whatever method is chosen to implement a decision to induce labor, uterine contractility, and maternal and fetal well-being must be monitored carefully.

Amniotomy alone is often inadequate to induce labor. When amniotomy is used to induce labor and fails to result promptly in adequate uterine contractility, oxytocic drugs should be administered. The administration of oxytocin without amniotomy is also associated with an unacceptable failure rate.

Prostaglandins are more likely than oxytocin to result in vaginal birth within a reasonable length of time after the start of induction, and to lower the rate of operative delivery associated with induction of labor. The extent to which this may reflect the greater mobility possible with some forms of prostaglandin administration, than with intravenously administered oxytocin, is unknown. These positive effects of prostaglandins must be balanced against their negative effects, troublesome gastro-intestinal symptoms or fever, although these are rarely seen with the newer formulations of prostaglandin E_2 that are now available.

If a decision has been made to use prostaglandins to induce labor, the best option appears to be vaginal administration of prostaglandin E_2 in a viscous gel. $PGF_{2\alpha}$ should no longer be used. There is too little evidence to allow any judgement about whether prostaglandins are more or less safe for the baby than oxytocin.

Sources

Effective care in pregnancy and childbirth

Thiery, M., Baines, C.J. and Keirse, M.J.N.C., The development of methods for inducing labour.

Keirse, M.J.N.C., Chalmers I. Methods for inducing labour.

Keirse, M.J.N.C., Van Oppen ACC. Comparison of prostaglandin and oxytocin for inducing labour.

Cochrane Library

Alfirevic, Z., Howarth, G. and Gausmann, A., Oral misoprostal for induction of labour with a viable fetus.

Boulvain, M. and Irion, O., Stripping/sweeping of the membranes for inducing labour or preventing post-term pregnancy.

Boulvain, M., Irion, O., Lohse, C. and Matonhodze, B., Mechanical methods to induce labour [protocol].

Hofmeyr, G.J. and Gulmezoglu, A.M., Vaginal misoprostol for cervical ripening and labour induction in late pregnancy.

Lumbiganon, P., Laopaiboon, M., Kuchaisit, C. and Chinsuwan, A., Oral prostaglandins (excluding misoprostol) for cervical ripening and labour induction when the baby is alive [protocol].

Tan, B.P. and Hannah, M.E., Oxytocin for prelabour rupture of membranes at or near term.

Prostaglandins for prelabour rupture of membranes at or near term.

Prostaglandins versus oxytocin for prelabour rupture of membranes at or near term.

Prostaglandins versus oxytocin for prelabour rupture of membranes at term.

Other sources

Cammu, H, and Haitsma, V. (1998). Sweeping of the membranes at 39 weeks in nulliparous women: a randomised controlled trial. *Br. J. Obstet. Gynaecol.*, 105, 41–4.

Hodnett, E.D., Hannah, M.E., Weston, J.A., Ohlsson, A., Myhr, T.L., Wang, E.E. *et al.* (1997). Women's evaluations of induction of labor versus expectant management for prelabor rupture of the membranes at term. TermPROM Study Group. *Birth*, 24, 214–20 .

MacKenzie, I.Z. and Burns, E. (1997). Randomised trial of one versus two doses of prostaglandin E_2 for induction of labour: 1. Clinical outcome. *Br. J. Obstet. Gynaecol.*, 104, 1062–7 .

Sanchez-Ramos, L., Kaunitz, A.M., Wears, R.L., Delke, I. and Gaudier, F.L. (1997). Misoprostol for cervical ripening and labour induction: a meta-analysis. *Obstet. Gynecol.*, 89, 633–42.

CHAPTER 41

Instrumental vaginal delivery

1 Introduction

When there is a valid indication for expediting the birth of the baby, instrumental vaginal delivery rather than cesarean section may be selected on the basis of a number of factors. These include the condition of the fetus and mother, progress in labor, dilatation of the cervix, the station of the presenting part, position and moulding of the fetal head, comfort, morale and co-operation of the mother, experience and attitudes of the operator, and the availability of the necessary equipment.

Few indications for instrumental delivery are absolute, and there are considerable regional and international differences in the rate of instrumental deliveries. Various care practices may help to achieve lower rates of assisted delivery. Among these are encouraging companionship in labor, active management of delay in the second stage of labor with oxytocin, and the use of upright posture for birth. When epidural analgesia is used, allowing time for the analgesic effect to wear off, and having a more liberal approach to the length of the second stage, will also reduce the need for assisted delivery.

There is considerable disagreement concerning the preferred method. In the English-speaking world, in general, forceps are the preferred instruments, although the use of vacuum extraction when instrumental delivery is required is increasing. The situation is the reverse in many European countries, where forceps are used less frequently than vacuum extraction.

2 Conditions for instrumental delivery

The operator is a major determinant of the success or failure of instrumental delivery. Unfavorable results are almost always caused by the user's unfamiliarity with either the instrument or the basic rules governing its use.

A fully dilated cervix is a prerequisite for instrumental vaginal delivery. The station and degree of moulding of the head must be carefully assessed and its position accurately known. The use of oxytocin may be better than too early instrumental delivery for dealing with a delay in second stage labor before the baby's head reaches the pelvic floor.

The common indications for instrumental delivery, such as fetal distress or delay in the second stage of labor, are likely to create anxiety in the mother and her partner. Some of this anxiety can be relieved by keeping them fully informed of the reasons for, and the nature of, the procedures that are undertaken.

Proper and effective analgesia should be provided before instrumental delivery is commenced. Less pain relief is needed, as a rule, for vacuum extraction than for forceps delivery. Vacuum extraction or outlet forceps delivery can usually be accomplished comfortably with local infiltration of the perineum or pudendal nerve block. Rotational forceps deliveries will often require a more profound form of anesthesia, such as epidural or spinal block.

The total force exerted on the fetal head during instrumental birth will depend on the type of instrument, the duration of the procedure, and on the number and strength of pulls. Some descent of the head should occur with each pull. Absence of descent with traction on a correctly positioned instrument should be regarded as a reason to abandon the procedure in favor of cesarean section.

Elective instrumental vaginal delivery has been compared with spontaneous vaginal birth in only a few small trials. Instrumental delivery results in significantly more perineal trauma (both episiotomy and laceration) than spontaneous birth. The alleged benefits of an elective 'lift out' forceps in terms of slightly fewer babies with low cord blood pH values have to be weighed against the more frequent problem of maternal vaginal and perineal trauma.

3 Equipment and techniques

3.1 Forceps

Since the introduction of forceps, numerous modifications have been made in attempts to improve their efficiency and safety. Forceps can be grouped on a functional basis into those whose primary function is to exert traction and those whose primary function is to correct malposition. No controlled trials of the use of different types of forceps have been reported. One trial evaluated the use of a forceps pad designed to reduce infant trauma; the use of the pad resulted in fewer babies having craniofacial markings.

3.2 Vacuum extraction

Various cup designs have been used to perform vacuum extraction. The metal cups most widely used are the Bird-modification ones. The posterior cup is designed to be inserted higher up in the vagina than the anterior cups. This is to allow correct placement over the occiput when the head is deflexed.

More recently, a number of soft cups have been developed, which follow the contour of the baby's head during application. They are less likely than metal cups to be associated with scalp trauma, though serious complications, such as subgaleal hemorrhage, have been reported. Being soft, they are easy to apply and unlikely to injure the mother. As they are cleaned and sterilized as one item, they present no problems with assembly or leakage. In addition, the opinions of both women and midwives about the instruments appear to be favorable.

All the vacuum cups are satisfactory for outlet and non-rotational midpelvic operations. Operators would be well advised to develop confidence in outlet and non-rotational midpelvic procedures before embarking on assisted deliveries where the head is malrotated. The basic technique is similar in all positions of the occiput, and experience gained with non-rotational procedures will prove invaluable when the more difficult rotational operations are attempted. In one small study, no advantage of graded over rapid creation of a vacuum was shown. The few trials that have been carried out comparing the various rigid cup designs to one another have not demonstrated any differences in outcome. Comparisons of soft with rigid vacuum extraction cups suggest that soft cups are less likely to achieve vaginal delivery, but result in significantly fewer fetal scalp injuries than metal cups.

The success rate with a metal cup is better than with a soft cup, especially for delivering a baby in an occiput-posterior position, where the 'OP' cup is very useful. Because soft cups are also more likely to fail with a large baby, a high head, or a large amount of caput, it is reasonable to limit their use to more straightforward deliveries. Despite these disadvantages, it is worth continuing to use soft cups when feasible because they are associated with less neonatal trauma.

The risk of injury to the infant is directly related to the number of pulls with the vacuum extractor. Sudden cup detachments may cause injury to the scalp of the infant. In one study, increasing asynclitism (oblique presentation of the fetal head) and increasing application to delivery time correlated significantly with cephalhematoma. No advantage has been shown with reduced vacuum pressure between contractions.

4 Comparison of vacuum extraction and forceps

4.1 Efficiency

With adequate experience and proper placement of the vacuum cup, most deliveries that require instrumental rotation of the head can be accomplished by vacuum extraction, thus avoiding the need for painful and potentially traumatic forceps rotations. This experience should not be difficult to obtain and should form part of all specialty training programs in obstetrics. Although the vacuum extractor is less likely than forceps to achieve a vaginal delivery with the chosen instrument, with backup of forceps when required, vacuum extraction is associated with a lower overall cesarean-section rate.

The mean time between the decision to deliver and delivery itself is similar for forceps and vacuum extraction, although the range of the decision-to-delivery interval is greater for forceps. This is at least in part due to the time required to institute the more complex forms of analgesia used for forceps delivery. The widely held belief that vacuum extraction is too slow to be useful when rapid delivery is required for fetal distress can firmly be laid to rest.

On balance, for most instrumental vaginal deliveries, vacuum extraction is to be preferred over forceps. Reserving one instrument for routine applications and the other for especially difficult situations would be ill-advised. Even moderately difficult extractions, whether by forceps or by vacuum extraction, should not be undertaken unless the operator has considerable expertise with the instrument chosen. In the absence of such expertise, delivery by cesarean section should be considered.

4.2 Effects on the mother

The vacuum extractor is significantly less likely to cause serious maternal injury than the forceps. Its use is associated with a lower usage of regional and general anesthesia, and with significantly less pain to the mother, both at delivery and in the puerperium.

4.3 Effects on the infant

Vacuum extraction is more likely to cause cephalhematoma than forceps, but forceps are more likely to cause other kinds of scalp and facial injuries. No significant differences between the instruments have been found in the number of babies requiring phototherapy. Perhaps because of the chignon caused by the rigid vacuum cup, mothers tend to be more worried by the immediate appearance of the baby delivered by vacuum extraction than with forceps.

The vacuum extractor appears to be associated with an increased incidence of retinal hemorrhages (although this latter result is largely influenced by a single study that was methodologically less sound than all other trials reviewed).

There is not enough information available to judge the relative effects of the two instruments on the risk of perinatal death or the long-term condition of the infants. In the only follow-up study of cohorts randomized to the two instruments, the incidence of problems was similar in the vacuum and forceps groups, but the numbers of infants studied was too small to exclude anything other than very dramatic differences in outcome.

Follow-up studies showed no significant differences in mothers' attitudes to the instruments or in infant readmissions to hospital.

5 Conclusions

Both a valid indication and the necessary conditions must be met before instrumental delivery is undertaken. The cervix must be fully dilated; effective analgesia must be in place; and the operator must be familiar with the chosen instrument. There is no justification for a 'difficult instrumental delivery'. Cesarean section would almost always be preferable.

Shortening of the second stage with elective instrumental delivery can result in a clinically unimportant gain in umbilical cord blood pH, but may lead to a considerable increase in maternal vaginal and perineal trauma.

Forceps delivery and vacuum extraction are to a large extent interchangeable procedures. The available evidence indicates that the use of forceps is more likely to result in maternal injury, and is more dependent on extensive analgesia or anesthesia than is vacuum extraction.

Sources

Effective care in pregnancy and childbirth

Vacca, A and Keirse, M.J.N.C., Instrumental vaginal delivery.

Cochrane Library

Johanson, R.B. and Menon, V.J., Vacuum extraction versus forceps for assisted vaginal delivery.

Soft vs rigid vacuum extractor cups for assisted vaginal delivery.

Pre-Cochrane reviews

Johanson, R., Forceps vs spontaneous vaginal delivery. Review no. 07087.

Obstetric forceps pad designed to reduce trauma. Review no. 07086.

O'Neil vs Malmstrom vacuum extraction. Review no. 03795.

New Generation vs original Bird vacuum extraction. Review no. 03259.

Silastic vs Mityvac vacuum extraction. Review no. 03258.

Renfrew, M.J., Vacuum extraction compared to normal delivery. Review no.06517.

Other sources

Bofill, J.A., Rust, O.A., Schorr, S.J., Brown, R.C., Roberts, W.E. and Morrison, J.C. (1997). A randomized trial of two vacuum extraction techniques. *Obstet. Gynecol.*, **89**, 758–62.

Chalmers, J.A. and Chalmers, I. (1989). The obstetric vacuum extractor is the instrument of first choice for operative vaginal delivery. *Br. J. Obstet. Gynaecol.*, **96**, 505–6.

Garcia, J., Anderson, J., Vacca, A., Elbourne, D.R., Grant, A.M. and Chalmers, I. (1985). Views of women and their medical and midwifery attendants about instrumental delivery using vacuum extraction and forceps. *J. Psychosom. Obstet. Gynaecol.*, **4**, 1–9.

Cesarean section

1 Introduction

The term 'cesarean section' refers to the operation of delivering the baby through incisions made in the abdominal wall and uterus. It has an enormous potential for the preservation of life and health, probably greater than that of any other major surgical operation.

The cesarean section rate varies considerably among countries, from about 5% to over 25% of all deliveries. The optimal rate is not known, but little improvement in outcome appears to occur when rates rise above a minimum level. Despite this, high rates of cesarean section persist in many parts of the world.

Many cesarean sections are carried out for unequivocal indications, such as placenta praevia or transverse lie. The majority of the operations, however, are carried out for rather ambiguous indications. Criteria for the diagnoses of dystocia (prolonged labour) and fetal distress, two of the most common reasons for performing a cesarean section, are by no means clear. No data are yet available to suggest what proportion of babies presenting as a breech would benefit from delivery by cesarean section. Previous lower segment cesarean section by itself is rarely an adequate indication for a repeat cesarean section.

The extent to which obstetricians differ in the use of this major operation to deliver babies suggests that different obstetricians and the societies in which they practise have different practice guidelines and expectations as to when cesarean section is indicated. It also suggests that other factors, such as the socio-economic status of the woman, the influence of malpractice litigation, women's expectations, financial considerations, and convenience for both the obstetrician and the woman may sometimes be more important than obstetrical factors in determining the decision to operate.

2 Anesthesia for cesarean section

When cesarean section is required, its safety depends on the care with which the anesthetic is administered and the operation performed. Cesarean section can be carried out under either regional (epidural or spinal block) or general anesthesia. Regional anesthesia has many advantages. It largely avoids the risk of regurgitation and aspiration of stomach contents associated with general anesthesia, allows the mother to remain awake, and permits early contact between mother and baby at birth. The main disadvantages of using regional anesthesia for cesarean section relate to the extensive block required for the operation. This may result in a drop in blood pressure, which may require treatment with intravenous fluids and vasopressors. The limited data available from controlled trials show only minor differences in the effects of epidural or spinal anesthesia for cesarean section; spinal resulting in a quicker onset of anesthesia, less shivering with the onset of block, more frequent hypotensive episodes, and no differences in other substantive outcomes.

Despite the increasing popularity of regional anesthesia, general anesthesia is sometimes required. Regional anesthesia is contraindicated if the mother has a coagulation disorder. If the reason for the cesarean section relates to a bleeding complication in the mother, the drop in blood pressure with regional anesthesia can be particularly dangerous. General anesthesia can usually be more rapidly administered, and is of value when speed is important, such as when the fetus is in serious jeopardy. Some women prefer to be asleep for the operation.

The disadvantages of general anesthesia relate to the serious problems that are sometimes associated with it, such as pulmonary aspiration, inadequate airway control, and neonatal depression. If not managed properly, these can lead to significant maternal and fetal morbidity, and sometimes death. Aspiration of acidic stomach contents can cause acid pneumonitis (Mendelson's syndrome), the severity of which depends on the acidity of the aspirate (see Chapter 29).

The most important measure in preventing pulmonary aspiration is occlusion of the esophagus by cricoid pressure. The maneuver requires an assistant who is knowledgeable and capable. It loses its effectiveness unless skilled help is available. Deaths from Mendelson's syndrome usually result from not applying cricoid pressure, relaxing the pressure before intubation, or applying pressure inefficiently. An equally important problem with general anesthesia arises when the anesthetist is unable to intubate the trachea. Deaths due to aspiration or failed intubation are largely preventable, and can be almost eradicated by improvements in clinical care.

Whatever form of anesthesia is chosen, the woman should be in a 15–20 degree lateral tilt position, instead of lying flat on her back. This results in improved neonatal Apgar scores, probably as a result of relieving the pressure of the pregnant uterus on the vena cava and the aorta.

3 Surgical technique

Details of operative technique vary from surgeon to surgeon, and few of these techniques have been evaluated in controlled trials.

Pulmonary embolism is an important cause of maternal morbidity and mortality with cesarean section. Evidence from other surgical fields shows that this risk can be reduced by the pre-operative use of low-dose heparin, and the available data show no evidence that the use of heparin increases the risk of bleeding with cesarean section.

One small trial compared the use of an antiseptic impregnated film with the usual antiseptic scrub technique for skin preparation prior to cesarean section. No differences in infection rates were demonstrated.

When a transverse rather than a vertical skin incision is used, average operating time is longer, and more women require blood transfusions. On the other hand, febrile morbidity occurs somewhat less frequently with the transverse skin incision, and most women find the transverse scar more acceptable cosmetically.

A modification of the Joel Cohen technique has been compared with the Pfannenstiel technique in one randomized trial. The technique involves a transverse incision through the skin and short transverse incision in the subcutaneous tissue and fascia, which is extended laterally by blunt dissection to minimize bleeding. The peritoneal and subcutaneous layers are not sutured. Blood loss and operating time were significantly reduced in the study group, although postoperative hemoglobin levels were similar.

The uterine incision should be made transversely in the lower uterine segment, except in extremely rare circumstances. The initial incision is made with a scalpel. Whether scissors or fingers should be used to extend the incision, and whether the suture material or technique used for closure influences the post-operative result, have not been adequately evaluated. No benefits have been demonstrated for the use of a hemostatic stapler for incising the uterus, although the number of women involved in the trials has not been large enough to rule out significant benefits or adverse effects of the technique.

Elective manual removal of the placenta at cesarean should be avoided, particularly in Rh-negative women or others where transplacental bleeding might increase the risk of iso-sensitization. The available information from controlled trials suggests that manual removal increases maternal blood loss.

The results of single-layer or two-layer closure of the uterine incision are similar, and the time saved by use of a single-layer closure may be worthwhile. A policy of repairing the uterine incision after bringing the uterus out through the abdominal wound seems to have little impact on blood loss compared to one of repairing it within the abdomen, although it may decrease the risk of infective morbidity. It would seem sensible to exteriorize the uterus for repair, if there is difficulty with intra-abdominal exposure. Non-closure of the visceral and/or parietal peritoneum reduces operating time but available evidence does not point to any other clear clinical advantage or disadvantage. There is no evidence of the impact of peritoneal non-closure on longer term outcomes, such as technical difficulties in performing future cesarean sections.

The few small trials that have been carried out on other minutiae of operative technique do not provide sufficient data to guide clinical policy.

4 Conclusions

Cesarean section is a major operation, with great potential benefit, but also with substantial risks for both mother and baby. The hazards can be kept to a minimum, first, by avoiding unnecessary operations, and, second, by meticulous attention to proper anesthetic and surgical techniques. Consensus by clinicians and consumers by means of evidence-based clinical guidelines and public education may result in more uniform and appropriate use of this major intervention.

Sources

Effective care in pregnancy and childbirth

Lomas, J. and Enkin, M.W., Variations in operative delivery rates.

Pearson, J. and Rees, G., Technique of caesarean section.

Cochrane Library

Enkin, M.W. and Wilkinson, C., Lateral tilt for caesarean section.

Absorbable staples for uterine incision at caesarean section.

Manual removal of placenta at caesarean section.

Single versus two layer suturing for closing the uterine incision at caesarean section.

Uterine exteriorization versus intraperitoneal repair at caesarean section.

Wilkinson, C. and Enkin, M.W., Peritoneal non-closure at caesarean section.

Other sources

Wallin, G. and Fall, O. (1999). Modified Joel-Cohen technique for caesarean delivery. *Br. J. Obstet. Gynecol.*, **106**, 221–6.

CHAPTER 43

Prophylactic antibiotics with cesarean section

1 Introduction
2 Effects on infection and febrile morbidity
3 Choice of antibiotic preparation
4 Route of administration
5 Potential adverse consequences of antibiotic prophylaxis
6 Conclusions

1 Introduction

Maternal morbidity after cesarean section has not been studied as systematically as the maternal mortality associated with the operation, but the problem is undoubtedly substantial. Febrile morbidity, caused by postoperative infection or by other factors, appears to follow cesarean section in at least one in five women. Serious infections, such as pelvic abscess, septic shock, and septic pelvic vein thrombophlebitis, are not rare.

Labour and ruptured membranes are the most important factors associated with an increased risk of infection, the risk rising with increased duration of each. Obesity appears to be a risk factor of particular importance for wound infection. At one time, extraperitoneal cesarean section was proposed to reduce infectious morbidity in women at high risk of infection, but this approach is now of historical interest only.

The first step toward reducing the infectious morbidity that is so common after cesarean section is to minimize the number of unnecessary operations. The second step requires attention to the many factors that reduce the risk of infection when the operation is justified, such as: minimizing the length of hospital admission before surgery; delaying shaving of the operation site until immediately before the operation; sterilizing swabs, instruments, the gloves worn by the operating team; cleaning the skin of the woman; air exchanges in the operating theatre; and paying attention to good surgical technique.

The potential for prophylactic antibiotics to reduce maternal morbidity after cesarean section has by now been investigated systematically. The benefits have been unequivocally demonstrated. Although the extent to which toxic or allergic effects of antibiotics may cause maternal morbidity is not well established, the information that is available provides clear guidelines for practice.

2 Effects on infection and febrile morbidity

Antibiotic prophylaxis markedly reduces the risk of serious postoperative infection, such as pelvic abscess, septic shock, and septic pelvic vein thrombophlebitis. A protective effect of the same order of magnitude is seen for endometritis. The degree of reduction in the risk of wound infection is slightly less but still substantial. The evidence for these benefits is overwhelming.

Prophylactic antibiotics reduce the relative risk of endometritis to a similar extent for women having planned (elective) cesarean sections, as for those having emergency procedures, whilst the impact on wound infection seems greater after emergency procedures. The absolute numbers of serious infections avoided by prophylactic administration are greater with emergency cesarean sections because the rates of infection are higher. Postoperative febrile morbidity has fewer sequelae than the more serious infections, but is important because of its higher incidence. Secondary effects, such as the economic impact of prolongation of hospital stay and interference with mother–infant contact, must also be considered.

3 Choice of antibiotic preparation

The risk of postoperative febrile morbidity is reduced to a comparable extent by broad-spectrum penicillins, such as ampicillin, and cephalosporins. The evidence from direct comparisons between broad-spectrum penicillins and cephalosporins suggests that they have similar effects on the risk of postoperative febrile morbidity. There is no convincing evidence that antibiotics with a broader spectrum of activity, such as second- and third-generation cephalosporins, are more efficacious than a first-generation cephalosporin.

Trials comparing different regimens show no clear advantage to a combination of antibiotics over single agents. Likewise, the use of three to five doses, rather than a single dose of antibiotics for prophylaxis of infection with cesarean section does not appear to confer any additional benefit.

4 Route of administration

Intra-operative irrigation with antibiotics has been shown to be more effective than irrigation with placebo in reducing the risk of postoperative febrile morbidity, but trials do not suggest that antibiotic irrigation is more effective than systemic administration.

5 Potential adverse consequences of antibiotic prophylaxis

Only a minority of the reports of controlled trials included information about adverse effects of the prophylactic agents used, and even in these reports the reference was usually rather casual. It is thus not surprising that the reported incidence of adverse reactions was very low – 1% or less. This is well below the rate of adverse reactions that one would expect of antibiotics, especially broad-spectrum antibiotics given intravenously.

Drug effects on the infant (which might include protective as well as unwanted effects) have not been studied systematically by the majority of investigators. Many clinicians prefer to prevent exposure of the baby to antibiotics by starting them after the umbilical cord has been clamped, as was done in most of the trials reported, even if there is some slight, as yet undetected, loss of prophylactic efficacy.

Antibiotics received by the mother can also reach the baby through breast milk. The drug levels involved seem likely to be very low, particularly if the course of prophylactic antibiotics has been relatively short.

An important argument of those who have objected to routine antibiotic prophylaxis has been their concern about the effects of this practice on the bacterial flora, namely replacement of non-pathogenic bacteria with pathogenic ones, and a rise in resistance of bacteria in the women and in the hospital environment generally. At least some antibiotics appear to cause these changes with relatively few doses.

There is some suggestion that certain prophylactic regimens, e.g. trimethoprim and sulfamethoxazole, may be less disruptive of flora, yet remain effective.

Adverse ecological effects on bacterial flora are difficult to quantify and predict, but are potentially of greater concern than adverse drug reactions in individual mothers and babies. Although routine culture of genital tract specimens to manage infections following cesarean section is not recommended, the hospital bacteriology laboratory should monitor and report on the susceptibility patterns of commonly isolated organisms to detect gradual changes in antibiotic resistance and advise on appropriate empiric treatment regimens.

6 Conclusions

Antibiotic prophylaxis can reduce the risk of serious infections. If the level of post-cesarean infectious morbidity is very low without a policy of antibiotic prophylaxis, the ratio of benefits to costs, in absolute terms, might argue against instituting such a policy. Such circumstances are rare, and the evidence justifies far wider adoption of antibiotic prophylaxis than currently exists. Although the incidence of adverse drug effects among women receiving prophylactic antibiotics has probably been underestimated, it is inconceivable that it could outweigh the reduction in serious maternal morbidity that can be achieved by a policy of antibiotic prophylaxis. Potential adverse drug effects in the baby may be lessened by beginning prophylaxis after the umbilical cord has been divided.

The risk of adverse ecological effects is likely to be reduced if the total load of antibiotics is reduced. The disadvantages of longer courses of antibiotics, in terms of an increase in the total antibiotic load and in the number of women experiencing side effects, and the additional financial cost, may outweigh the advantages of greater prophylactic efficacy compared with shorter or single-dose regimens.

In regard to choice of antibiotic, the broad-spectrum penicillins are as effective as the cephalosporins. No strong case for using a second- or third-generation cephalosporin, or adding aminoglycosides to broad-spectrum penicillins, can be made.

Withholding prophylactic antibiotics from women having cesarean section will increase the chances that they will experience serious morbidity. Further trials which include no-treatment controls would be unethical.

Sources

Effective care in pregnancy and childbirth

Enkin, M., Enkin. E, and Chalmers. I., Prophylactic antibiotics in association with caesarean section.

Cochrane Library

Hopkins, L. and Smaill, F., Antibiotic prophylaxis regimens and drugs for caesarean section.

Smaill, F. and Hofmeyr, G.J., Antibiotic prophylaxis for caesarean section.

Other sources

Mugford, M., Kingston, J. and Chalmers, I. (1989). Reducing the incidence of infection after caesarean section: implications of prophylaxis with antibiotics for hospital resources. *BMJ*, **299**, 1003–6.

Care after childbirth

CHAPTER 44

Immediate care of the newborn infant

1 Introduction

The vast majority of newborn babies require little more than a clear airway and adequate warmth to support the first few minutes of adaptation to extra-uterine life. The success of human evolution and the exceptionally high survival rate of human infants attest to this. Unless specific problems need urgent attention, babies should be given to their mothers as soon after birth as the mother is ready.

2 Immediate care of the normal newborn infant

2.1 Welcoming the newborn infant

In his book *Birth without Violence*, Frederick Leboyer described a number of measures designed to minimize 'the shock of the newborn's first separation experiences': the use of a dark delivery room, delayed clamping of the umbilical cord, gentle massage, and a warm bath for the infant. Controlled trials of these specific measures have not shown any effects, either adverse or beneficial, on infant health, neurobehavioral status in the first few days of life, or subsequent development. The fact that no long-term advantages of the specific measures advocated by Leboyer have been demonstrated does not obviate the need for treating the newborn with the regard and respect due to any human being, including gentleness and avoidance of excessive noise in the environment.

2.2 Ensuring a clear airway

The practice of routine suctioning to remove secretions from the newborn infant's oral and nasal passages has not been assessed in any clinical trials, and its value is uncertain. Possible benefits of the practice include improved air exchange, reduced likelihood of aspiration of secretions, and, perhaps, reduced acquisition of any pathogens present in the amniotic fluid or birth canal. Potential hazards include cardiac arrhythmias, laryngospasm, and pulmonary artery vasospasm.

Most healthy babies require no suction, they can usually clear their own airways. If nasal and pharyngeal suctioning is required, care should be taken to minimize pharyngeal stimulation. Suction bulbs, rather than catheters should be used, because suction bulbs are less likely to induce cardiac arrhythmias.

The practice of routine suctioning of the stomach was introduced following an untested suggestion that the respiratory distress of infants of diabetic women often resulted from regurgitation and aspiration that might have been prevented by gastric suctioning. As the passage of the tube during the immediate neonatal period may produce brady-cardia or laryngospasm and disruption of prefeeding behavior, there is no justification for routine gastric suctioning.

2.3 Maintaining body temperature

The recommendation that all babies be kept warm immediately after birth is based on a large body of evidence about thermal physiology of both newborn animals and humans. Newborns can maintain their body temperature in a cool environment only by greatly increased energy expenditure. Even vigorous newborns exposed to cold delivery rooms may experience marked drops in body temperature and develop metabolic acidosis during the first two hours of life.

Babies should be dried with prewarmed towels, giving particular attention to drying the head. They should be held by their mothers, preferably in skin-to-skin contact, and covered with a dry warm blanket. They may be held by the father or companion, or placed under a radiant warmer or in an incubator, if the mother is unable to hold her baby.

2.4 Initiation of breastfeeding

For several decades in developed countries the usual practice was to separate the mother from her baby soon after birth. After a brief visit with his or her mother, the baby was transferred to a nursery. Bottles of water or glucose water were routinely given for the first and subsequent early feeds.

These unhelpful routines were phased out when research identified the beneficial properties of colostrum. Further changes came with the growing belief that early contact between mother and infant would enhance the mother's attachment to her baby. Results of the small controlled trials comparing early versus late contact, including timing of breastfeeding, are inconclusive. The implications of this are that mothers should have contact with their babies as soon after birth as they wish, and for as long as they wish.

Babies exhibit wide ranges in normal behavior. Some, but not all, are ready to feed immediately after birth. Interventions aimed at either delaying or speeding-up the time of the first feed should be avoided (see also Chapter 46).

2.5 Prophylactic administration of vitamin K to prevent hemorrhagic disease

The natural population incidence of hemorrhagic disease in early infancy due to vitamin K deficiency is not known, because infants at high risk have been given prophylactic intramuscular vitamin K at birth. Oral or no prophylaxis has been reserved for healthy term infants. In the 1950s, before prophylaxis was given, fully breastfed infants were said to have an incidence of about 4 per 1000 births, with most being classic hemorrhagic disease of the newborn occurring within the first 10 days of life. The incidence may have been high because of the relatively common occurrence of birth trauma and because the practice of delaying breastfeeding denied infants colostrum with its relatively high vitamin K content. Classic hemorrhagic disease, occurring predominantly from the umbilicus and gut or into the skin, can be totally prevented with a single dose of vitamin K given at birth.

The main concern now is adequate prophylaxis for late hemorrhagic disease, a rarer but more serious disorder, which is largely confined to infants who are fully breastfed. The concentration of vitamin K in cow's milk or infant formula is considerably greater than in human milk. Late hemorrhagic disease usually presents at 2–12 weeks of age, and is often fatal or leaves serious morbidity due to intracranial hemorrhage. In 40–60% of cases, there is another underlying problem, such as malabsorption or liver disease, contributing to the vitamin K deficiency.

Recent data indicate that the rate of the late vitamin K deficiency bleeding is about 1 in 17 000 without prophylaxis, in the range of 1 in 25 000 to 1 in 70 000 in infants who have had a single oral dose of 1–2 milligrams at birth, and 1 in 400 000 after a single intramuscular injection at birth.

Although intramuscular vitamin K is the most reliable and effective prophylaxis, giving an intramuscular injection at birth is invasive and painful. There has been considerable debate as to whether it is associated with cancer or leukemia, and although not completely resolved, the weight of evidence favors no association. Very similar rates of protection against classical and late hemorrhagic disease can be achieved by giving repeated oral doses, either 1 milligram weekly or 25 micrograms daily. Undertaking this form of oral prophylaxis requires that parents accept responsibility for ensuring the course is completed.

2.6 Prophylactic measures to prevent eye infections

The Credé procedure of instilling silver nitrate routinely into the eyes of all newborn babies, introduced in 1881, was credited with the control of gonococcal ophthalmia of the newborn in the last century. As a result, many countries have a legal requirement that one of a list of approved chemical agents be instilled routinely into the eyes of all newborn infants, with the aim of preventing infectious conjunctivitis. No controlled trials have been carried out to ascertain whether or not this is a more effective means of preventing blindness than careful observation of the newborn, followed by adequate treatment of any conjunctivitis that might appear. In circumstances where the incidence of bacterial ophthalmia is high, routine chemical prophylaxis may be useful.

In these circumstances, the next question concerns the choice of the most effective and least harmful agent. Silver nitrate results in more chemical conjunctivitis and provides no greater protection than tetracycline or erythromycin against gonococcal ophthalmia. It is ineffective against *Chlamydia* (which in many areas is the most common cause of neonatal ophthalmia). It should no longer be used. Both tetracycline and erythromycin provide protection against chlamydia, as well as gonococcal conjunctivitis.

Topical agents applied to the eyes of newborn infants may decrease eye openness and inhibit visual responses. This may disrupt the visual interaction between mother and baby during the first hour of life. If topical agents are necessary, their use should be delayed for an hour after birth. Mothers and babies should be able to enjoy the immediate closeness of the first hour or so after birth before chemical agents are applied.

3 Prophylactic measures in newborns considered to be at above-average risk

3.1 Suctioning of infants who have passed meconium before birth
For infants who have passed meconium before birth, suctioning the nostrils, mouth, and pharynx before delivery of the chest may prevent postnatal aspiration of meconium in the pharynx. This procedure is sufficiently safe to be recommended, even though its effectiveness in preventing severe meconium aspiration is unproven.

Four controlled trials, involving 2800 infants, have compared a policy of routine versus no (or selective) endotracheal intubation and aspiration in the immediate management of vigorous term meconium-stained babies at birth. Contrary to what was commonly believed, routine endotracheal suctioning conferred no benefits and increased the risk of meconium aspiration syndrome. Based on current evidence, routine intubation of these infants should be abandoned, and reliance placed on nasal and pharyngeal suction.

3.2 Elective tracheal intubation for very-low-birthweight infants

Although some neonatologists advocate immediate intubation of all very-low-birthweight infants, whether or not signs of respiratory depression or respiratory distress are present, the available evidence does not warrant such a policy. Because of the potential hazards of intubation, routine delivery room intubation of infants below 1500 g with no signs of respiratory distress or respiratory depression is not justified on the basis of current evidence.

3.3 Prophylactic administration of surfactant to immature infants

A number of surfactant preparations, both synthetic and derived from animal sources, are available and in general use. There is clear evidence from large trials that prophylactic administration of surfactant to preterm newborns at high risk of developing respiratory distress syndrome (intubated infants less than 30 weeks gestation) is beneficial. Compared to therapeutic administration, prophylactic administration of surfactant improves respiratory function, and decreases the incidence of respiratory distress symptoms, pneumothorax, bronchopulmonary dysplasia, and death. No significant untoward effects of prophylactic surfactant administration have been noted.

4 Immediate care of ill newborn infants

The availability of professionals skilled in neonatal resuscitation has increased with the growth of neonatology as a specialty. This means that the birth of a very preterm asphyxiated or otherwise high-risk neonate is now more likely to be attended by someone who is experienced in giving care to such infants. A proportion of ill and high-risk infants will continue to present as unpredicted emergencies, however, and it will often fall to a midwife, nurse, general practitioner, or trainee obstetric specialist to initiate and continue neonatal resuscitation.

Whenever possible, a person skilled in resuscitation who can devote all of his or her attention to the infant should be in attendance at high-risk deliveries. Basic resuscitation equipment (a radiant warmer, resuscitation bags and masks, endotracheal tubes, laryngoscope, stethoscope, oxygen source and tubing) should be readily available for every delivery room. Those attending births at home should ensure that there is a means of keeping the baby warm, and that they carry resuscitation bag and masks, a stethoscope, and possibly an oxygen source. Because the need for resuscitation is not recognized prior to the birth of approximately half of all infants requiring resuscitation, the presence and proper working order of this equipment should be verified before each delivery.

While anesthesia bags are likely to be required for the optimal resuscitation of severely asphyxiated infants, their hazards if used improperly (e.g. the application of dangerously high airway pressures) make them unsuitable for routine use by inexperienced caregivers. Likewise, the hazards of umbilical artery catheters and trochars for endotracheal tubes should preclude their use in delivery rooms, except by highly experienced resuscitators.

4.1 Resuscitation

Artificial ventilation should be initiated promptly for infants with a heart rate less than 100 beats/minute after birth, and oxygen should be administered to any infant with generalized cyanosis. Regardless of heart rate or colour, artificial ventilation should also be commenced for infants with inadequate chest excursion and poor breath sounds, especially small preterm infants likely to have surfactant deficiency.

Proper ventilation of the infant is the single most important aspect of neonatal resuscitation, and the heart rate is the most useful and easily measured criterion for its success. Caregivers who do not frequently intubate newborn infants should initiate resuscitation using a face mask, and consider intubation only when the heart rate does not increase with properly performed bag and mask ventilation.

Before intubation, attention should be given to the following points: proper positioning of the head ('sniffing position'); ensuring that the upper airway is clear; using sufficient pressure to produce adequate chest excursions; and administering an adequate inspired oxygen concentration. Observing distension of the throat as the resuscitation bag is squeezed indicates that a proper head position and clear airway (allowing delivery of gas to the level of the glottis) has been established. The careful use of an anesthesia bag may be required to deliver more pressure or a greater oxygen concentration, than can be delivered by self-inflating bags. Applying excessive pressure to the infant's head through the face mask may cause persistent bradycardia.

4.2 Oxygen

Supplemental oxygen (100% concentration of the warm and humidified gas) is usually recommended for artificial ventilation of neonates who have not established effective spontaneous respiration by one minute of age. The need for 100 % oxygen has been challenged, and some recent trials are investigating the benefits and risks of lower concentrations of oxygen. Outside a hospital setting, positive pressure ventilation with air may be more practical and is reported to be effective.

Some concern has been expressed that blowing oxygen across the face of a newborn infant might result in bradycardia, but most concern has been focused on whether the risk of severe retinopathy would be appreciably increased in immature infants who experience short periods of exposure to high blood-oxygen levels. There is no satisfactory evidence, however, to suggest that the risk is any greater than that associated with the relatively high blood-oxygen levels that occur at birth in all babies with the onset of air breathing.

4.3 Cardiac massage

Cardiac massage through the intact chest wall of the newborn baby can be life-saving when used for infants born with an absent heart beat. The procedure is not without hazard; it may cause rib fractures and trauma to the liver or lung.

Little information of the kind needed to recommend precise indications and methods is available. Current recommendations are to perform cardiac massage either by using both thumbs with the hands encircling the chest, or by using the tips of the middle finger and either the index or ring finger of one hand positioned directly above the chest. The sternum should be depressed one-half to three-quarters of an inch (1.5 cm), 120 times per minute.

4.4 Naloxone

Naloxone hydrochloride is a narcotic antagonist, believed to be virtually free of side-effects. It may be administered as an adjunctive measure *after* assisted ventilation has been established, if depression is thought to be the result of a narcotic drug given to the mother before birth. It is probably wise not to give naloxone to the newborn of a narcotic-dependent mother for fear of precipitating withdrawal illness in the baby.

Apart from concern about the potential importance of endogenous opioid substances in newborn infants, mothers have reported less optimal ratings of infant behavior among naloxone-treated infants than among controls. Administration of naloxone should, therefore, be restricted to infants who have been exposed to narcotics during labour and who also require active resuscitation in the immediate neonatal period.

4.5 Sodium bicarbonate

Randomized trials have failed to detect any benefit from either rapid or slow administration of sodium bicarbonate to asphyxiated neonates. Potential hazards include a transient rise in $PaCO_2$ and fall in PaO_2; a sudden expansion of blood volume; a reduction in cerebral blood flow; and an increased incidence of intracranial hemorrhage.

In the absence of any demonstrated benefits of giving sodium bicarbonate in the immediate postnatal period, its use cannot be recommended.

4.6 Blood volume expanders

The only clear-cut indication for the use of blood volume expanders in the early neonatal period is the combination of unmistakable signs of shock with evidence of acute blood loss, including fetomaternal hemorrhage. In this circumstance, shock may be treated with repeated infusions of blood volume expanders (usually 5–10 ml) and the infant's response assessed after each infusion. The volume expander may be Ringer's lactate, saline, or in extreme emergency due to blood loss, heparinized placental blood. In the past, 5% albumin solutions have been used and are often still used for this purpose, but meta-analysis comparing colloid with electrolyte solutions for shock in adults clearly showed that mortality was higher with the use of albumin solutions, and this may be the case with newborns as well.

Volume expanders have also been used in the presence of hypotension unaccompanied by other signs of shock or blood loss. This practice is of far more dubious validity.

5 Indications for withholding or discontinuing resuscitation

The issue of when to withhold or discontinue resuscitation is the most difficult treatment decision to be made in the delivery room. Much of the information needed to define appropriate indications for using intensive care is lacking. Better data are required on the effect of intensive care on mortality and the quality of life of survivors, and the cost of care for severely impaired or malformed infants.

Ultimately, decisions to withhold or withdraw aggressive care involve value judgements about what is considered an acceptable outcome and an acceptable cost. Although much has been written to express the views of health-care professionals, lawyers, and ethicists concerning aggressive care of extremely high-risk infants, little has been done to explore the views of the parents who, apart from the child, have most at stake in such decisions. The problem may be compounded in developing countries, where neonatal intensive care facilities are limited.

Given the limited amount of useful information for reaching decisions about instituting or withholding aggressive neonatal care, a liberal policy of resuscitation must be recommended whenever doubt exists. This allows the physician time to gather important information about the infant, and the distressed parents time and opportunity to participate more effectively in joint decisions about subsequent treatment.

6 Conclusions

The vast majority of infants need only a vigilant caregiver, warmth, a clear airway, and a gentle welcome. Mothers should have contact with their babies as soon as possible after birth, for as long as they wish. Initiation of breastfeeding should happen when the baby and mother are ready.

Many high-risk newborns can be successfully cared for by rather simple means.

Nasal and pharyngeal suction should be carried out on babies who have passed meconium *in utero*. Endotracheal intubation and suction should not be carried out routinely on vigorous, term babies who are meconium-stained at birth. There is no justification for routine suctioning of the stomach or for routine intubation of all very low-birthweight infants in the delivery room.

The great majority of babies who are depressed at birth require only appropriate ventilation without the need of drugs, volume expanders, or other adjuncts. The most common serious error in neonatal resuscitation is the failure to recognize and correct hypoventilation, a problem that is preventable with sufficient training and experience. Each hospital must establish appropriate methods to facilitate the most effective care for asphyxiated or depressed neonates. Whenever feasible, the birth of high-risk infants should be attended by a caregiver experienced in neonatal resuscitation.

In the absence of further evidence, breastfed babies should receive supplemental vitamin K routinely to prevent hemorrhagic disease of the newborn. Although the evidence is not conclusive, it is probably best to administer vitamin K to formula-fed babies as well.

Where not required by law, observation for, and prompt treatment of, ophthalmia may be as effective as routine prophylaxis and save many babies from unnecessary medication. If eye prophylaxis is required, erythromycin causes less chemical conjunctivitis than silver nitrate and is more effective against chlamydia infection. Silver nitrate should not be used. There is no evidence to suggest that topical ophthalmic preparations must be given immediately after birth.

Sources

Effective care in pregnancy and childbirth

Berger, H., Clinical examination of the newborn infant.

Tyson, J., Silverman, W. and Reisch, J., Immediate care of the newborn infant.

Effective care of the newborn infant

Tyson, J., Immediate care of the newborn infant.

Cochrane Library

Alderson, P., Bunn, F., Lefebvre, C., Li Wan Po, A., Li, L., Roberts, I. *et al.*, Human albumin solution for resuscitation and volume expansion in critically ill patients.

Bunn, F., Alderson, P. and Hawkins, V., Colloid solutions for fluid resuscitation.

Flenady, V.J. and Woodgate, P.G., Radiant warmers versus incubators for regulating body temperature in newborn infants.

Halliday, H.L., Endotracheal intubation at birth for prevention of mortality and morbidity in vigorous, meconium-stained infants born at term.

Puckett, R.M. and Offringa, M., Vitamin K for preventing haemorrhagic disease in newborn infants [protocol].

Renfrew, M.J. and Lang, S., Early versus delayed initiation of breast-feeding.

Schierhout, G., Roberts, I. and Alderson, P., Colloid versus crystalloids for fluid resuscitation in critically ill patients.

Soll, R.F. and Morley, C.J., Prophylactic versus selective use of surfactant for preventing morbidity and mortality in preterm infants.

Other sources

Leboyer, F. (1975). *Birth without violence.* New York: Knopf.

von Kries, R. (1998). Neonatal vitamin K prophylaxis: the Gordian knot still awaits untying. *BMJ*, **316**, 161–2.

von Kries, R. and Hanawa, Y. (1993). Neonatal vitamin K prophylaxis. Report on Scientific and Standardization Subcommittee on Perinatal Haemostasis. *Thromb. Haemostas.*, **69**, 293–5.

Mother and baby

1 Introduction

A new mother needs both emotional support and practical help in the days following childbirth. The form that this help takes, and the way it is given, varies from culture to culture and from time to time. The shift from home to hospital, as the usual place of birth in the twentieth century, has influenced the pattern of mother–baby interaction in at least two ways. First, a woman who gives birth in unfamiliar surroundings, attended by caregivers who she does not know, may feel inhibited and behave differently towards her newborn child than she might at home among familiar faces. Second, institutional rules and policies may obstruct spontaneous social interaction between a new mother and her baby.

2 Restriction of early mother–infant contact

The only justification for practices that restrict a woman's autonomy, her freedom of choice, and her access to her baby, would be clear evidence that these restrictive practices do more good than harm.

Evidence about the adverse consequences of routine separation of mothers and their newborn infants in the early postnatal period, accumulated during the thirty years or more during which this practice was widespread. Several controlled trials have compared the effects of institutional policies that restrict interaction between mothers and their newborn babies in the early hours after birth with policies that encourage interaction at that time. Maternal affectionate behavior was significantly less evident among mothers whose contact with their baby had been restricted than among mothers whose care encouraged liberal contact.

Trials have also compared standard hospital practices with attempts to encourage mother–infant interaction after the immediate postnatal period. The additional interaction in these trials ranged from a small amount of caretaking in the intensive-care nursery by mothers of preterm infants, to full rooming-in for mothers of normal infants. The few statistically significant differences that were observed suggest that restrictive policies were associated with less affectionate maternal behavior and more frequent feelings of incompetence and lack of confidence. Perhaps most important of all, the results of one well-conducted study suggests that, compared with a policy of rooming-in, the routine hospital policy of separating mothers from their babies led to an increase in the subsequent risk of child abuse and neglect among socially deprived, first-time mothers.

Hospital policies can affect subsequent breastfeeding patterns among women who wish to breastfeed their babies. In all trials that have addressed this question, the proportion of women who discontinued breastfeeding in the first 3 months was substantially higher among women who had been subjected to more restrictive policies.

Maternal caretaking behavior is so essential to the newborn baby that a variety of biological and social mechanisms must have evolved to promote it. The mutually reinforcing affectionate behavior that occurs during early postnatal mother–infant contact is only one such mechanism. It is not the only mechanism. Most mothers who are constrained from early contact with their babies, whether through illness, misguided hospital policies, or personal preference, are likely to overcome any effects of this separation in the longer term.

3 Control of infection

Many of the regulations and routines in hospital postpartum care were instituted as attempts to prevent or contain cross-infection. As hospital nurseries began to fill up with members of the baby boom that followed the Second World War, staphylococcal skin disease among neonates became the major infectious problem. A variety of measures were taken in attempts to deal with this problem, including isolation, segregation, rules of dress and entry to the nursery, medicated bathing, and special treatment of the umbilical cord.

The inflexible use of central nurseries, in which a number of babies were kept in close proximity to each other but apart from their mothers, may actually have increased the risk of infection. A study performed almost 50 years ago showed lower rates of colonization and infection in babies who spent between 8 and 12 hours a day with their mothers, than in babies who were kept in a nursery and were rarely in contact with their mothers. The results of this controlled study had little impact on the then almost universal policy of routinely separating mothers and babies. Instead, the problem of cross-infection and nursery epidemics of staphylococcal infection was addressed with more technological approaches. The use of gowns, hats, and masks in nurseries became routine, despite the lack of any evidence from controlled trials that they reduced infant colonization and infection rates.

As segregation and isolation failed to control neonatal infection, the mainstay of infection prophylaxis shifted to regimens of treatment of the umbilical cord and medicated bathing. Questions about various regimens for umbilical cord care have been addressed in studies that compared application of an antiseptic with no antiseptic, antibiotics versus antiseptics, powders versus no powders, and closed versus open dressings. Studies of bathing have compared medicated bath water with unmedicated bath water, and routine daily bathing while in hospital with an initial bath only. All the studies were conducted in developed countries, on healthy term infants. Under these circumstances there is no evidence of benefit from any form of cord care beyond keeping the cord clean, and the available evidence suggests that routine bathing (medicated or otherwise) of babies is not justified.

Hospital practices vary widely. With the increasingly widespread practice of 24-hour rooming-in for healthy mothers and babies, normal newborn nurseries have become obsolete in some hospitals. In those hospitals that retain newborn nurseries, however, many restrictive and costly practices remain in force. Gowning rules persist in almost three-quarters of newborn nurseries, despite the lack of evidence that this ritual has any beneficial effect. Many hospitals invoke concern about infection as a reason for restricting or forbidding siblings to visit, although studies using concurrent and historical control groups have been unable to detect any adverse effect of this on infant colonization rates.

It would be extremely dangerous to take a cavalier attitude to the undoubted reality of hospital-spread infection among new mothers and babies. Means for preventing or containing such infections must be kept under constant review. But maintaining or instituting restrictive measures without assessing whether or not they accomplish these ends is not an appropriate response. Unrestricted contact between mothers and babies, as with 24-hour rooming-in, is believed to be protective, in that the infants become colonized with the organisms of their mothers rather than the antibiotic-resistant organisms prevalent in hospitals.

4 Routine observations

Making and recording regular measurements of temperature, pulse, blood pressure, fundal height, and observations of lochia and the various wounds that a woman may sustain during childbirth, is still common practice in the days following childbirth. The intensity of this screening activity varies arbitrarily and depends more on the hospital in which a mother happens to give birth, and on the length of time she spends in it, than on her individual needs. While it is prudent to observe women in this way when they are known to be at increased risk of either infection or hemorrhage, it is difficult to justify this as a routine for all women.

5 Drugs for relief of symptoms

The postpartum period is often accompanied by a number of discomforts. Pain in the perineum and breasts (discussed in other chapters) is common. After-pains (uterine spasms) can also cause pain and distress in the first 4 days after birth. Women not infrequently count these symptoms among the most unpleasant memories they have of childbirth.

In most hospitals, medication for such discomforts tends to be under the direct control and supervision of hospital personnel. This policy is valid in the case of dangerous drugs, drugs that might interact with other medications, or those that would normally be available only on a doctor's prescription. It does not make sense for drugs that outside hospital, are readily available without a prescription. Because these medications are usually for the relief of symptoms, it would be more reasonable for women to use them when they feel the need to do so.

In many hospitals, non-prescription drugs intended for the relief of symptoms are still administered routinely and at set times. Professional belief in the value of early and regular bowel evacuation, for example, has led to some rather obsessional concerns on this matter. Laxatives, stool softeners, enemas, and anal ointments, remain routine components of postpartum care in some hospitals. In the puerperium, as at other times, routinely prescribed laxatives and medicated enemas do result in earlier bowel movements, and bulk-forming laxatives are less likely to cause unpleasant cramps and diarrhea than are irritant laxatives. This cannot be regarded, however, as justification for administering any of these preparations routinely.

In an attempt to provide a more rational basis for care (including self-care), a number of hospitals have developed programs to provide mothers with information about the drugs they may use, and have given them access to their own supply of medications. These descriptive studies all suggest that women are usually pleased with these arrangements and that staff time is used more efficiently after their introduction.

Routine medications for 'non-symptoms', such as oral ergometrine with the aim of hastening uterine involution, should not be used without evidence of a beneficial effect on substantive outcomes.

6 Length of hospital stay

How long should a healthy woman and baby remain in hospital after childbirth? The generally accepted 'correct' length of postnatal stay has varied greatly from time to time and varies equally widely among institutions today. It appears to be determined more by fashion and the availability of beds than by any systematic assessment of the needs of recently delivered women and their new babies.

The period of 'lying in' in industrialized societies had its institutional foundations with the establishment of charitable lying-in hospitals in the mid-eighteenth century. In these first maternity hospitals, women were, quite literally, confined to bed for a period of 28 days following delivery! By the 1950s, the usual hospital lying-in period was 12–14 days but, since then, it has fallen in most countries and frequently it is no more than 1–2 days.

Several formal early discharge programs, often with strict inclusion criteria, have been instituted as a deliberate change from standard hospital policies. The most common impetus for initiating such programs seems to have been the needs of the institution (because of a shortage of beds or personnel), although some programs appear to have been inspired by the preferences of childbearing women.

Both randomized trials and observational studies have shown that few women or babies are re-admitted to hospital after early discharge. These low re-admission rates demonstrate that early discharge from hospital is feasible and that healthy mothers and babies who have help at home, and follow-up care and guidance available, may safely go home within a few hours of birth.

Although no adverse consequences of early postnatal discharge from hospital have been demonstrated in terms of maternal and child health, there is also no evidence that such programs save money or resources, unless beds are closed as a result. If home support is provided, the costs of support given to women discharged early have been estimated to be about the same as the savings in hospital costs that result from earlier discharge. Also, when healthy women go home earlier, those remaining in hospital are, on average, more sick, require more intensive care, and involve additional work and strain for the staff. Early hospital discharge programs inevitably put an additional load on the primary care sector and on the family or friends of the woman. The additional resources required to cope with this load must be assessed in any credible attempt to assess the costs of early discharge from hospital.

Demands for early discharge programs have been made by a variety of activists who believe themselves to be speaking on behalf of child-bearing women. When such programs have been instituted, they have not always been popular. The extent to which women who give birth in hospital want early discharge may have been overestimated, and may depend on the support available at home.

Women's physical, social, and psychological circumstances after delivery vary greatly. Professionals should be as flexible as possible in response to this variation; this may be easier in situations where there is continuity of care. Choice may well be the crucial issue. Some women may feel that their hospital stay was too long, while others feel it was too short. Perhaps a more extended escape from duties at home would have helped some women to recover from childbirth more effectively.

Although early discharge from hospital is feasible and safe, it is neither clearly beneficial (in either health or economic terms) nor wanted by the majority of women. Firm decisions about when a woman should go home after childbirth should be delayed until after she has given birth and, as far as possible, be based on her individual needs and preferences, rather than on any predetermined formula.

7 Support and education

7.1 General support and education

Fragmentation of care is almost inevitable when the care of mothers is the responsibility of midwives or postpartum nurses and obstetricians, while care of the babies is carried out by nursery nurses and pediatricians. Consistent advice and continuity of care are prerequisites for effective support to mothers and their newborn babies. This is easier to achieve if mother and baby are accommodated together or, at the very least, if the same people are looking after both of them. The postpartum stay in hospital presents clear opportunities for imparting information that may be of help to new mothers. Although there is little agreement on what should be the content of formal postpartum educational programs, a number of studies, several of them controlled trials, have addressed the methods of postpartum education. These studies have dealt with educational programs including subjects ranging from contraception, through feeding and immunization advice, to information about child safety. Although the demonstrable effects of teaching were rarely as dramatic as the investigators had hoped, this body of research shows that postpartum educational programs can, and do, favorably affect parental behavior and health outcomes.

7.2 Support for mothers with special needs

Providing a hospital telephone service to offer advice or information by postpartum nursing staff to new parents is believed to be of benefit, but the only controlled study of this practice did not evaluate it in terms of effects on mothers' or babies' well-being, and there have been no economic evaluations of this practice.

Eleven controlled trials have evaluated the effectiveness of additional home-based support for mothers and babies who were believed to be at risk because of social disadvantage (related to poverty, ethnicity, social isolation, marital status, and/or age). In most studies, the additional support involved regular home visits by a specially trained, experienced mother from the community. The mothers who received home-based support were less likely to have infants with incomplete well-child immunizations, and their babies were less likely to be hospitalized in the first year of life, suggesting that home-based support for families with special needs may help to prevent childhood injury and serious illness.

8 Unhappiness after childbirth

Lack of social and psychological support during the days and weeks after birth is one of the main reasons that unhappiness after childbirth is such a common problem, estimated to occur in 7–30% of women in developed countries. This has traditionally been seen as a medical subject, labeled 'postpartum depression'. There is no persuasive evidence to support traditional explanations of postpartum depression. No biochemical explanation of women's unhappiness after childbirth has been uncovered, and psychoanalytic explanations of postpartum depression cannot be validated empirically. Mothers of young children are often depressed and are no less likely to be so 6 months or a year after giving birth, than in the first few weeks or months following childbirth. Sociological and psychological studies have provided strong evidence of a relationship between some social conditions and postpartum depression. The social conditions linked with depression are only rarely 'out of the ordinary'; more often, they correspond to social expectations about what normal womanhood and normal motherhood must be.

Because many of the social factors that lead to postpartum unhappiness are rooted in society's expectations of new mothers, the solutions lie mainly in social change. There is considerable scope, however, for professionals to reduce the difficulties and unhappiness experienced by women after childbirth. In particular, they should be more ready to listen to women, to learn about their social circumstances, and to provide them with information that will lead to more realistic predictions about the experience of pregnancy, childbirth, and early parenthood.

If, in spite of the best efforts being made to prevent the problem, women do become seriously depressed, then encouraging them to talk about their feelings to a non-judgmental person has been shown in controlled trials to increase their chances of early recovery.

9 Conclusions

The restriction of early postnatal mother–infant interaction, which has been such a common feature of the care of women giving birth in hospitals, has undesirable effects. Disruption of maternal–infant interaction in the immediate postnatal period may set some women on the road to breastfeeding failure and, possibly, alter their subsequent behavior towards their children. Nevertheless, for mothers who, for whatever reason, cannot have early contact with their babies, other mechanisms are likely to overcome any effects of this separation.

Most of the restrictive practices perpetuated in some hospitals are ineffective and possibly harmful. Unless or until new evidence appears to the contrary, mothers should have unrestricted access to their babies. Caps and masks should be abolished, and aprons and gowns used only by those who wish to protect their own clothing from the various kinds of messes that babies make. Bathing the baby should be seen, not as a measure for preventing infection, but as an opportunity for a mother to interact with, and gain confidence in, handling her child.

There is no evidence to warrant the use of routine prophylactic medications or medicated bathing to prevent infection of the umbilical cord.

The standard hospital setting, with its orientation towards sickbed protocols and procedures, and its division of care along the lines of the separate medical disciplines of obstetrics and pediatrics, is not conducive either to helping the new mother develop the skills and self-confidence she needs to care for herself and her new baby, or to enhancing her sense of personal worth and self-esteem. It is unlikely that any single scheme of care will prove to be right for all women. Treating the new mother as a responsible adult by giving her accurate and consistent information, letting her make her own decisions, and supporting her in those decisions, is the essence of effective postpartum care, regardless of where it given.

Postnatal follow-up programs for mothers and babies that offer home based social support and continuity of caregiver, and which are sensitive to the social circumstances of families, provide important benefits for socially disadvantaged mothers and their children.

Depression in the postpartum period is a common and serious complication in developed countries. It appears to be related to social rather than hormonal or psychological factors, and there is evidence that women benefit from additional support and counselling, alone or in conjunction with medical therapy.

Sources

Effective care in pregnancy and childbirth

Romito, P., Unhappiness after childbirth.

Rush, J., Chalmers, I. and Enkin, M.W., Care of the new mother and baby.

Thompson, M. and Westreich, R., Restriction of mother–infant contact in the immediate post-natal period.

Cochrane Library

Hiller, J.E. and Griffith, J., Education for contraceptive use by women after childbirth.

Hodnett, E.D. and Roberts, I., Home-based social support for socially disadvantaged mothers.

Lawrie, T.A., Herxheimer, A. and Dalton, K., Oestrogens and progestogens for preventing and treating postnatal depression.

Ray, K. and Hodnett, E.D., Caregiver support for postpartum depression.

Stamp, G. and White, G., Psychosocial support for preventing postpartum depression [protocol].

Zupan, J. and Garner, P., Topical umbilical cord care at birth.

Other sources

Carty, E.M. and Bradley, C.F. (1990). A randomized, controlled evaluation of early postpartum hospital discharge. *Birth*, 17, 199–204.

Dalby, D.M., Williams, J.I., Hodnett, E. and Rush, J. (1996). Postpartum safety and satisfaction following early discharge. *Can. J. Pub. Health*, 87, 90–4.

Rush, J. and Kitch, T. (1991). A randomized, controlled trial to measure the frequency of use of a hospital telephone line for new parents. *Birth*, 18, 193–7.

Tulman, L. and Fawcett, J. (1991). Recovering from childbirth: looking back six months after delivery. *Heal. Care Wom. Int.*, 12, 341–50.

Breastfeeding

1 Introduction

Breastfeeding is important for both mother and baby. Women who breastfeed their babies usually do so both because they believe it is best for their babies and because they find it satisfying and enjoyable. However, many women encounter problems and stop breastfeeding before they wish to do so, especially in the early days and weeks. As well as depriving the baby of the benefits of breastfeeding, this also causes distress for the mother and her family.

There have been attempts in several countries, some of them successful, to increase the number of women who initiate breast-feeding. Women who start to breastfeed should also be supported in breastfeeding their babies for as long as they wish. Promotional campaigns to encourage breastfeeding are likely to fall short of important objectives if women are not also supported in continuing to breastfeed.

Many elements of care during pregnancy and childbirth can foster or jeopardize the successful establishment and maintenance of breast-feeding. Efforts to provide social and psychological support, for example, may increase the likelihood that mothers will breastfeed their babies successfully. In contrast, sedative and analgesic drugs given during labour can alter the behavior of the newborn infant, and compromise its crucial role in the initiation of lactation. The establishment of lactation may be jeopardized at the time of birth in other ways as well. Routine gastric suctioning and administration of silver nitrate eye drops in the immediate postnatal period can prejudice the infant's role in establishing lactation. Separating babies from their mothers, whether because of entrenched hospital routines or for necessary treatment of the baby, reduces the likelihood that breastfeeding will be established successfully.

Antenatal care practices, the time of the first feed, positioning, feeding frequency and duration, supplements for babies and mothers, and support for breastfeeding mothers, can all affect the establishment and maintenance of breastfeeding.

2 Antenatal preparation

Most women who decide to breastfeed make this decision either before or early in pregnancy. Those who choose to bottle-feed tend to make up their minds later in pregnancy. This effect is not mediated by knowledge alone. Giving women well-designed, well-written, and well-illustrated information about breastfeeding, increases their knowledge of the subject and can increase the numbers of women starting and continuing to breastfeed. It is likely, however, that other influences, such as her own previous experiences, and the attitudes and experiences of her family, friends, and caregivers, will also have an important role in this decision. For example, involvement of family, friends, and caregivers in health education programs can further assist in increasing the numbers of women starting and continuing to breastfeed.

Regular, face-to-face contact and advice from local women with previous breastfeeding experience, or trained health professionals, is also likely to increase the numbers of women starting and continuing to breastfeed. Research studies to assess the efficacy of peer-support programs, particularly for women in socially deprived communities, have shown an increase in the numbers of women who initiate breastfeeding.

Antenatal information given to women who have already decided to breastfeed may also be beneficial. The available data suggest that antenatal classes may be effective in promoting breastfeeding, but more evidence is needed to find out which elements of the information, and what kind of classes, women find helpful.

Research studies to assess the efficacy of antenatal nipple 'conditioning' have not shown any significant differences, either objective or subjective, among the different methods of conditioning: the use of Massé cream, expression of colostrum, or no form of preparation. Two trials have assessed the effects of antenatal treatment for women with inverted or non-protractile nipples. Neither of the two treatments tested – Hoffman's nipple stretching exercises and breast shells – were shown to have any beneficial effect on the duration of breastfeeding.

3 Early versus later suckling

Early contact between mother and baby has beneficial effects on breastfeeding, in addition to other important benefits. It is difficult to separate the effects of early suckling *per se* from the effects of other early mother–baby interactions, such as touching, gazing, and skin-to-skin contact. Feeding within the first 2 hours after birth increases the duration of breastfeeding when compared to a delay of 4 hours or more. No research has demonstrated a 'critical period' for the first feed in terms of breastfeeding success; that is, there is no evidence to suggest that her breastfeeding will suffer if a mother does not feed her baby immediately after birth. There are, therefore, no research-based grounds for replacing old dogma ('no baby should breastfeed until 4 hours after birth') with new dogma ('all babies should feed immediately after birth'), or for encouraging a mother to breastfeed her baby before she and the baby are ready. Babies have a wide range of behavior following spontaneous birth, and are not all ready to feed at the same time. Unless or until more evidence is available, interventions aimed either at delaying or speeding up the time of the first feed should be avoided.

The first *feed* after birth (as opposed to the immediate post-delivery nuzzle at the breast) should be given in privacy, at a time when the baby is receptive, and after the mother and baby have been made comfortable. Skilled professional help would be useful at this time. If possible, it should be done while the father, or someone else whom the mother has found supportive, is still present. The baby's behavior and needs can be explained to the new parents. A brief explanation of the importance of correct positioning and the concept of supply and demand can be given before the mother positions the baby properly at the breast. This can be followed by a little more information, on the importance of unrestricted feeding, on potential problems, and on how (and why) to summon help.

4 The importance of correct positioning

Positioning of the baby at the breast plays a crucial role, both in the prevention of sore nipples and in the successful establishment of breastfeeding, and professionals should know how a mother can be helped to position her baby properly at the breast. A woman's ability to position her baby at her breast, so that feeding is pain-free and effective, is a learned and predominantly physical skill, which the mother must acquire from observation and practice. Industrialized societies, on the whole, do not provide women with the opportunity to observe other breastfeeding women before they attempt breast-feeding themselves. This deficiency is compounded by the frequent lack of experienced breastfeeding mothers in the woman's immediate social sphere and the regrettable lack of skill demonstrated by some health professionals in this essential area.

Professionals must understand the underlying mechanisms of suckling and acquire the skill and experience to help a mother to position her baby correctly before they can be of real value to the mother. The fragmentation of postnatal care, and a general lack of understanding of breastfeeding techniques, has prevented many professionals from acquiring these skills.

When the baby is properly attached to the breast (see Figure 1), feeding should be pain-free, although the mother may need a short time to accustom herself to the new sensation of her breast and nipple being stretched. The nipple, together with the areola and some of the surrounding breast tissue, is drawn out into a teat by the suction created within the baby's mouth. Breaking this suction causes the nipple to recoil abruptly. The teat thus created extends as far back as the junction of the baby's hard and soft palate, with the nipple itself forming only about one-third of the teat. At its base, the teat is held between the upper gum and the tongue, which covers the lower gum. It lies in a central trough formed by the raised edges of the baby's tongue, which directs the expressed milk backwards into the pharynx, using a roller-like, peristaltic movement. The peristaltic action begins as the front edge of the tongue curves upwards, closely followed by the

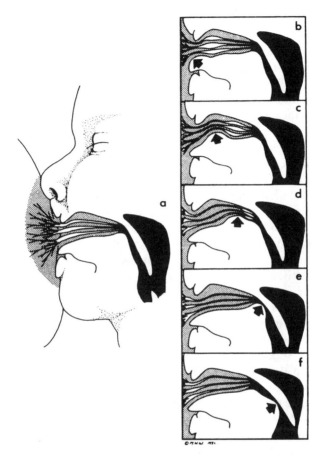

Fig. 1 (a–f) Diagrams of accurate positioning of the baby on the breast (from Woolridge 1986).

raising of the lower jaw, which follows the tongue's movement with pressure from the lower gum. This wave of compression moves progressively backwards beyond the tip of the nipple, thus directing the milk into the pharynx and on into the esophagus. Meanwhile, a fresh cycle of compression by the tongue has been initiated from its tip.

Thus the breast tissue opposed to the baby's lower jaw and tongue is the critical region in the transfer of milk. The tongue applies peristaltic force to the underside of the teat; the hard palate simply provides the necessary resistance to the tongue's action. Once sufficient breast tissue has been formed into the teat, there should be virtually no movement of this teat in and out of the baby's mouth. Friction from the tongue against the nipple should be minimal; and the gums should not come in contact with the nipple at all. If the baby is incorrectly positioned at the breast and is unable to form a teat out of the breast tissues as well as the nipple, then the nipple is likely to incur frictional damage as the teat is repeatedly drawn in and out of the mouth between the tongue and gums by the cyclical application of suction.

The mother needs to be taught how to elicit and use the two components of the baby's rooting reflex: the moving of the head towards the source of stimulation when the skin around the mouth is touched; and the accompanying gaping of the mouth preparatory to receiving the breast. She should be shown how to move the baby towards the breast and 'plant' the lower rim of the baby's mouth around and predominantly under the nipple area at the moment that the baby's mouth gapes widely. This should be accompanied by moving the baby close to the breast as it takes a good mouthful of breast tissue. The mother cannot rely, as her helper does, on seeing where the baby's lower lip and jaw are in relation to her nipple, for she has a poor view of the underside of the breast, the critical area of attachment. Observation of the baby's sucking pattern, as well as the sensations that the mother herself experiences, will serve to confirm that the baby is properly positioned; she should feel no pain other than perhaps her sudden 'intake of breath' as she becomes accustomed to the sensation of feeding, and the baby should feed strongly and rhythmically within a short while (see Figure 2).

Anything that interferes with the baby's ability to gape and grasp the breast can cause problems, and probably pain for the mother. Factors may include the baby being sleepy as a result of drugs used in labour, jaundice (and phototherapy), and tongue tie, which prevents the baby from using its tongue effectively to grasp and milk the breast. Early diagnosis of the problem and sensitive support for such mothers and babies is needed until the problem is resolved.

More widespread acquisition and use of the skills needed to achieve correct positioning of the baby on the breast would probably do more than anything else to reduce the frequency of the problems currently experienced by so many breastfeeding mothers.

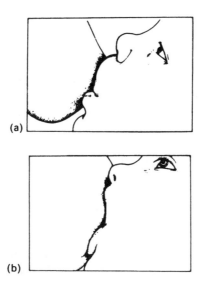

(a)

(b)

Fig. 2 (a) Baby incorrectly positioned at breast. (b) Baby correctly positioned at breast. (From Fisher 1981.)

5 The importance of flexibility

A baby needs to eat and sleep according to his or her own individual rhythms, rather than those imposed by arbitrary regimens. Babies usually wish to feed infrequently in the first day or so, but more frequently between the 3rd and 7th day. The frequency then tends to decrease more slowly over the next few days. Although a few babies are content to feed as infrequently as six times a day, most babies want to be fed more often than this. The interval between feeds, for the first few weeks of life at least, is variable, ranging from 1 to 8 hours. Babies who are permitted to regulate the frequency of their feeds themselves gain weight more quickly, and remain breastfed for longer than those who have external limitations imposed on them. There are no data providing any justification for the imposition of breastfeeding schedules, and the frequency of feeds should not be restricted.

Similar comments apply to the duration of feeds. The fact that limitation of suckling time is still being advocated in some books addressed both to mothers and to professionals reflects the deeply ingrained belief that the nipples need to be 'toughened' to permit pain-free feeding. As the previous section described, positioning of the baby at the breast is a key element in preventing pain during feeding. Mothers and professionals may still be told, however, that the baby should be permitted to feed for only 2 minutes at each breast for the first day, increasing the time by 2–3 minutes daily, so that at the end of the first week the baby has reached a maximum of 10 minutes on each side. These admonitions are based on the unwarranted belief that this practice will 'break the nipples in gradually', prevent their exposure to prolonged sucking, and thus prevent nipple pain and bleeding. Controlled studies show that this is not the case. Comparison of restricted and unrestricted duration of feeds show no significant differences between the two groups in the proportion of women who develop painful or bleeding nipples, but significantly more mothers in the regulated groups give up breastfeeding altogether by 6 weeks.

The still commonly given advice to limit suckling time to 10 minutes on each breast has repercussions beyond its failure to prevent nipple damage. The composition and the rate of flow of milk changes over time. The fat content increases and the flow rate decreases as the feed progresses. Thus, at the start of a feed the baby takes a large volume of low-calorie foremilk; this changes to a smaller volume of high-calorie hindmilk at the end of the feed. Babies feed for differing lengths of time at the breast if left undisturbed. The length of the feed is probably determined in response to the effectiveness and rate of milk transfer between mother and baby. While many babies will terminate a feed spontaneously in under 10 minutes, those who have a slow rate of intake may well take longer than this. Even though the volume of milk that they consume after the first 10 minutes may not be very great, it may be sufficiently high in calories to make a significant contribution in energy value. The external imposition of a time limit for feeding will thus result in some babies having their calorie intake significantly curtailed.

Babies are driven to feed by the need to obtain calories, and thus take much larger volumes of low-calorie milk than they would of high-calorie milk, in an attempt to gain the required number of calories. Babies who are taken from the first breast before they spontaneously terminate the feed, may take a much larger volume of milk from the second breast than they might otherwise have done, in order to try to 'make up' their calories. For the same reason these babies may also require feeding much more frequently than they would have if they were allowed to finish feeding spontaneously.

In addition, interference with spontaneous feeding patterns may result in the baby being deprived of essential vitamins. Vitamin K, for example, is especially concentrated in colostrum and hindmilk, and this may partly explain the increased incidence of hemorrhagic disease of the newborn in breastfed babies. The duration of feeds, therefore, should not be limited. There is still a need, in some institutions, for more intensive policy discussions and in-service training to ensure that a policy that supports and encourages flexible breastfeeding is translated effectively into practice.

6 'Supplementing' the baby

There is no evidence to support the widespread practice of giving breastfed babies supplementary feeds of water, glucose, or formula. A healthy baby has no need for large volumes of fluid any earlier than these become available physiologically from the breast. There is equally no evidence to support the widespread belief that giving additional fluids to breastfed babies prevents or helps to resolve physiological jaundice. In the only randomized, controlled trial to have examined the question, there was no statistically significant reduction in mean plasma bilirubin levels associated with giving water supplements, nor any evidence that babies receiving extra fluids were any less likely to develop 'breast milk jaundice' or require phototherapy.

The practice of giving breastfed babies formula while lactation is becoming established is also misconceived. Women whose babies receive routine supplements are up to five times more likely to give up breastfeeding in the first week and twice as likely to abandon it during the second week, as women whose babies are not supplemented and who are encouraged to feel that their own colostrum and milk are sufficient.

Those hospitals that allow breastfeeding mothers to be given free samples of formula also prejudice the chances of successful establishment and maintenance of breastfeeding. This policy increases the chance that breastfeeding will have been abandoned within a few weeks of birth.

7 'Supplementing' the mother

Advice given to breastfeeding women concerning their own fluid intake has been inconsistent and has led to confusion and misinformation. The results of controlled studies provide no evidence that increased fluid intake by breastfeeding mothers will result in improved lactation. Some women find it unpleasant to drink when they are not thirsty because it makes them feel 'turgid' and unwell. Women with perineal and labial trauma may have their discomfort increased by the diuresis associated with greater fluid intake. Urging women to drink more than their thirst dictates is not justified.

8 Oral contraceptives

Combined estrogen/progestogen contraceptives may affect the composition of breast milk. Their effect on milk volume is not clear, probably because of limitations in the methods used to estimate milk volume. What is clear is that their use increases the incidence of both breastfeeding failure and supplementation with breast-milk substitutes. This does not appear to be the case with the use of progesterone only 'mini-pills'.

All the evidence from controlled trials suggests that combined estrogen/progestogen contraceptives are unsuitable for women who wish to breastfeed their babies. This finding is particularly important in parts of the world in which breast-milk substitutes pose a threat to infant life and health. Lactation itself, particularly if breastfeeding is unrestricted, has a contraceptive effect. In developing countries, breastfeeding prevents more pregnancies than all other methods of contraception combined. For contraceptive effectiveness, breastfeeding must be exclusive, and cannot be considered, by itself, to be a reliable contraceptive. Women who wish to enhance the contraceptive effect of lactation should use means other than combined estrogen/progestogen preparations.

9 Supporting breastfeeding mothers

Many women who wish to breastfeed begin to do so, but discontinue long before their babies are 4 months old. Perhaps the most important factor in the efforts to increase the rate of breastfeeding is that those who attempt it should succeed. Many of the problems that confront women who are trying to breastfeed are avoidable. Fewer women would experience these problems if all breastfeeding women had access to accurate information, and appropriate and practical help and support when they need it. More pregnant women would then know of others who had breastfed successfully, and be more confident that they themselves will succeed.

A number of controlled trials have assessed the effects of various forms of support for breastfeeding mothers. The duration of breastfeeding can be increased by regular and frequent face-to-face contact; providing support by telephone alone seems to be less effective. Advice and support for mothers who wish to breastfeed can be important in helping them to achieve their objectives. If the advice given is flawed, however, it is unlikely to be helpful.

10 Nipple trauma

The most widely held explanation for the prevalence of nipple pain in industrialized cultures is the supposed thinness or sensitivity of the nipple epithelium. This probably explains the widespread belief, unsupported by the studies that have examined the question, that women with fair skin or red hair are more likely to experience problems.

A number of treatments, including ointments, tinctures, and sprays have been used for the prevention or treatment of nipple damage. None that have been evaluated have been shown to be of benefit. The use of a nipple shield for any length of time, even by those who find its use acceptable, may add to a mother's problems by suppressing her milk production.

The only factor that has been shown to both prevent and treat nipple trauma is good positioning of the baby at the breast.

11 Problems with milk flow

If the milk is not removed as it is formed (as regulated by the baby's need to go to the breast) the volume of milk in the breast will exceed the capacity of the alveoli to store it comfortably. Over-distension of the alveoli with milk causes the milk secreting cells to become flattened, drawn out, and even to rupture. If severe, this will cause secondary vascular engorgement. Once the alveoli become distended, further milk production begins to be suppressed.

Engorgement results from limitations on feeding frequency and duration, and from problems with positioning the baby at the breast. A number of different treatments have been advocated. Some, such as the use of moist heat or ice packs, have not been evaluated. In the past, treatment of severe engorgement has included both administration of stilbestrol and binding of the breasts, two measures also advocated for suppression of lactation in women who do not wish to breastfeed. Controlled evaluations of the effects of oxytocin failed to find any beneficial effect of oxytocin in relieving engorgement. Two early studies seem to indicate that manual expression, started antenatally and continued postnatally, will help to relieve engorgement and increase the duration of breastfeeding; both of these studies, however, were carried out under conditions where feeding was restricted and engorgement was, as a result, very common.

Placebo-controlled trials of oral proteolytic enzymes suggest that they may provide effective relief for women with breast pain, swelling, and tenderness. The evidence is not yet sufficiently strong to recommend this form of treatment.

Application of plant products directly onto the breast has also been advocated for the relief of engorgement. The plant remedy most commonly used is raw cabbage leaves. The only randomized, controlled trial to evaluate the use of cabbage leaves compared to women who had 'routine care' found no difference in the relief of engorgement. The women who applied the cabbage leaves, however, were more likely to be breastfeeding exclusively at 6 weeks and to breastfeed for longer. Both groups of women carried out a 'breast exercises' program.

Allowing the baby unrestricted access to the breast while properly positioned still appears to be the most effective method of treating, as well as of preventing, breast engorgement.

The other common difficulty caused by milk flow problems is mastitis. Milk flow can be limited by restriction of feeding, by a badly positioned baby, or when some obstacle is placed in the way of milk draining from one section of the breast. This obstacle can result from such factors as blocked ducts, reduction in the normal frequency of feeding, compression from fingers holding the breast, bruising from trauma or rough handling, or because a brassiere is too small or too tight. In consequence, the milk collects in the alveoli and the pressure in the alveoli rises. The distension of the alveoli can often be felt as a tender lump in the breast tissue. If this distension is not relieved the pressure may force substances from the milk through the cell walls into the surrounding connective tissue, setting up an inflammatory reaction. The mother develops a swollen, red, and painful area on her breast, a rise in her pulse and temperature, and an aching, flu-like feeling, often accompanied by shivering attacks and rigors. At this stage the process is not infectious, and the problem can be resolved by relieving the obstruction. If this is not speedily accomplished, bacterial infection may supervene, and may ultimately give rise to a breast abscess.

Perhaps understandably, the immediate response of the professional confronted with the symptoms of localized breast tenderness, redness, and fever in breastfeeding women is often the prescription of antibiotics. What begins as a non-infectious, inflammatory process may, if not treated appropriately, rapidly progress to an infectious process; delay in treating an infectious process will adversely affect the outcome. Nevertheless, a substantial proportion of women with mastitis do not have an infection.

For women with milk stasis simply continuing to breastfeed, ensuring unlimited feeds, gives the best results. Expression of breast milk alone has not been shown to confer any advantage. The outcome for women with non-infectious mastitis is best with continuation of breastfeeding supplemented by breast-milk expression. For women with infectious mastitis, antibiotics are necessary, and for them expression of breast milk improves the outcome.

12 Problems with milk supply

The most common reason given for discontinuing breastfeeding is 'insufficient milk'. There is little information, however, about the extent to which this insufficiency is physiological and inevitable, as opposed to iatrogenic and thus preventable. Objective evidence of insufficient milk is hard to obtain, but it is likely that the high reported incidence reflects over-diagnosis of the problem; countries with high rates of initiation and continuation of breastfeeding, such as Scandinavia, report much lower rates of 'insufficient milk'. Observations in traditional societies suggest that less than 1% of women would be physiologically incapable of producing an adequate milk supply.

It is important to be able to diagnose the occurrence and etiology of insufficient milk accurately. Accurate measurement of milk production is possible with expensive and sophisticated research techniques, but the only clinically available method for this measurement is weighing of the baby before and after feeds, then calculating the breast milk intake by the difference in weights. Such 'test weighing', which is grossly inaccurate, has been used to estimate the baby's intake in cases of anxiety about milk supply, and is a routine practice in some hospitals.

The rationale for test weighing is to determine whether babies are taking 'too much' or 'too little' milk. If too little they may be given supplements; if too much the duration of breastfeeding may be curtailed. The hazards of these inappropriate responses to an inherently inaccurate test have already been discussed. In the one study mounted to examine this question directly, the effect of routine test weighing and supplementary feeding was compared with a policy of neither weighing nor supplementing. Mothers in the test-weigh group were five times more likely to stop breastfeeding in the first week, and twice as likely to stop in the second week as those in the group whose babies were not test weighed.

The decision to give a healthy term breastfed baby supplementary feeds as a result of information gained by assessing milk intake is based on the unwarranted assumption that it is possible to know how much breast milk an individual baby needs. It would be more relevant to monitor the general condition of a baby (health, contentment/behavior, colour and consistency of stools, colour of urine, and frequency of urination) and note his or her progress, especially the change in body weight over time.

The best means of preventing the occurrence of insufficient milk is unrestricted feeding by a well-positioned infant, while giving good practical and emotional support to the breastfeeding mother. This is also the basis for the treatment of insufficient milk and is likely to solve the problem in a high proportion of, but not all, mothers.

Although the true incidence is unknown, professionals should remain alive to the possibility that physiological milk insufficiency may occur. Babies may become seriously undernourished because of a dogged, but mistaken, belief that the problem will always be resolved by practical help with feeding. When mothers and babies do not respond to the fundamental elements of good breastfeeding practice, other treatments should be considered.

In the past, when a baby's life depended on breast milk, many remedies were sought for those who seemed unable to produce enough milk. In addition to some rather bizarre prescriptions, a variety of herbal infusions, such as the seeds of fennel (*Foeniculom vulgare*) and the flowers of goat's rue (*Galega officinalis*) were, and still are, recommended to increase milk production. We have been unable to identify any controlled evaluation of the effects of these preparations. Four main types of drugs have, however, been evaluated in attempted treatment of insufficient milk: dopamine antagonists, iodine, thyro-tropin-releasing hormone, and oxytocin. Since dopamine has been shown to have a critical role in the mechanisms that control prolactin production, several researchers have experimented with drugs that block dopamine receptors, including metoclopramide (Maxalon), sulpiride (Dolmatil), and domperidone (Motilium). There is some evidence that these drugs may be of use for women who are temporarily unable to feed their babies. Of all of them, domperidone seems to be most likely to be useful. Further research is required to clarify this. None of these drugs has been tested as part of a regimen that also provides supportive care.

As the let-down reflex, which is primed by oxytocin release from the posterior pituitary, is essential for successful breastfeeding, some investigators have reasoned that to give oxytocin may improve problems with milk supply. A variety of outcomes have been studied, but the most crucial information concerns weight changes in the baby. The trials conducted have produced conflicting results, and to date there is no strong evidence that oxytocin administration has a beneficial effect on milk supply.

13 Conclusions

Those who care for women during pregnancy and childbirth have a crucial role to play in enabling a woman to breastfeed successfully. Now that sound, research-based information is readily available to them, the professional ignorance that may have been understandable in the past is no longer tolerable. If the potential for helping women to breastfeed their babies is to be realized, professionals must reject many of the historical practices in this field and pass on to women only those practices that have been demonstrated to be effective.

Those who are most likely to be closely involved with mothers at the time that breastfeeding is becoming established, should have a clear understanding of how a baby breastfeeds. They should recognize that, although separation of babies from their mothers after birth jeopardizes the successful establishment of lactation, there is no evidence to suggest that the timing of the first feed, in itself, is crucial to success. Interventions aimed either at delaying or speeding up the time of the first feed should be avoided.

Professionals should know how a mother can be helped to position her baby properly at the breast. They should impose no restrictions on the duration or frequency of feeds, and neither offer nor recommend additional fluids or formula for healthy breastfed babies. Free samples of formula given to women in hospital can be particularly detrimental to successful breastfeeding.

Normal lactating women with access to adequate fluid can depend on their thirst to regulate fluid intake effectively. Urging women to drink more than their thirst dictates has no justification.

Use of combined estrogen/progestogen contraceptives compromises lactation. Women who wish to enhance the contraceptive effect of lactation should use means other than hormonal methods containing estrogens and progestogens.

Women can be helped to establish and maintain breastfeeding in a number of ways, but the experimentally-derived evidence suggests that continuity of personal support from an individual who is knowledgeable about breastfeeding is most effective.

The main reasons women give for discontinuing breastfeeding are nipple trauma, breast engorgement, mastitis, and insufficient milk. The majority of these problems can be prevented by unrestricted breastfeeding by a baby who has been well-positioned from the first feed on, and by giving mothers practical and emotional support.

If a woman does sustain nipple trauma, she should continue to breastfeed, express milk if necessary, and receive help with positioning. Discontinuing breastfeeding, and the application of any of a variety of preparations to the nipple, does not help. Indeed, some of these interventions have been shown to prejudice the success of breastfeeding.

Problems with milk flow can result in engorgement and possibly in mastitis. If mastitis does not resolve rapidly with good feeding and expression, then antibiotic treatment should be instituted. In all cases of engorgement and mastitis, however, the key to successful treatment is good drainage of the breast. This is best achieved by unlimited feeds by a well-positioned baby.

Mothers and health professionals who suspect insufficient milk as a result of signs and symptoms in the baby or the mother, face a challenging problem. Identifying the problem and its cause is always difficult and often impossible. Until diagnostic precision improves, the basis of the treatment offered when insufficient milk is suspected remains unrestricted breastfeeding by a well-positioned baby, together with practical and emotional support for the mother. Only when mothers and babies do not respond to the fundamental elements of good breastfeeding practice, should other treatments be considered.

Sources

Effective care in pregnancy and childbirth

Inch, S., Antenatal preparation for breastfeeding.

Inch, S., Garforth S. Establishing and maintaining breastfeeding.

Inch, S., Renfrew M. Common breastfeeding problems.

Cochrane Library

Fairbank, L., Lister-Sharpe, D., Renfrew, M.J., Woolridge, M.W., Sowden, A.J.S. and O'Meara, S., Interventions to promote the initiation of breastfeeding [protocol].

Martin, L.A., Renfrew, M.J. and Woolridge, M.W., Additional foods and fluids for breastfed full-term infants [protocol].

Renfrew, M.J. and Lang, S., Feeding schedules in hospitals for newborn infants.

Interventions for influencing sleep patterns in exclusively breastfed infants.

Oxytocin for promoting successful lactation.

Breastfeeding and discharge times.

Interventions for improving breastfeeding technique.

Early versus delayed initiation of breastfeeding.

Early versus late discharge from hospital after childbirth.

Cabbage leaves for breast engorgement.

Sikorski, J. and Renfrew, M.J., Support for breastfeeding mothers.

Pre-Cochrane reviews

Renfrew, L., Single daily bottle use in early postpartum period. Review no. 07908.

Renfrew, M.J., Antenatal breastfeeding education. Review no. 04171.

Antenatal expression of colostrum. Review no. 04028.

Antenatal breastfeeding classes vs individual teaching. Review no. 07144.

Postnatal anticipatory guidance for mothers on infant feeding. Review no. 04177.

Provision of formula supplements to breastfed newborns. Review no. 04175.

Provision of free formula samples to breastfeeding mothers. Review no. 04172.

Combined estrogen/progestogen contraceptive in breastfeeding mothers. Review no. 04376.

Chlorhexidine/alcohol nipple spray. Review no. 04176.

Oral sulpiride for women with poor lactation. Review no. 04187.

Other sources

Renfrew, M.J., Woolridge, M.W. and Ross McGill, H., *Enabling women to breastfeed. A structured review of practices which promote or inhibit breastfeeding.* The Stationery Office, London. (In press.)

Perineal pain and discomfort

1 Introduction

Postnatal perineal pain is a distressing problem for mothers, which can negatively affect their functioning and early experiences of motherhood. Perineal pain and/or dyspareunia may persist for long periods of time. A UK survey found that after spontaneous vaginal birth, 10% of women experienced pain for more than 2 months; the percentage increased to 30% for those who had an assisted vaginal delivery. Other studies have found that some women continue to have pain and dyspareunia more than a year after childbirth.

Perineal damage may be obvious, in that suturing has been necessary, bruising is evident, or hemorrhoids are visible. Sometimes the trauma is not visible; a new mother with an intact perineum and no obvious signs of injury may also suffer considerable perineal discomfort.

Avoiding perineal damage when possible, and proper repair when trauma occurs (see Chapters 32 and 36), are the primary approaches to preventing or reducing these problems. When pain occurs despite the use of measures to prevent it, a wide range of secondary measures and active treatments are available for alleviation of perineal pain.

2 Local applications

2.1 Non-pharmacological applications

Sprays, gels, creams, solutions, ice packs, baths, and douches are all commonly recommended for the relief of perineal discomfort after vaginal birth, but they have received little, if any formal evaluation.

Cooling with ice or sprays is often used in postnatal care, in the belief that pain and edema are reduced. Ice packs in the puerperium give immediate symptomatic relief by numbing the perineum, but this relief is usually short-lived, and there is no evidence of any longer term benefit. Sprays have also been reported to relieve perineal discomfort, probably by a cooling effect, although they occasionally cause a stinging discomfort.

There is evidence from a randomized trial that cold sitz baths are more often effective than warm sitz baths in relieving perineal discomfort, but the differential effect is limited to the first half-hour after bathing and the cold baths are not popular with women.

The warmth of a hot bath may give some comfort in the immediate puerperium. In a recent survey, over 90% of women reported that bathing had relieved perineal discomfort. This observation was uncontrolled, however, and there is no knowing whether a similar proportion of women would have gained relief if they had not bathed at all, or had taken a shower instead.

The growing popularity of herbal substances, either locally applied or in the form of aromatic oils, probably reflects both a belief in the safety of 'natural' remedies and their increased availability from many retail outlets. Witchhazel soaked into gauze swabs or other pads and applied directly to the perineal tissues is commonly recommended for the relief of pain, but a randomized trial showed no evidence that it was any more effective than tap water. Only one controlled trial of aromatherapy for perineal pain has been reported, and it found that lavender oil added to bath water did not affect perineal pain in the first 10 days after childbirth.

Salt added to bath water is one of the oldest claimed remedies for perineal and other trauma, and is still very popular. The salt is believed to soothe discomfort and to promote healing, although a precise mode of action is unclear. Claims that it has antiseptic or antibacterial properties have not been confirmed. There is no consensus as to the type of salt preparation or quantity that should be used. Recommendations about the quantity range from a heaped tablespoon in a small bath to 3 lb in 30 gallons of water (about 10 g/l). In a large controlled trial, the addition of salt to the bath water had no detectable effect either on perineal pain or on perineal wound healing.

2.2 Local antiseptics

The addition of antiseptic solutions, particularly 'Savlon' concentrate, to the bath water was studied in the large trial mentioned above. Women were asked to add Savlon to a daily bath for the first 10 days after birth. There was no evidence that this addition improved symptomatic relief from bathing or that it reduced perineal discomfort. Similarly, a study comparing antiseptic solution with unmedicated tap water for 'jug douching', also showed no differential effect on symptoms, healing, or infection rates.

The use of vaginal creams containing sulphonamides, once recommended for routine use in the postpartum period, has been evaluated in two controlled studies. The results suggested that minor benign cervical abnormalities, such as erosion or ectropion, were less common in the women who had used the sulphonamide creams and that these women used fewer vaginal douches. Equal proportions of women in each group had resumed sexual intercourse by 6 weeks after birth.

2.3 Local anesthetics

Local anesthetics are commonly applied as sprays, gels, creams, or foams. Double-blind comparisons of local anesthetics show them to be clearly more effective for relief of perineal pain than placebo. Aqueous 5% lignocaine spray or lignocaine gel appears to be the first choice of agent and formulation.

2.4 Combinations of local anesthetics and topical steroids

Based on the assumption that much of the pain from perineal trauma arises from local edema and inflammation, a local anesthetic (pramoxine) has been combined with a steroid (hydrocortisone) as a single topical agent. Early uncontrolled studies gave very encouraging results, but two well-controlled studies produced conflicting findings.

The first study reported better pain relief in the pramoxine/hydrocortisone group, whereas the other reported more edema and a greater use of oral analgesia with the use of the combined agents, particularly after the third day. Wound breakdown was also more common in the group treated with the combination cream in this study. As steroids are known to impair wound healing, the latter finding is biologically plausible. It would not seem sensible to use this combination without further assessment in the context of a controlled trial.

3 Local physiotherapies

3.1 Relief of pressure on the perineum
A variety of simple aids may be used during sitting or lying as a means of relieving pressure on the sore perineum. When a mother is resting in bed, a wedge or pillow may be used to support her on her side. These should be covered with a waterproof fabric so that they can be easily cleaned. Rubber or foam rubber rings have been widely advocated in the past, especially for mothers needing to sit comfortably to feed their babies. These rings have largely been withdrawn from use as they are believed to compress venous return, thereby increasing the risk of thrombosis in women already at higher risk postpartum. The fact that they are no longer supplied in hospital does not prevent many women from buying their own, or substituting children's swimming rings. The popularity of this simple measure suggests that it gives relief to many women. This suggests that further research into its safety would be worthwhile.

3.2 Ultrasound and pulsed electromagnetic energy
Developments in the physical treatments of soft tissue injuries have led to the increased use of electrical therapies for the traumatized perineum. Two such treatments have become popular: ultrasound and pulsed electromagnetic energy.

Evidence about the effectiveness of therapeutic ultrasound for other soft-tissue injuries is not wholly consistent and the precise mode of action is not fully understood. Although the treatment of pain is not a primary indication for the use of therapeutic ultrasound, proponents suggest that pain is decreased as the resolution of the inflammatory process is accelerated and compression of pain-sensitive structures by hematoma and edema is reduced. Ultrasound therapy requires constant operator attendance during treatment, and hence is costly in physiotherapist's time. The transducer is applied directly to the skin and must be moved during transmission as a safeguard against tissue damage; conduction is aided by a jelly or cream.

Similar benefits have been claimed for pulsed electromagnetic energy, on the basis of observational studies of treatment for soft tissue injury. The interrupted transmission of the energy allows high-intensity waves to be used while minimizing local heat. One possible advantage of pulsed electromagnetic energy is its ease of application. It may be transmitted through a sanitary pad or towel, thus avoiding the need for constant operator attendance (although this is not always supported as good practice).

Three studies have compared ultrasound with pulsed electromagnetic energy and/or placebo treatments for acute perineal pain, and one study compared ultrasound versus placebo for persistent perineal pain. No studies have assessed safety and none reported whether there were adverse effects of treatment. Participants receiving active ultrasound were more likely to report improvement with treatment, compared to those receiving placebo, but there were no other differences between groups, i.e. no differences in pain, edema, bruising, use of analgesia, or dyspareunia. Compared to those who received pulsed electromagnetic energy, women who were treated with ultrasound were less likely to have perineal pain at 10 days and 3 months, and more likely to have bruising at 10 days. At present there is insufficient evidence to draw valid conclusions about important benefits or harms of either of these expensive modalities in the treatment of perineal trauma. Further use of these techniques should only be in the context of a properly controlled trial.

3.3 Pelvic floor exercises

The usual rationale for advising postnatal exercises of the pelvic floor muscles is the belief that the exercises will reduce the risk of urinary stress incontinence and genital prolapse. In the only large controlled trial in which the effects of postnatal exercises on incontinence rates have been assessed, the rate of incontinence (3 months after birth) among women who had received intensive instruction and reinforcement for pelvic floor exercises was similar to that among women who had received the usual level of information and no special reinforcement. Although no beneficial effects of postnatal exercises on subsequent incontinence rates were detected, women who received the intensive postnatal exercise program and reinforcement were significantly less likely to have perineal pain at 3 months. These results suggest that the use of these exercises would be a worthwhile measure to help relieve persistent perineal pain.

4 Treatments taken by mouth

4.1 Herbal preparations

A number of herbal preparations, aimed at relieving perineal symptoms, are available. For example, arnica (Leopard's Bane) supplied as tablets and comfrey as a tablet or a tea, are claimed to reduce bruising. *Arnica montana* has been evaluated in one small double-blind trial, the results of which were inconclusive.

4.2 Proteolytic enzymes

Some of the pharmacologically active proteolytic enzymes occur naturally. Ananase, for example, is an extract of Hawaiian pineapple plants. Three such enzyme preparations (bromolain, chymotrypsin alone, and chymotrypsin plus trypsin) have been evaluated in controlled trials. Although the trials individually gave somewhat conflicting results, an overview of the results shows significant decreases in edema, in pain on sitting, and in pain on walking by the third day. These results suggest that oral proteolytic agents may have an important effect on perineal discomfort. Nevertheless, the trials vary in terms of quality, prevalence of outcomes, and estimates of treatment effect, so this conclusion can be only tentative. Firm conclusions must await the results of better controlled studies.

4.3 Oral analgesics

A bewildering choice of pharmacologically active preparations can be taken by mouth to relieve perineal pain. Despite the large number of randomized trials, in which these agents have been evaluated, the experimental evidence is not helpful. There are two main reasons for this. First, most trials show that the active preparations are superior to placebo but fail to distinguish clinically important differences between alternative analgesics. Second, many of the drugs included in the trials are no longer commercially available.

A number of factors must be considered when making a choice of oral analgesic preparations. One is the severity of the pain being treated. Another is whether the formulation is likely to cause constipation, which is particularly important to avoid when treating perineal pain. Some oral preparations can cause stomach upset, and this too should be avoided if possible. Whether the drug or drugs are carried in breast milk and if so, whether this has any potential danger for the baby is a further important consideration. In addition, some drugs have more serious, albeit rare, adverse effects. Finally, the relative costs of the alternative preparations should be taken into account.

On the basis of these criteria, paracetamol (acetaminophen) is probably the drug of choice for mild perineal pain. It has useful analgesic properties and is largely free of unwanted side-effects. Of the other non-steroidal anti-inflammatory drugs, ibuprofen would seem to be the most appropriate, if an alternative to paracetamol is required for treating perineal pain. Unlike some of the other non-steroidal anti-inflammatory drugs, it appears to be largely free of unwanted side-effects, and very little is excreted in breast milk. Aspirin is less satisfactory because it can cause gastric irritation, prolongs bleeding time, and poses a potential risk to the baby because of its carriage in breast milk.

The choice of analgesics is less satisfactory when perineal pain is insufficiently relieved by paracetamol or ibuprofen. It would seem sensible as a first step to consider the additional use of local therapies, such as heat and local anesthetics. If stronger analgesia is still required there is no obvious first choice. Individuals differ in their susceptibility to different analgesic formulations.

Codeine derivatives are less suitable for perineal pain than for other types of pain because they predispose to constipation. The opioid dextropropoxyphene may cause dependence and cannot be recommended. For this reason the combinations of paracetamol (acetaminophen) with a stronger opioid analgesic may have a special place for the relief of perineal pain. One option is to give paracetamol in combination with lower doses of codeine or dihydrocodeine than would be the case if the latter were being used on their own. Although it seems reasonable to combine the two types of analgesia, it is uncertain whether the analgesic effect is greater than that of paracetamol on its own.

5 Conclusions

Cooling with crushed ice, witchhazel, or tap water, gives short-term symptomatic relief from perineal pain and discomfort. Locally applied anesthetics, such as aqueous 5% lignocaine spray or lignocaine gel, are also effective and their effect may last longer. Adding a steroid to such local anesthetics may do more harm than good. The addition of salt, lavender oil, or antiseptic solution to bathwater has no additional effect on perineal pain or healing.

The quality of personal care during the puerperium is likely to be a major determinant of postpartum perineal discomfort. On the basis of currently available evidence, the therapeutic effects noted from physiotherapies, such as therapeutic ultrasound, pulsed electromagnetic energy, and the teaching of postnatal exercises, may derive from the personal attention involved, rather than from the treatment modalities themselves. Further research is needed to investigate factors, such as dosage and timing of these treatments.

Paracetamol (acetaminophen) is the oral analgesic of choice for mild perineal pain. If paracetamol in conjunction with the local therapies fails to control the pain, a non-steroidal anti-inflammatory agent such as ibuprofen is a useful alternative. The oral proteolytic enzymes may also be considered for relatively intractable perineal pain, although their effectiveness has still not been clearly established. There is no obvious oral analgesic for more severe pain that is inadequately controlled by paracetamol. The tendency for codeine derivatives to cause constipation makes these drugs less suitable for perineal pain than for pain in other sites.

Until recently, the prevention and treatment of perineal pain following childbirth, using approaches other than systemic analgesia, have been the subject of little formal evaluative research. Yet, postpartum perineal pain is so common that alternative strategies can be readily compared in randomized controlled trials. Such trials are needed if more effective treatments for this common problem are to be developed.

Sources

Effective care in pregnancy and childbirth

Grant, A. and Sleep, J. Relief of perineal pain and discomfort after childbirth.

Cochrane Library

Hay-Smith, E.J.C., Therapeutic ultrasound for postpartum perineal pain and dyspareunia.

Pre-Cochrane reviews

Kaufman, K., Adding Savlon concentrate to bath water for perineal trauma. Review no. 03796.

Adding salt to bath water for perineal trauma. Review no. 03691.

Intensive postnatal pelvic floor exercises. Review no. 05563.

Warm vs cold sitz baths. Review no. 05564.

Local heat vs local cold for perineal injury. Review no. 05565.

Pramoxine/hydrocortisone for perineal pain. Review no. 05569.

Pramoxine/hydrocortisone vs local anesthetic for perineal pain. Review no. 05570.

Pramoxine/hydrocortisone vs ice for perineal pain. Review no. 05571.

Pramoxine/hydrocortisone vs witchhazel for perineal pain. Review no. 05572.

Witchhazel vs ice for perineal pain. Review no. 05573.

Local anesthetic for perineal pain. Review no. 05575.

Alcoholic vs aqueous lignocaine for perineal pain. Review no. 05577.

Lignocaine vs cinchocaine for perineal pain. Review no. 05576.

Oral proteolytic enzymes for perineal trauma. Review no. 03204.

Other sources

Bansal, R.K., Tan, W.M., Ecker, J.L., Bishop, J.T. and Kilpatrick, S.J. (1996). Is there a benefit to episiotomy at spontaneous vaginal delivery? A natural experiment. *Am. J. Obstet. Gynecol.*, 175, 897–901.

Dale, A. and Cornwell, S. (1994). The role of lavender oil in relieving perineal discomfort following childbirth: a blind randomized controlled trial. *J. Adv. Nurs.*, 19, 89–96.

Glazener, C.M. (1997). Sexual function after childbirth: women's experiences, persistent morbidity and lack of professional recognition. *Br. J. Obstet. Gynaecol.*, 104, 330–5.

Greenshields, W. and Hulme, H. (1993) *The Perineum in Childbirth*. London: National Childbirth Trust.

Hofmeyr, G. .J, Piccioni, V. and Blauhof, P. (1990). Postpartum homoeopathic Arnica montana: a potency-finding pilot study. *Br. J. Clin. Pract.*, 44, 619–21.

Robson, K.M., Brant, H.A. and Kumar, R. (1981). Maternal sexuality during first pregnancy and after childbirth. *Br. J. Obstet. Gynaecol.*, **88**, 882–9.

CHAPTER 48

Breast symptoms in women who are not breastfeeding

1 Introduction

Women may not breastfeed their newborn baby for many reasons, ranging from personal choice to stillbirth. Sometimes the choice may be difficult for a woman. For example, HIV-infected women face enormous conflict between the wish to nurture a child who may die in childhood or be orphaned, and the knowledge that the child may be infected with HIV during breastfeeding. Whatever the reason, the decision not to breastfeed results in considerable breast pain and engorgement during the days after childbirth, until lactation becomes spontaneously suppressed. A number of approaches have been adopted in attempts to hasten the suppression of lactation and reduce the symptoms that accompany it.

2 Non-pharmacological approaches

Until the 1950s, when a number of pharmacological alternatives were promoted, tight binding of the breasts and fluid restriction were the most common approaches to the suppression of lactation. Both are still frequently adopted. Almost no formal investigation of these methods has been undertaken, although the results of one small randomized trial showed that breast pain was less frequent in women who restricted their fluid intake in addition to just wearing brassieres.

Non-pharmacological methods of inhibiting lactation have been implicitly compared with pharmacological methods in trials of different drug agents. In general, the drugs studied were found to be more effective than non-pharmaceutical methods in controlling symptoms during the first week postpartum; by the second week there is no difference; by the third week symptoms are more frequent in women who have received medication. It is probable, therefore, that there may be short-term disadvantages but longer term benefits, of non-pharmacological approaches to suppress lactation.

3 Pharmacological approaches

3.1 Sex hormones

Stilbestrol, now rarely used, reduces the incidence of continuing lactation, breast pain, and engorgement, during the first week postpartum, but these short-term benefits are more than counter-balanced by long-term adverse effects. More women given stilbestrol than women given placebo required additional treatment after discharge from hospital, and four times as many in the stilbestrol-treated group reported abnormal vaginal bleeding after the end of treatment.

There does not appear to be much difference in effect with the use of different estrogens or combinations. Trials comparing the effects of different estrogens show that stilbestrol suppresses lactation and pain more effectively than quinestrol. Chlorotrianisene, another stilbestrol analog, has also been shown to reduce lactation, breast pain, and engorgement in placebo-controlled trials.

Various combinations of an estrogen and testosterone have been shown to have dramatic short-term effects on lactation, breast pain, and breast engorgement. The only trial in which long-term effects have been reported, shows a recurrence of pain and engorgement by the end of the second week.

The risk of thrombo-embolic complications is increased with estrogen use, although the absolute level of risk is low. Withdrawal bleeding after hormonal treatment is reported by about 15% of women, irrespective of the type of drug used.

3.2 Bromo-ergocriptine (bromocriptine)

Although the short-term beneficial effects of bromo-ergocriptine, compared with placebo, have been well established, only limited data are available on effects during the second week, when the beneficial effects are much less dramatic. Rebound lactation is common. As serious adverse cardiovascular and cerebrovascular effects have been reported in women treated with bromo-ergocriptine for suppression of lactation, the drug is now rarely used.

3.3 Cabergoline

Cabergoline has been compared with a placebo and with bromocriptine in three trials. The results indicate that a single dose of cabergoline is as effective and results in fewer side-effects and less rebound lactation than a twice daily dose of bromocriptine for 14 days. Cabergoline should be the drug of choice if pharmacological suppression of lactation is chosen, although more information is needed about the best dose and timing of administration.

3.4 Other drugs

Pyridoxine has been compared with placebo in three studies; the few data available show little effect on continued lactation.

In the early 1960s, the effects on lactation and breast symptoms of spraying synthetic oxytocin intranasally was studied in at least three trials, one of them unpublished. None of these studies provided any evidence that the treatment was effective.

4 Conclusions

The available evidence suggests that physical methods of lactation suppression, such as breast binding, are as effective or more effective than pharmacological methods in the longer term, although they are associated with more pain in the first week after childbirth. Women should be informed of these relative advantages and disadvantages when a method to suppress lactation is chosen.

If they decide to use one of the pharmacological approaches, the available evidence suggests that cabergoline should be the drug of choice.

Cabergoline and newer drugs that may be developed, should be compared formally with physical methods of suppressing lactation in controlled trials with adequate sample sizes and duration of follow-up.

Women's views of the relative merits and disadvantages of the alternative methods should be an essential element in the evaluation, and more serious attention should be given to documenting the frequency of short- and long-term adverse reactions.

Sources

Effective care in pregnancy and childbirth

Parazzini, F., Zanaboni, F., Liberati, A. and Tognoni, G., Relief of breast symptoms in women who are not breastfeeding.

Cochrane Library

Brocklehurst, P., Interventions for reducing mother-to-child transmission of HIV infection.

Pre-Cochrane reviews

Renfrew, M.J., Breast binder vs fluid limitation for lactation suppression. Review no. 03878.

Stilbestrol for lactation suppression. Review no. 03379.

Quinestrol for lactation suppression. Review no. 03380.

Chlorotrianisene for lactation suppression. Review no. 03382.

Estrogen/testosterone combination for lactation suppression. Review no. 03381.

Bromocriptine for lactation suppression. Review no. 03384.

Pyridoxine for lactation suppression. Review no. 03385.

Intranasal oxytocin for lactation suppression. Review no. 03888.

Cabergoline (ergot derivative) for lactation suppression. Review no. 05723.

Other sources

Dunn, D.T., Newell, M.L., Ades, A.E. and Peckham, C.S. (1992). Risk of human immunodeficiency virus type 1 transmission through breastfeeding. *Lancet*, **340**, 585–8.

Henschel, D. and Inch, S. (1996). *Breastfeeding: a Guide for Midwives.* The Royal College of Midwives p.83.

Hofmeyr, G.J. and McIntyre, J. (1997). Preventing perinatal infections. *BMJ*, **315**, 199–200.

CHAPTER 49

Loss and grief in the perinatal period

1 Introduction

Attitudes towards neonatal illness, childhood impairment, and peri-natal death have changed greatly over the past few decades. Improvements in perinatal and infant mortality have been accompanied by ever-increasing expectations by parents that their children will be born safely and will survive. When things do go wrong, it comes as a great shock. Parents may suffer much more than the sense of loss of the healthy baby they had anticipated. They may also lose their faith in modern medicine and doctors, and the belief in their own ability to produce a normal baby. In a similar way it is often shattering for care-givers to witness the apparent failure of their skills.

To compound the difficulties further, those who live in industrialized societies have lost day to day familiarity with death and bereavement, and the mourning rituals that used to play an important part in dealing with the psychological needs of the bereaved. They have thus become poorly equipped to cope with this tragic situation.

Grieving will follow the birth of an ill or impaired baby, as well as after a baby's death. The two components of normal grief are the acute symptoms (episodes of restlessness, angry pining, and anxiety), set against a background disturbance consisting of chronic low mood, loss of purpose in life, social withdrawal, impaired memory and concentration, and disturbances of appetite and sleep. These symptoms occur as bereaved people go through the process of coming to terms with the reality of their loss, and of psychologically withdrawing from their relationships with the impaired or dead child. This process, which is necessary to let them continue with their own lives in a positive manner, may take months or years to complete. A successful outcome depends on the personalities and life experiences of the people concerned; on the circumstances of the impairment or death; and on the effectiveness of the supportive network surrounding them.

2 Perinatal loss

2.1 Illness and impairment

The reaction of parents to a newborn baby who is gravely ill or impaired is a form of grief reaction to the loss of the healthy child that they had expected. The initial phase is marked by shock and panic ('I can't look after a handicapped child'), denial ('He's not my baby'), grief, guilt, and anger. This is followed by a phase of bargaining ('I will look after him if he can be taught to be clean and dry'); and finally acceptance, when parents cope with the reality of the situation. Some parents remain in a state of chronic sorrow. It is important for caregivers to form an effective alliance with the parents, on which plans for care can be based.

In addition to a grief reaction, most parents of ill or impaired babies suffer high levels of anxiety, which appear to be increased by contact with the baby. This does not mean that separation of mother and baby is to be recommended. On the contrary, close contact between parents and the baby, with support from caregivers, will allow parents to form a relationship with a real child. If the mother planned to breastfeed, she can be encouraged to initiate lactation by expressing her milk.

Providing this milk for her baby may help in the development of her relationship with the child, and demonstrate her own unique role in caring for the baby.

Apart from the emotional stress of the situation, parents have the physical and financial stress of visiting their baby in hospital, particularly if the baby has recurrent medical crises and needs care over a long period of time. Some parents withdraw emotionally and physically from their baby before the medical staff have given up hope of the baby's survival. This is termed 'anticipatory mourning'. It can be precipitated by giving an excessively gloomy prognosis, or even by a casual remark indicating a possible bad prognosis. It carries with it a risk of rejection if the baby does eventually survive.

2.2 Perinatal death

Grief after perinatal death is not different from that following the death of any loved person. There are, however, some special features to be considered.

Bereaved parents may feel anxious and angry, and direct blame at their caregivers, other members of the family, or themselves. This may be due in part to the suddenness of the death, and is probably compounded when there is no 'scientific' explanation for what has gone wrong. Parents desperately seek for a cause for the baby's death. It is easier for those who have an explanation, such as malformations or extreme immaturity. 'Empty arms' is another common and distressing symptom after the phase of numbness has passed. Mothers are frequently tormented by hearing their dead baby cry. Some bereaved parents experience negative feelings towards other babies and are fearful of losing control, while others long to hold a baby – any baby – however painful this might be. Many mothers do not expect to lactate once the baby has died and find the fact that they do upsetting. Most mothers experience a great loss of self esteem, a sense of having failed, both as a woman and as a wife.

Most parents will not have been bereaved before, and are likely to have difficulty coping with the complicated registration and funeral procedures. Many are unprepared for the emotional turmoil of their grief reaction, and may feel they should be 'over it' after a few weeks. This view may be reinforced by well-meaning friends, relatives, and even medical practitioners, who may advise the couple to go ahead with another pregnancy long before they have recovered sufficiently from their loss. There is evidence that fathers recover from their grief more quickly than mothers. This in itself may lead to problems with their relationship, particularly if the couple are not used to sharing their feelings, or if one of them is blaming the other for the baby's death. Sexual and marital difficulties are common. Another difficult area is the reaction of other young children in the family to the loss of the baby. They may be confused about what has happened to the baby, and even feel responsible for the disappearance. Behavioral changes are common; they may take the form of over-activity, naughtiness, regression, problems at school, and other emotional problems. These reactions are usually fairly short-lived (a few weeks or months) unless the emotional state of the parents is such that there is an absence of normal warmth in family relationships for an extended period, or serious difficulties develop in the relationships between the mother and her living children.

It may be particularly difficult to work through one's grief when a baby is stillborn. There is no real object to mourn. The baby has never lived outside the womb and there are no memories to help. The problems are accentuated if the stillborn baby is rapidly removed from the delivery room before the parents have a chance to see or hold him or her, and if the hospital, for whatever reason, takes over the funeral arrangements without involving the parents.

Long-term follow up studies show that a significant proportion, up to a fifth of women interviewed, still suffer from serious psychological symptoms for years after losing a baby. Although it is not possible to identify with great confidence those most at risk of developing problems, the most frequently reported markers are not seeing or holding the baby, having an unsupportive partner or social network, and embarking immediately on another pregnancy.

There may be problems with parental relationships when babies have been conceived too quickly after a loss. If the dead child has not been adequately mourned before the start of a new pregnancy, mourning may be postponed until after the birth of the next baby, when it can reappear as 'postpartum depression'. The new baby's identity can become confused with that of the idealized baby, causing great emotional problems. The new child may never be able to live up to the parents' expectations, and may become the focus of any unresolved anger that the parents have as a result of their loss. The survivor of a twin pregnancy may be involved in similar problems if the dead twin is not properly mourned at the time.

3 Care by hospital staff

The maternity unit staff play a vital role in the care of bereaved parents. A program of care should encourage the parents to see, hold, and name their baby, and to hold a funeral. Arrangements should be made for them to see senior obstetrical, midwifery, and pediatric staff to discuss what went wrong, obtain genetic and obstetrical counseling, and receive the autopsy results. Providing informed, compassionate care will help the recovery process after a perinatal death.

Effective care for most families can and should be provided by the maternity unit staff. These professionals and the family doctor are in a position to help bereaved families by facilitating the establishment of normal grieving from the start. Special bereavement counseling services are not often required.

3.1 Communication

Good care hinges upon good communication. Parents frequently comment on communication failures when describing their experiences. Caregivers must give bereaved parents opportunities to talk about the loss of their baby, and even more importantly, listen sympathetically to their expressions of grief. The senior obstetrical, midwifery, or pediatric staff must help parents with their search for a cause of death and create opportunities for discussing this with them.

Seeing both parents together helps to strengthen their relationship, as they share the experience of their baby's loss, and prevents misunderstandings and inconsistencies in explanation. Arranging for the same caregivers to attend regularly to the parents also helps this. Any information given in the first few days of the loss will probably need to be repeated later, as the initial shock passes. A follow-up interview a few weeks later seems to be the best way of dealing with this.

Good communication among professionals about the loss of the baby is necessary to prevent painful situations, such as a member of staff being unaware that the baby has died, and asking the mother about the baby. The primary-care team should be informed about the baby's loss immediately, so that they can make contact with the family as soon as, or even before, the mother is discharged. Parents may want the support of their own religious adviser, and the hospital should check on this and contact him or her if required.

3.2 Immediate and early care when the baby is dead or dying

For mourning to begin, parents must be enabled to face their fear of death and dying, so that they can experience the painful reality of their loss. This involves encouraging them to have as much contact as possible with their baby, both before and after death. It is particularly important for parents of a stillborn baby to see, hold, and name their baby.

When an intra-uterine death is suspected, the fears for the baby's condition should not be denied, but shared with the parents, together if at all possible. If the mother is at an outpatient clinic or doctor's office, efforts should be made to contact her partner or a friend or family member, so that she is not left to travel home alone and unsupported. The technicians in the ultrasound scanning room have an important role to play when the confirmatory scan is done. They need to be sympathetic to the situation and allow the mother to be accompanied by anyone she chooses (see Chapter 27).

Most women are frightened at the prospect of delivering a dead baby, as well as shocked by their loss. It helps if caregivers take time to explain carefully what will happen, that adequate pain relief will be available, and what the baby will look like at birth. This is usually successful in overcoming any reluctance that the parents may have about seeing or holding their baby. It may help to show a malformed or macerated baby to the parents wrapped up at first.

A few parents will not be able to cope with seeing and holding the baby at the time of birth. A photograph should be taken and kept in the medical notes for possible use later, and further opportunities for seeing the baby should be offered to parents over the next few days, as they often change their minds. Photographs and other mementoes of the baby, such as a lock of hair, a piece of the umbilical cord, or a print of the baby's hand or foot are important, as they provide tangible evidence of the reality of the baby's existence and loss. They should be available for parents as keepsakes, if they wish.

When the baby lives long enough to be transferred to a neonatal unit, it is again important for caregivers to keep parents as fully informed as possible about the baby's condition, and to encourage them to share in the care. Photographs of the baby are helpful, particularly for fathers to keep at home, or if the mother is too unwell to visit the unit. In a randomized trial of the use of routine photographs of sick neonates in the first week of life, there was a significant increase in visiting by the parents of the photographed babies, compared with the non-photographed group.

When the baby's condition is known to be terminal, it is important to involve the parents in the decision to cease life-support, and then to let them take their dying baby in their arms, if at all possible, free of all equipment that has been necessary until then. In describing this, authors quote parents saying such things as, 'It was all I could do for her to hold her in my arms as she died'. Some parents may wish to take the baby home to die; they should be supported in this decision. Feelings of guilt about removing the baby from the life-support system have not been reported.

Many parents like to help with the laying out of the baby's body, and this should be encouraged. Often they have selected special clothes or toys to be placed in the coffin with the baby. Supporting the parents' contact with the reality of the death of their baby in these ways will facilitate their grief reaction. They will need privacy to express their grief, and this should be provided, however busy the unit happens to be.

The choice of site for the aftercare of the mother is important, as mothers differ in their requirements at this time. Some want to be on their own, far away from the sound of babies crying; others long to return to familiar faces on the ward. It is helpful if as much flexibility as possible is offered to them and if, at least for the first night, partners are allowed to remain with them. Ideally, the hospital should provide a couch in the mother's room so that the parents can share their grief together. Lactation and help with its suppression is an important issue for the mother whose baby has died. If the mother is physically fit to return home immediately and wishes to do so, it is important to ensure that she has a supportive network of family, friends, and professionals before she goes home.

3.3 Autopsy

Consent for an autopsy and chromosome studies should always be requested after a perinatal death. These investigations may provide information about the cause of death, help parents with their grief, and assist the planning of future pregnancies. Most parents agree to an autopsy, although it is often a painful decision for them. Having consented, parents cherish great hopes that the results will provide answers to their questions about why the baby died. It is important that they receive the results in a form that makes sense to them. The best person to do this would be a senior member of staff who can interpret the pathological findings.

3.4 Death registration and funeral arrangements

Knowledge of the legal procedures required when a baby dies or is still-born is fundamental to good care. It is necessary to be familiar with the registration and funeral arrangements operating in one's own locality, as these are often complicated and baffling for parents still suffering from the shock of their baby's death. Religious practices vary greatly as well, and an awareness of these and sensitivity to the wishes of individual parents is crucial. The funeral may involve considerable expense; helping those in financial difficulties, besides encouraging them to attend, are therapeutic aspects of care.

Many units have leaflets outlining their own procedures and giving helpful advice for parents.

3.5 Follow-up

Most mothers will be discharged home within a few days of their baby's death, still too shocked by it to grasp properly what has happened and why. Careful and supportive follow-up is extremely important. Parents should be able to contact the staff who cared for them by telephone after they leave the hospital. Some units are able to offer home visits by their social worker. An appointment should be made for both parents to see a senior member of staff 2–6 weeks later, as soon as the chromosome studies and autopsy results are available, and some form of perinatal mortality conference has taken place. Caregivers should be aware that returning to the hospital is likely to be traumatic for the parents.

The next pregnancy will inevitably be an extremely anxious time, and the mother will need extra support during pregnancy and in the first few months after the birth.

4 Care in the community

4.1 Health professionals

The general practitioner, health visitor, community midwife, and other primary health-care workers will form the professional supportive network once the mother has returned home. These professionals can help by continuing to support parents in the expression of their grief and putting them in touch with local support groups for parents who have lost a child.

The general practitioner or midwife can watch for signs of patho-logical grief reactions, and refer the parents for specialist help if necessary. These pathological reactions can take the form of an inhibited reaction, with no sign of any sense of loss, or a prolonged reaction, with unremitting symptoms of depression, severe anxiety or the appearance of psychosomatic illness. There may be drug or alcohol abuse.

Unremitting anger is another feature of a pathological grief reaction. General practitioners and midwives may need to deal with anger focused on the maternity unit. To do so, they must ensure that the parents have good relationships with the obstetrical, midwifery, and pediatric staff, and are fully informed about the course of events that led to the baby's loss. The parents may blame the general practitioner or midwife, as well as the maternity unit. When this happens, it is essential that he or she meets with the family as soon as possible, so that they can ventilate their feelings and, hopefully, re-establish their relationship. Many parents remain angry simply because they were denied any compassionate response to their situation: no one said, 'I'm so sorry your baby died'.

The general practitioner or health visitor will probably be the person to whom the family will turn to for help in coping with the reactions of their other children to the baby's death. Parents may need help to allow their children to express their feelings about so painful a subject. It must be remembered that young children will use play as a vehicle for doing so. Explaining death to children under 5 year of age is difficult because they are not yet able to grasp the concept. Even simple statements like, 'The baby's gone' will be interpreted literally and lead to questions about where the baby has gone and when a visit can be made. The parents will need to add more information as the child's capacity for understanding develops.

4.2 Self-help groups

Self-help can be effective in providing the right kind of support for parents facing many different kinds of problems, and perinatal bereavement is no exception. It is important though, that the people running the group have recovered sufficiently from their own loss to be able to help others, and that they have access to professionals for help and advice as and when necessary. Parents can benefit from sharing their experiences together, from discovering that they are not alone in their suffering, and from learning that time does help to heal the wounds. Not everyone can cope with group support, and it is unwise to rely on a local self-help group to meet the needs of all bereaved families. While it is invaluable to give parents the telephone number or address of a local contact, this should not replace follow-up by the hospital staff, general practitioner, and health visitor.

5 The role of specialist counselors

5.1 Routine counseling
Three small trials have been conducted, which evaluated routine counseling for bereaved parents by caregivers trained in grief work, compared to standard care. The studies did not produce conclusive evidence of effectiveness, primarily because the dropout rates of participants were high. More research is needed in this important area.

5.2 Counseling for prolonged grief reactions
Prevention of prolonged grief reactions through appropriate care is not always successful. About one in five families will show reactions that are detrimental to their health and are likely to be accompanied by problems in family relationships. Little is known about the factors that precipitate prolonged grief reactions or the most effective measures of preventing or decreasing their severity. The help of specialist counselors trained in grief work will be needed in these situations, either to advise other colleagues giving care, or to take over responsibility for care themselves. The treatment required is often protracted, and antidepressant drugs and psychiatric surveillance may be necessary for severe depressive symptoms. Child and family psychiatrists may be particularly helpful in dealing with the relationship problems within families.

Specialist counselors can also be useful in supporting the staff of the unit (through regular staff meetings, case discussions, or training sessions) and can offer help and advice to self-help groups. The training of caregivers in the care of families who lose their baby, or who are faced with a baby with a severe impairment, deserves as much emphasis as the development of their technical expertise.

6 Conclusions

Much can be done to help a bereaved family cope with their loss and recover from their grief. The extent to which this is accomplished will depend on the importance that is attached to training in this area, and on the attitudes of individual professionals, both in the maternity unit and in the community. Parents need the opportunity to have contact with their ill child, and support for the mother to lactate if she wishes. Parents of stillborn or dying babies should similarly be encouraged to touch and hold their baby. Photographs of their baby will provide tangible evidence of the reality of the baby's existence and loss. Giving photographs to parents of sick babies has also been shown to increase their visits to their babies in the first week of life.

The practical aspects of death registration and funeral arrangements for babies should receive careful attention. Time must be spent, listening as well as talking, with parents whose baby has died or is impaired. The senior members of staff need to play a central role in caring for the parents, sharing their experience and expertise with more junior caregivers. The primary health-care team must accept the role of monitoring and supporting the parents during the ongoing bereavement process.

The provision of adequate support will almost certainly lead to improved rapport with grieving families. It will help professionals to cope better with their own grief, because they feel more able to help. Most importantly, it may help families to emerge from their grief able to resume normal functioning.

Sources

Effective care in pregnancy and childbirth

Forrest, G., Care of the bereaved after perinatal death.

Cochrane Library

Chambers, H.M. and Chan, F.Y., Support for women/families after perinatal death.

Other sources

Fox, R., Pillai, M., Porter, H. and Gill, G. (1997). The management of late fetal death: a guide to comprehensive care. *Br. J. Obstet. Gynaecol.*, **104**, 4–10.

Schneiderman, G., Winders, P., Tallett, S. and Feldman, W. (1994). Do child and/or parent bereavement programs work? *Can. J. Psychiat.*, **39**, 215–8.

Stinson, K., Lasker, J., Lohmann, J. and Toedter, L. (1992). Parents' grief following pregnancy loss: a comparison of mothers and fathers. *Fam. Rel.*, **41**, 218–23.

Synopsis

CHAPTER 50

Effective care in pregnancy and childbirth: a synopsis

The underlying thesis of this book is that evidence from well-controlled comparisons provides the best basis for choosing among alternative forms of care in pregnancy and childbirth. This evidence should encourage the adoption of useful measures and the abandonment of those that are useless or harmful.

In this final chapter we have tried to summarize the main conclusions reached in earlier chapters. This summary takes the form of six tables which list, respectively:

(1) beneficial forms of care;

(2) forms of care that are likely to be beneficial;

(3) forms of care with a trade-off between beneficial and adverse effects;

(4) forms of care of unknown effectiveness;

(5) forms of care that are unlikely to be beneficial;

(6) forms of care that are likely to be ineffective or harmful.

Tables 1 and 6 are based on clear evidence from systematic reviews of randomized controlled trials. Tables 2 and 5 are based on information from reviews of controlled trials or good observational evidence, but for which the conclusions can not be as firmly based as those for Tables 1 and 6. Table 3 lists forms of care with both beneficial and adverse effects, which women and caregivers should weigh according to their individual circumstances and priorities; and Table 4 lists forms of care for which there are insufficient data, or data of inadequate quality on which to base a recommendation.

We have tried to be explicit about our criteria for choosing which table to use for each intervention, but there is inevitably some subjectivity in our choice. We worked from two basic principles: first, that the only justification for practices that restrict a woman's autonomy, her freedom of choice, and her access to her baby, would be clear evidence that these restrictive practices do more good than harm; and second, that any interference with the natural process of pregnancy and childbirth should also be shown to do more good than harm. We believe that the onus of proof rests on those who advocate any intervention that interferes with either of these principles.

A tabulated summary such as this is necessarily selective. Nuances discussed in the chapters cannot find full expression in summary tables. Nevertheless, we hope that the explicit form in which these conclusions have been stated will be useful, and that the advantages of this summary approach will outweigh its drawbacks.

The inclusion of a particular form of care in Tables 1 or 2 does not imply that it should always be adopted in practice. Research based on the study of groups may not always apply to individuals, although it should be relevant to guide broad policies of care. Forms of care listed in Tables 5 and 6 may still be useful in particular circumstances, although, once again, they should be discouraged as a matter of policy. Practices listed in Table 3 will require careful consideration by the individuals concerned, while those in Table 4 should usually be avoided except in the context of trials to better evaluate their effects.

Some of the conclusions that we have reached will be controversial, but they must be judged in the light of the methods we used to assemble and review the evidence on which they are based. While we have made great efforts to ensure that the data presented are comprehensive and accurate, it is possible that errors and misinterpretations have crept in. We conclude by reiterating the invitation extended to readers in our first edition, to bring omissions and mistakes to our attention for inclusion and correction in *The Cochrane Library* and in later editions of this book. Correspondence should be addressed to the Cochrane Pregnancy and Childbirth Group, Liverpool Women's Hospital NHS Trust, Crown Street, Liverpool, UK L8 7SS.

TABLE 1   487

Table 1 Beneficial forms of care

Effectiveness demonstrated by clear evidence from controlled trials.	Chapter
Basic care	
Women carrying their pregnancy record to enhance their feeling of being in control	3
Pre- and peri-conceptional folic acid supplementation to prevent recurrent neural tube defects	5, 6
Folic acid supplementation (or high folate diet) for all women envisaging pregnancy	5, 6
Assistance (especially behavioral strategies) to stop smoking during pregnancy	5
Balanced energy and protein supplementation when dietary supplementation is required	6
Vitamin D supplementation for women with inadequate exposure to sunlight	6
Iodine supplementation in populations with a high incidence of endemic cretinism	6
Screening and diagnosis	
Doppler ultrasound in pregnancies at high risk of fetal compromise	12
Pregnancy problems	
Antihistamines for nausea and vomiting of pregnancy that is resistant to simple measures	13
Local imidazoles for vaginal candida infection (thrush)	13
Local imidazoles instead of nystatin for vaginal candida infection (thrush)	13
Magnesium sulphate rather than other anticonvulsants for treatment of eclampsia	15
Administration of anti-D immunoglobulin to Rh-negative women whose newborn baby is not Rh-negative	18
Administration of anti-D immunoglobulin to Rh-negative women at 28 weeks of pregnancy	18
Antiretroviral treatment of HIV-infected pregnant women to prevent transmission to fetus	19
Antibiotic treatment of asymptomatic bacteriuria	19
Antibiotics during labor for women known to be colonized with group B streptococcus	19

Table 1 (continued)

Effectiveness demonstrated by clear evidence from controlled trials.	Chapter
Tight as opposed to too strict or loose control of blood sugar levels in pregnant diabetic women	20
External cephalic version at term to avoid breech birth	22
Corticosteroids to promote fetal maturity before preterm birth	25
Offering induction of labor after 41 completed weeks of gestation	26

Childbirth

Physical, emotional and psychological support during labor and birth	28, 35, 41
Continuous support for women during labor and childbirth	28
Agents to reduce acidity of stomach contents before general anesthesia	29
Complementing fetal heart-rate monitoring in labor with fetal acid-base assessment	30
Oxytocics to treat postpartum hemorrhage	33
Prophylactic oxytocics in the third stage of labor	33
Active versus expectant management of third stage of labor	33

Problems during childbirth

Absorbable instead of non-absorbable sutures for skin repair of perineal trauma	36
Polyglycolic acid sutures instead of chromic catgut for repair of perineal trauma	36

Techniques of induction and operative delivery

Prostaglandins to increase cervical readiness for induction of labor	39
Amniotomy plus oxytocin for induction of labor instead of either amniotomy alone or oxytocin alone	40
Vacuum extraction instead of forceps when operative vaginal delivery is required	41
Antibiotic prophylaxis (short course or intraperitoneal lavage) with cesarean section	43

Care after childbirth

Use of surfactant for very preterm infants to prevent respiratory distress syndrome	44
Support for socially disadvantaged mothers to improve parenting	45

TABLE 1   489

Table 1 (continued)

Effectiveness demonstrated by clear evidence from controlled trials.	Chapter
Consistent support for breastfeeding mothers	46
Personal support from a knowledgable individual for breastfeeding mothers	46
Unrestricted breastfeeding	46
Local anesthetic sprays for relief of perineal pain postpartum	47
Cabergoline instead of bromocriptine for relief of breast symptoms in non-breastfeeding mothers	48

Table 2 Forms of care likely to be beneficial

The evidence in favour of these forms of care is strong, although not established by randomized trials	Chapter
Basic care	
Adequate access to care for all childbearing women	3
Social support for childbearing women	3
Financial support for childbearing women in need	3
Legislation on paid leave and income maintenance during maternity or parental leave	3
Midwifery care for women with no serious risk factors	3
Continuity of care for childbearing women	3
Antenatal classes for women and their partners who want them	4
Advice to avoid excessive alcohol consumption during pregnancy	5
Avoidance of heavy physical work during pregnancy	5
Screening and diagnosis	
Ultrasound to resolve questions about fetal size, structure, or position	8
Selective use of ultrasound to assess amniotic fluid volume	8
Selective use of ultrasound to estimate gestational age in first and early second trimester	8, 9
Ultrasound to determine whether the embryo is alive in threatened miscarriage	8, 14
Ultrasound to confirm suspected multiple pregnancy	8, 17
Ultrasound for placental location in suspected placenta praevia	8, 21

Table 2 (continued)

The evidence in favour of these forms of care is strong, although not established by randomized trials	Chapter
Second trimester amniocentesis to identify chromosomal abnormalities in pregnancies at risk	9
Transabdominal instead of transcervical chorion villus sampling	9
Genetic counseling before prenatal diagnosis	9
Clinical history to assess risk of pre-eclampsia	10
Regular monitoring of blood pressure during pregnancy	10
Testing for proteinuria during pregnancy	10
Uric acid levels for following the course of pre-eclampsia	10
Fundal height measurements during pregnancy	12

Pregnancy problems

Ultrasound to facilitate intra-uterine interventions	8, 9
Antacids for heartburn of pregnancy if simple measures are ineffective	13
Bulking agents for constipation if simple measures are ineffective	13
Local metronidazole for symptomatic trichomonal vaginitis after the first trimester	13
Antibiotics for symptomatic bacterial vaginosis	13
Antiplatelet agents to prevent pre-eclampsia	15
Antihypertensive agents to control serious hypertension in pregnancy	15
Calcium to prevent pre-eclampsia, for women at high risk or with low calcium in diet	6, 15
Balanced protein/energy supplementation for impaired fetal growth	6, 16
Ultrasound surveillance of fetal growth in multiple pregnancies	17
Screening all pregnant women for blood group iso-immunization	18
Anti-D immunoglobulin to Rh-negative women after any uterine bleeding, intrauterine procedure, or abdominal trauma during pregnancy	18, 21
Intra-uterine transfusion for a severely affected iso-immunized fetus	18
Advice to not breastfeed for HIV infected women to prevent transmission to baby	19, 46
Routine screening for, and treatment of, syphilis in pregnancy	19
Rubella vaccination of seronegative women postpartum	19
Screening for and treatment of chlamydia in high prevalence populations	19

TABLE 2   491

Table 2 *(continued)*

The evidence in favour of these forms of care is strong, although not established by randomized trials	Chapter
Cesarean section for active herpes (with visible lesion) in labor with intact membranes	19
Prepregnancy counseling for women with diabetes	20
Specialist care for pregnant women with diabetes	20
Home instead of hospital glucose-monitoring for pregnant women with diabetes	20
Ultrasound surveillance of fetal growth for pregnant women with diabetes	20
Allowing pregnancy to continue to term in otherwise uncomplicated diabetic pregnancies	20
Careful attention to insulin requirements postpartum	20
Encouraging diabetic women to breastfeed	20
Checking for clotting disorders with severe placental abruption	21
Vaginal instead of cesarean delivery for placental abruption in the absence of fetal distress	21
Vaginal instead of cesarean birth for a dead fetus after placental abruption	21
Repeat ultrasound scanning of a low-lying placenta in late pregnancy	21
Delaying planned cesarean section for placenta praevia until term	21
Cesarean section for placenta praevia covering any portion of the cervical os	21
Ultrasound examination for vaginal bleeding of undetermined origin	21
External cephalic version for transverse or oblique lie at term	22
Tocolysis for external cephalic version of breech, particularly if unsuccessful otherwise	22
External cephalic version for breech in early labor if the membranes are intact	22
Corticosteroid administration after prelabor rupture of the membranes preterm	23
Vaginal culture after prelabor rupture of the membranes preterm	23
Antibiotics for prelabor rupture of the membranes with suspected intrauterine infection	23
Not stopping spontaneous labor after prelabor rupture of the membranes preterm	23

Table 2 (continued)

The evidence in favour of these forms of care is strong, although not established by randomized trials	Chapter
Elective delivery for prelabor rupture of the membranes preterm with signs of infection	23
Amnio-infusion for fetal distress thought to be due to oligohydramnios in labor	23, 30
Betamimetic tocolysis to allow effective preparation for preterm birth	24
Short-term indomethacin to stop preterm labor	24
Offering induction of labor as an option after fetal death	27
Prostaglandin or prostaglandin analogs for induction of labor after fetal death	27

Childbirth

Respecting women's choice of companions during labor and birth	28
Respecting women's choice of place of birth	28
Presence of a companion on admission to hospital	29
Giving women as much information as they desire	29
Freedom of movement and choice of position in labor	29
Change of mother's position for fetal distress in labor	30
Intravenous betamimetics for fetal distress in labor to 'buy time'	30
Respecting women's choice of position for the second stage of labor and giving birth	32
Guarding the perineum versus watchful waiting during birth	32
Intramyometrial prostaglandins for severe postpartum hemorrhage	33

Problems during childbirth

Regular top-ups of epidural analgesia instead of top-ups on maternal demand	34
Maternal movement and position changes to relieve pain in labor	34
Counter-pressure to relieve pain in labor	34
Superficial heat or cold to relieve pain in labor	34
Touch and massage to relieve pain in labor	34
Attention focusing and distraction to relieve pain in labor	34
Music and audio-analgesia to relieve pain in labor	34
Epidural instead of narcotic analgesia for preterm labor and birth	34, 37
Amniotomy to augment slow or prolonged labor	35

TABLE 2   **493**

Table 2 (continued)

The evidence in favour of these forms of care is strong, although not established by randomized trials	Chapter
Continuous subcuticular suture for perineal skin repair	36
Primary rather than delayed repair of episiotomy breakdown	36
Delivery of a very preterm baby in a center with adequate perinatal facilities	37,44
Presence of a pediatrician at a very preterm birth	37, 44
Trial of labor after previous lower segment cesarean section	38
Trial of labor after more than one previous lower segment cesarean section	38
Use of oxytocic agents when indicated for labor after a previous cesarean section	38
Use of epidural analgesia in labor when needed after previous cesarean section	38
Techniques of induction and operative delivery	
Assessing the state of the cervix before induction of labor	39
Transverse instead of vertical skin incision for cesarean section	42
Low-dose heparin with cesarean section to prevent thrombo-embolism	42
Transverse lower segment uterine incision for cesarean section	42
Care after birth	
Keeping newborn babies warm	44
Prophylactic vitamin K to the baby to prevent hemorrhagic disease of the newborn	44
Nasopharyngeal suctioning of infants who have passed meconium before birth	44
Presence of someone skilled in neonatal resuscitation at birth of all infants likely to be at risk	44
Oxygen for resuscitation of distressed newborn infants	44
Cardiac massage for infants born with absent heart beat	44
Naloxone for infants with respiratory depression due to narcotic administration before birth	44
Encouraging early mother–infant contact	45
Allowing mothers access to their own supply of symptom-relieving drugs in hospital	45
Consistent advice to new mothers	45

Table 2 (continued)

The evidence in favour of these forms of care is strong, although not established by randomized trials	Chapter
Offering choice in the length of hospital stay after childbirth	45
Telephone service of advice and information after women go home from hospital after birth	45
Psychological support for women depressed after childbirth	45
Encouraging early breastfeeding when mother and baby are ready	46
Skilled help with first breastfeed	46
Flexibility in breastfeeding practices	46
Antibiotics for infectious mastitis in breastfeeding women	46
Breast binding and fluid restriction for suppression of lactation	48
Support and care programmes for bereaved parents	49
Encouraging parental contact with a dying or dead baby	49
Providing parents with prompt, accurate information about a severely ill baby	49
Encouraging autopsy for a dead baby and discussing the results with the parents	49
Help with funeral arrangements for a dead baby	49
Self-help groups for bereaved parents	49

Table 3 Forms of care with a trade-off between beneficial and adverse effects

Women and caregivers should weigh these effects according to circumstances, priorities, and preferences	Chapter
Basic care	
Continuity of caregiver for childbearing women	3
Legislation restricting type of employment for pregnant women	3
Screening and diagnosis	
Formal systems of risk scoring	7
Routine ultrasound in early pregnancy	8
Chorion villous sampling versus amniocentesis for diagnosis of chromosomal abnormalities	9

TABLE 3   495

Table 3 *(continued)*

Women and caregivers should weigh these effects according to circumstances, priorities, and preferences	Chapter
Serum alpha-fetoprotein screening for neural-tube defects	9
Triple-test screening for down syndrome and neural-tube defects	09
Pregnancy problems	
Corticosteroids to promote fetal maturity before preterm birth in diabetic pregnancy	20, 25
Routine elective cesarean for breech presentation	22
Induction of labor for prelabor rupture of the membranes at term	23
Oral betamimetics to maintain uterine quiescence after arrest of preterm labor	24
Cervical cerclage for women at risk of preterm birth	24
Betamimetic drugs to stop preterm labor	24
Induction instead of surveillance for pregnancy after 41 weeks gestation	26
Expectant care versus induction of labor after fetal death	27
Childbirth	
Continuous electronic monitoring (with scalp sampling) versus intermittent auscultation during labor	30
Midline versus mediolateral episiotomy, when episiotomy is necessary	32
Prophylactic ergometrine/oxytocin (syntometrine) versus oxytocin alone in the third stage of labor	33
Problems during childbirth	
Routine preloading with intravenous fluids before epidural analgesia	34
Narcotics to relieve pain in labor	34
Inhalation analgesia to relieve pain in labor	34
Epidural analgesia to relieve pain in labor	34
Epidural administration of opiates to relieve pain in labor	34
Early amniotomy in spontaneous labor	35
Techniques of induction and operative delivery	
Mechanical methods for cervical ripening or induction of labor	39, 40
Endocervical versus vaginal prostaglandin for cervical ripening before induction of labor	39

Table 3 (continued)

Women and caregivers should weigh these effects according to circumstances, priorities, and preferences	Chapter
Oral prostaglandin E₂ for induction of labor with a ripe cervix	40
Natural prostaglandins versus oxytocin for induction of labor	40
Soft versus rigid vacuum extractor cups	41
Regional versus general anesthesia for cesarean section	42
Epidural versus spinal anesthesia for cesarean section	42
Ampicillin versus broader spectrum antibiotics for cesarean section	43
Care after childbirth	
Prophylactic antibiotic eye ointments to prevent eye infection in the newborn	44
Prophylactic versus 'rescue' surfactant for very preterm infants	44

Table 4 Forms of care of unknown effectiveness

There are insufficient or inadequate quality data upon which to base a recommendation for practice	Chapter
Basic care	
Formal preconceptional care for all women	5
Fish oil supplementation to improve pregnancy outcome	6, 15
Prostaglandin precursors to improve pregnancy outcome	6, 15
Calcium supplementation to improve pregnancy outcome	6, 15, 24
Magnesium supplementation to improve pregnancy outcome	6, 15, 24
Zinc supplementation to improve pregnancy outcome	6
Antigen-avoidance diets to reduce risk of an atopic child	6
Screening and diagnosis	
Placental grading by ultrasound to improve perinatal outcome	8, 12
Measuring placental proteins for pre-eclampsia	10
Doppler ultrasound of uterine artery for pre-eclampsia	10
Measuring hematocrit and platelets for following the course of pre-eclampsia	10
Fetal biophysical profile for fetal surveillance	12

TABLE 4   497

Table 4 (continued)

There are insufficient or inadequate quality data upon which to base a recommendation for practice	Chapter
Pregnancy problems	
Accupressure for nausea and vomiting of pregnancy if simple measures are ineffective	13
Vitamin B6 for nausea and vomiting of pregnancy if simple measures are ineffective	13
Ginger for nausea and vomiting of pregnancy	13
Acid suppressing drugs for heartburn	13
Rutosides for hemorrhoids	13
Rutosides for varicose veins	13
Exercise and education programs for backache	13
Increased salt intake for leg cramps	13
Oral magnesium for leg cramps	13
Progestogens for threatened miscarriage with a live fetus	14
Human chorionic gonadotrophin (HCG) for threatened miscarriage with a live fetus	14
Steroids for women with auto-antibodies and recurrent miscarriage	14
Evacuation versus 'wait and see' following spontaneous miscarriage	14
Medical versus surgical evacuation following spontaneous miscarriage	14
Hospitalization for women with pregnancy-induced hypertension	15
Bed rest for women with pre-eclampsia	15
Antihypertensive drugs for mild to moderate hypertension	15
Antioxidant vitamins C and E to prevent pre-eclampsia	15
Magnesium sulphate for pre-eclampsia	15
Interventionist versus expectant management for severe early onset pre-eclampsia	15
Plasma volume expansion for pre-eclampsia	15
Hospitalization and bed-rest for impaired fetal growth	16
Abdominal decompression for impaired fetal growth	16
Betamimetics for impaired fetal growth	16
Oxygen treatment for impaired fetal growth	16
Hormone treatment for impaired fetal growth	16
Calcium channel blockers for impaired fetal growth	16

Table 4 (continued)

There are insufficient or inadequate quality data upon which to base a recommendation for practice	Chapter
Plasma volume expanders for impaired fetal growth	16
Hospitalization and bed-rest for triplet and higher order pregnancy	17
Antiviral agents for women with a history of recurrent genital herpes	19
Prophylactic antibiotics for prelabor rupture of membranes at term or preterm	23
Postpartum prophylactic antibiotics after prelabor rupture of membranes	23
Bed-rest to prevent preterm birth	24
Progestogens to prevent preterm birth	24
Calcium antagonists to stop preterm labor	24
Antibiotic treatment in preterm labor	24
Oxytocin antagonists to stop preterm labor	24
Sweeping of the membranes to prevent post-term pregnancy	26,40
Nipple stimulation to prevent post-term pregnancy	26

Childbirth

Pre-admission assessment to determine if labor is in the active phase	29
Routine amnioscopy to detect meconium-stained amniotic fluid in labor	30
Routine artificial rupture of the membranes to detect meconium-stained amniotic fluid in labor	30
Short periods of electronic fetal monitoring as a screening test on admission in labor	30
Fetal stimulation tests for fetal assessment in labor	30
Maternal oxygen administration for fetal distress in labor	30
Institutional routines for repeating blood pressure measurements in labor	31
Nipple stimulation to prevent postpartum hemorrhage	33
Misoprostol in the third stage of labor to prevent postpartum hemorrhage	33
Early versus late clamping of the umbilical cord at birth	33
Methods for delivery of the placenta in the third stage of labor	33
Injecting oxytocin in the umbilical vein in the third stage of labor	33
Injecting oxytocin in the umbilical vein for retained placenta	33

TABLE 4   499

Table 4 (continued)

There are insufficient or inadequate quality data upon which to base a recommendation for practice	Chapter
Problems during childbirth	
Abdominal decompression to relieve pain in labor	34
Immersion in water to relieve pain in labor	34
Acupuncture to relieve pain in labor	34
Acupressure to relieve pain in labor	34
Transcutaneous electrical nerve stimulation to relieve pain in labor	34
Intradermal injection of sterile water to relieve pain in labor	34
Aromatherapy to relieve pain in labor	34
Hypnosis to relieve pain in labor	34
Continuous infusion versus intermittent top-ups for epidural analgesia	34
Free mobility during labor to augment slow labor	35
Early use of oxytocin to augment slow or prolonged labor	35
'Active management' of labor	35
Cervical vibration for slow or prolonged labor	35
Histoacryl tissue adhesive for perineal skin repair	36
Cesarean section for very preterm delivery	37
Cesarean section for preterm breech delivery	37
Immediate versus delayed clamping of the umbilical cord of preterm infants	37
Techniques of induction and operative delivery	
Oxytocin by automatic-infusion systems versus 'standard regimens' for induction of labor	40
Misoprostol orally or vaginally for induction of labor	40
Use of hemostatic stapler for the uterine incision at cesarean section	42
Single- versus two-layer closure of the uterine incision at cesarean section	42
Systemic versus intraperitoneal prophylactic antibiotics at cesarean section	43
Care after childbirth	
Tracheal suctioning for meconium in babies without respiratory depression	44
Routine use of antiseptics on the umbilical cord stump	45

Table 4 (continued)

There are insufficient or inadequate quality data upon which to base a recommendation for practice	Chapter
Oral proteolytic enzymes for breast engorgement in breastfeeding mothers	46
Cabbage leaves for breast engorgement in breastfeeding mothers	46
Dopamine agonists to improve milk supply in breastfeeding mothers	46
Oxytocin nasal spray to improve milk supply in breastfeeding mothers	46
Oral proteolytic enzymes for perineal pain postpartum	47
Ultrasound and pulsed electromagnetic energy for perineal pain	47
Rubber rings and similar devices to prevent pressure for perineal pain	47
Cabergoline versus physical methods of suppressing lactation	48

Table 5 Forms of care unlikely to be beneficial

The evidence against these forms of care is not as firmly established as for those in Table 6	Chapter
Basic care	
Reliance on expert opinion instead of on good evidence for decisions about care	2
Routinely involving doctors in the care of all women during pregnancy and childbirth	3
Routinely involving obstetricians in the care of all women during pregnancy and childbirth	3
Not involving obstetricians in the care of women with serious risk factors	3
Fragmentation of care during pregnancy and childbirth	3
Social support for high-risk women to prevent preterm birth	3, 24
Antenatal breast or nipple care for women who plan to breastfeed	46
Advice to restrict sexual activity during pregnancy	5
Prohibition of all alcohol intake during pregnancy	5
Imposing dietary restrictions during pregnancy	6
Routine vitamin supplementation in late pregnancy in well nourished populations	6

TABLE 5   501

Table 5 *(continued)*

The evidence against these forms of care is not as firmly established as for those in Table 6	Chapter
Routine hematinic supplementation in pregnancy in well-nourished populations	6
High-protein dietary supplementation	6, 16
Restriction of salt intake to prevent pre-eclampsia	6, 15
Screening and diagnosis	
Routine use of ultrasound for fetal measurement in late pregnancy	8, 12
Reliance on edema to screen for pre-eclampsia	10
Angiotensin-sensitivity test to screen for pre-eclampsia	10
Cold-pressor test to screen for pre-eclampsia	10
Roll-over test to screen for pre-eclampsia	10
Isometric exercise test to screen for pre-eclampsia	10
Measuring uric acid as a diagnostic test for pre-eclampsia	10
Screening for 'gestational diabetes'	11
Routine glucose challenge test during pregnancy	11
Routine measurement of blood glucose during pregnancy	11
Insulin plus diet treatment for 'gestational diabetes'	11
Diet treatment for 'gestational diabetes'	11
Routine fetal movement counting to improve perinatal outcome	12
Routine use of Doppler ultrasound screening in all pregnancies	12
Measurement of placental proteins or hormones (including estriol and human placental lactogen)	12
Routine cervical assessment for prevention of preterm birth	24
Pregnancy problems	
Calcium supplementation for leg cramps	13
Screening for, and treatment of, vaginal candidal colonization without symptoms	13
Screening for, and treatment of, vaginal trichomonas colonization without symptoms	13
Screening for, and treatment of, bacterial vaginosis without symptoms	13
Bed-rest for threatened miscarriage	14
Immunotherapy for recurrent miscarriage	14
Antithrombotic agents to prevent pre-eclampsia	15

Table 5 (continued)

The evidence against these forms of care is not as firmly established as for those in Table 6	Chapter
Reducing salt intake to prevent pre-eclampsia	15
Diazoxide for pre-eclampsia or hypertension in pregnancy	15
Ketanserin for severe hypertension in pregnancy	15
Diuretics for pregnancy-induced hypertension	15
High protein dietary supplementation for impaired fetal growth	16
Hospitalization and bed-rest for uncomplicated twin pregnancy	17
Cervical cerclage for multiple pregnancy	17
Prophylactic betamimetics for multiple pregnancy	17
Routine cesarean section for multiple pregnancy	17
Routine screening for mycoplasmas during pregnancy	19
Screening for toxoplasmosis during pregnancy	19
Treatment of group B streptococcus colonization during pregnancy	19
Cesarean section for non-active herpes simplex before or at the onset of labor	19
Amniotomy in HIV-infected women	19, 35
Elective delivery before term in women with otherwise uncomplicated diabetes	20
Elective cesarean section for pregnant women with diabetes	20
Discouraging breastfeeding in women with diabetes	20
Vaginal or rectal examination when placenta praevia is suspected	21
Postural techniques for turning breech into cephalic presentation	22
External cephalic version before term to avoid breech presentation at birth	22
X-ray pelvimetry to diagnose cephalopelvic disproportion	22
Computer tomographic pelvimetry to predict cephalopelvic disproportion	22
Cesarean section for macrosomia without a trial of labor to prevent shoulder dystocia	22
Induction of labor to prevent cephalopelvic disproportion	22
Amniocentesis for prelabor rupture of the membranes preterm	23
Prophylactic tocolytics with prelabor rupture of the membranes preterm	23
Regular leucocyte counts for surveillance in prelabor rupture of the membranes	23

TABLE 5   503

Table 5 (continued)

The evidence against these forms of care is not as firmly established as for those in Table 6	Chapter
Home uterine activity monitoring for prevention of preterm birth	24
Magnesium sulphate to stop preterm labor	24
Betamimetics for preterm labor in women with heart disease or diabetes	24
Hydration to arrest preterm labor	24
Diazoxide to stop preterm labor	24
Adding thyrotrophin releasing hormone (TRH) to corticosteroids to promote fetal maturation	25

Childbirth

Withholding food and drink from women in labor	29
Routine intravenous infusion in labor	29
Routine measurement of intra-uterine pressure during oxytocin administration	31, 35
Wearing face masks during labor or for vaginal examinations	31
Frequent scheduled vaginal examinations in labor	31
Routine directed pushing during the second stage of labor	32
Pushing by sustained bearing down during the second stage of labor	32
Breath holding during the second stage of labor	32
Early bearing down during the second stage of labor	32
Arbitrary limitation of the duration of the second stage of labor	32
'Ironing out' or massaging the perineum during the second stage of labor	32
Routine manual exploration of the uterus after vaginal birth	32
Injectable prostaglandins in the third stage of labor	33
Encouraging early suckling to prevent postpartum hemorrhage	33

Problems during childbirth

Injecting saline into the umbilical vein for retained placenta	33
Biofeedback to relieve pain in labor	34
Sedatives and tranquilizers to relieve pain in labor	34
Caudal block to relieve pain in labor	34
Paracervical block to relieve pain in labor	34
Intrapartum X-ray to diagnose cephalopelvic disproportion	35

Table 5 (continued)

The evidence against these forms of care is not as firmly established as for those in Table 6	Chapter
Diagnosing cephalopelvic disproportion without ensuring adequate uterine contractions	35
Relaxin for slow or prolonged labor	35
Hyaluronidase for slow or prolonged labor	35
Vitamin K to the mother to prevent intraventricular hemorrhage in the very preterm infant	37
Phenobarbitone to the mother to prevent intraventricular hemorrhage in the very preterm infant	37
Delivery of a very preterm infant without adequate facilities to care for a very preterm baby	37
Elective forceps delivery for preterm birth	37, 41
Routine use of episiotomy for preterm birth	37
Trial of labor after previous classical cesarean section	38
Routine manual exploration of the uterus to assess a previous cesarean section scar	38
Techniques of induction and operative delivery	
Relaxin for cervical ripening before induction of labor	39
Nipple stimulation for cervical ripening before induction of labor	39
Extra-amniotic instead of other prostaglandin regimens for cervical ripening	39
Instrumental vaginal delivery to shorten the second stage of labor	41
Routine exteriorization of the uterus for repair of the uterine incision at cesarean section	42
Care after childbirth	
Silver nitrate to prevent eye infection in newborn babies	44
Elective tracheal intubation for very low-birthweight infants who are not depressed	44
Routine suctioning of newborn babies	44
Medicated bathing of babies to reduce infection	45
Wearing hospital gowns in newborn nurseries	45
Restricting sibling visits to babies in hospital	45
Routine measurements of temperature, pulse, blood pressure, and fundal height postpartum	45

TABLE 5   505

Table 5 (continued)

The evidence against these forms of care is not as firmly established as for those in Table 6	Chapter
Limiting use of women's own non-prescription drugs postpartum in hospital	45
Administering non-prescription symptom-relieving drugs at regularly set intervals	45
Prohibition of oral contraceptives for diabetic women	20
Nipple shields for breastfeeding mothers	46
Switching breasts before babies spontaneously terminate the feed	46
Oxytocin for breast engorgement in breastfeeding mothers	46
Antibiotics for localized breast engorgement (milk stasis)	46
Discontinuing breastfeeding for localized breast engorgement (milk stasis)	46
Combinations of local anesthetics and topical steroids for relief of perineal pain	47
Relying on these tables without referring to the rest of the book	50

Table 6 Forms of care likely to be ineffective or harmful

Ineffectiveness or harm demonstrated by clear evidence	Chapter
Basic care	
Dietary restriction to prevent pre-eclampsia	6, 15
Screening and diagnosis	
Contraction stress cardiotocography to improve perinatal outcome	12
Nipple-stimulation test cardiotography to improve perinatal outcome	12
Non-selective use of non-stress cardiotocography to improve perinatal outcome	12
Pregnancy problems	
Adrenocorticotrophic hormone (ACTH) for severe vomiting of pregnancy	13
Saline cathartics for constipation	13
Lubricant oils for constipation	13
Diethylstilbestrol during pregnancy	14
Elective delivery for prelabor rupture of the membranes preterm	23
Ethanol to stop preterm labor	24
Progestogens to stop preterm labor	24
Childbirth	
Routine enema in labor	29
Routine pubic shaving in preparation for childbirth	29
Electronic fetal monitoring without access to fetal scalp sampling during labor	30
Prophylactic intrapartum amnio-infusion for oligohydramnios	30
Rectal examinations to assess labor progress	31
Requiring a supine (flat on back) position in the second stage of labor	32
Routine use of the lithotomy position for the second stage of labor	32
Routine or liberal episiotomy for birth	32
Ergometrine instead of oxytocin prophylaxis in the third stage of labor	33
Problems in childbirth	
Glycerol-impregnated catgut for repair of perineal trauma	36

TABLE 6   507

Table 6 (continued)

Ineffectiveness or harm demonstrated by clear evidence	Chapter
Techniques of induction and operative delivery	
Oral prostaglandins for cervical ripening	39
Estrogens for cervical ripening or for induction of labor	39
Oxytocin for cervical ripening before induction of labor	39
Care after childbirth	
Sodium bicarbonate for asphyxiated babies	44
Routine restriction of mother–infant contact	45
Routine nursery care for babies in hospital	45
Antenatal Hoffman's exercises for inverted or flat nipples	46
Antenatal breast shells for inverted or flat nipples	46
Limitation of suckling time during breastfeeding	46
Nipple creams or ointments for breastfeeding mothers	46
Routine supplements of water or formula for breastfed babies	46
Samples of formula for breastfeeding mothers	46
Encouraging fluid intake beyond demands of thirst for breastfeeding mothers	46
Combined estrogen–progesterone oral contraceptives for breastfeeding mothers	46
Test weighing of breastfed infants	46
Witchhazel for relief of perineal pain	47
Adding salt to bath water for treating perineal pain	47
Antiseptic solutions added to bath water for perineal pain	47
Hormones for relief of breast symptoms in non-breastfeeding mothers	48
Bromocriptine for relief of breast symptoms in non-breastfeeding mothers	48

Index